Handbook of Occupational Therapy

Handbook of Occupational Therapy

Editor: Abraham Miller

MURPHY & MOORE
www.murphy-moorepublishing.com

www.murphy-moorepublishing.com

MURPHY & MOORE

Cataloging-in-Publication Data

Handbook of occupational therapy / edited by Abraham Miller.
p. cm.
Includes bibliographical references and index.
ISBN 978-1-63987-292-3
1. Occupational therapy. 2. Therapeutics, Physiological. 3. Medical rehabilitation. 4. Medical care. I. Miller, Abraham.
RM735 .H36 2022
615.851 5--dc23

Murphy & Moore Publishing,
1 Rockefeller Plaza,
New York City, NY 10020, USA

ISBN 978-1-63987-292-3 (Hardback)

Contents

Preface

Every book is initially just a concept; it takes months of research and hard work to give it the final shape in which the readers receive it. In its early stages, this book also went through rigorous reviewing. The notable contributions made by experts from across the globe were first molded into patterned chapters and then arranged in a sensibly sequential manner to bring out the best results.

The usage of assessment and intervention in order to recover, maintain and develop meaningful activities of individuals or communities is termed as occupational therapy. People who suffer from disabilities, injuries and mental health ailments are treated under this branch of health care. Children and young adults with disabilities require occupational therapy for participating in social situations and attending schools. This field makes use of concepts and knowledge from a variety of other fields such as medicine, speech-language pathology, physical therapy, audiology, social work and psychology. The order of actions in which occupational therapy functions is known as the occupational therapy process. It mainly consists of evaluation, intervention and outcomes. This book discusses the fundamentals as well as modern approaches of occupational therapy. Also included herein is a detailed explanation of the various concepts and applications of occupational therapy in health practice. The readers would gain knowledge that would broaden their perspective about this field.

It has been my immense pleasure to be a part of this project and to contribute my years of learning in such a meaningful form. I would like to take this opportunity to thank all the people who have been associated with the completion of this book at any step.

Editor

1

Life Skills in Occupational Therapy

Hatice Abaoğlu, Özge Buket Cesim, Sinem Kars and Zeynep Çelik

Abstract

Occupational therapy is a health profession that uses the purposeful activities to achieve multiple and complex rehabilitation aims. The main goals of the occupational therapy are to support the reintegration of individuals in daily living skills as well as to increase their independence and autonomy. Interventions of occupational therapists have primarily focused on self-care, productivity, and leisure time activities. Since the life skills includes a wide range of abilities that enable a person to perform personal care and more complicated tasks such as traveling, shopping, community participation etc., occupational therapists provide life skills training programs to meet the needs of the clients. This chapter aims to contribute to the current understanding and practices of life skills from an occupational therapy perspective. The chapter starts with a brief discussion of the importance of life skills in occupational therapy. After this introduction, the first part takes a look at the definition of life skills and identifies core components of life skills. The second part describes assessment and interventions of life skills. The third one gives an overview about school life skills programs for children and adolescents. Finally, the last part explains some life skills programs in people with disadvantages.

Keywords: life skills, independent living, occupational therapy, people with disadvantages

1. Introduction

Today, depending on social, moral, ethical, or religious values, the lifestyles of societies are changing rapidly. Achieving essential life skills is crucial in order to adapt to changing environmental conditions and meet the demands. Life skills contribute to the development of self-efficacy, self-confidence, and self-esteem by helping people to understand and respond different situations [1, 2].

Occupational therapy has a key role in the lives of people who deal with disabling or potentially disabling conditions. Occupational therapy interventions are in accordance with the needs, interests, and values that are of importance to the clients. To this end, occupational therapists offer a unique and holistic approach to enhance or enable participation in daily life activities. They use therapeutic activities by identifying client problems, goals, and treatment focus to improve independence in life skills and to promote quality of life [3, 4].

In occupational therapy field, a skill is defined as a performance component acquired through training and practice. Skills contribute people to function as part of the community in which they belong [5]. Occupational therapists assist the clients to create individualized goals through life skills training. These goals include achieving skills such as banking/budgeting, shopping, meal preparation and planning, coping with stress, community access, assertiveness, and self-advocating. As life skills educators, occupational therapists use a client-centered approach to assess occupational performance areas and associated environmental factors. Life skills training can be given in the client's home or in various community areas, such as banks, markets, streets, as individual trainings, or group workshops that provide opportunities for the clients to learn from each other where appropriate [6].

2. Life skills and core components

Life skills are those abilities that help to deal with challenges in life and to promote physical, mental, and emotional well-being and competence. There are a wide range of life skills and definitions are usually broad and generic. Life skills can be cognitive, behavioral, emotional, personal, interpersonal, or social. As such, the term "life skills" is often not precisely defined. According to World Health Organization (WHO), life skills are defined as "abilities for adaptive and positive behavior that enable individuals to deal effectively with the demands and challenges of everyday life." The five main life skills areas defined by WHO Department of Mental Health are decision-making and problem-solving; creative thinking and critical thinking; communication and interpersonal skills; self-awareness and empathy; and coping with emotions and stress. UNICEF defines life skills as "psychosocial and interpersonal skills that help people make informed decisions, communicate effectively, and develop the coping and self-management skills needed for a healthy and productive life" [7, 8].

These definitions are meant to apply on various topic related to health in general population. Life skills include knowledge, behavior, attitudes, and values that are desirable and necessary for life roles. If we consider explanation of life skills, we could say that life skills may be different across cultures. Nevertheless, the research studies and literature of life skills indicate that there are specific life skills. They comprise a set of core skills that improve people's well-being and help them to be active and productive in the community. These skills may generally be classified in three basic dimensions: (a) cognitive skills, (b) emotional skills, and (c) communication and interpersonal skills (**Figure 1**) [9, 10].

Cognitive skills are decision-making, problem-solving, creative thinking, and critical thinking. Decision-making is important for health management through choosing different options

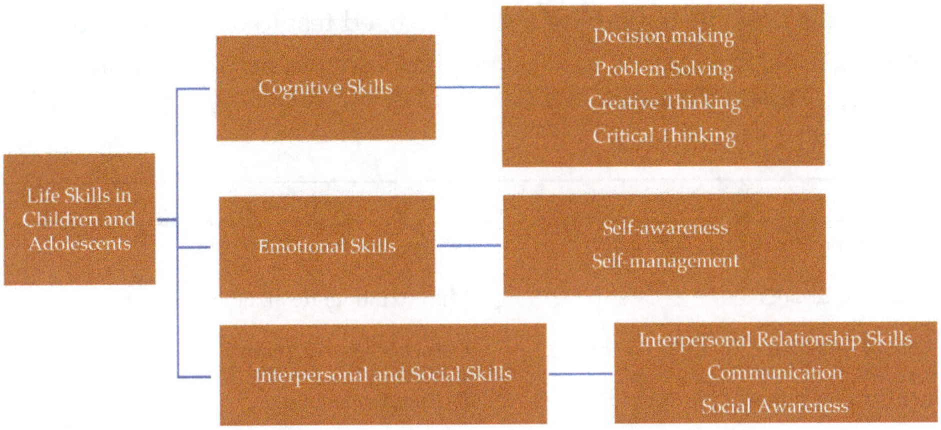

Figure 1. Life skill categories for children and adolescents.

about health status. Problem-solving is critical for coping with the problems which may cause stress in daily life. Creative thinking promotes problem-solving and decision-making and helps to provide adaptation and flexibility to daily life. Critical thinking analyses and assesses information such as attitudes and values which affects behavior [10–12].

Emotional skills compromise of self-awareness and self-management. Self-awareness includes self-esteem, self-evaluation, our likes and dislikes, and our weaknesses and strengths. Briefly, self-awareness is about our recognition of ourselves. Self-management includes time management, relaxation, and coping skills about stress and emotions such as anger [10, 11].

Interpersonal and social skills are interpersonal relationship skills, communication, and social awareness. Interpersonal relationship skills may be able to make good relationships with friends and family members which provide mental and social well-being. Communication is important for expression of ourselves verbally or nonverbally in certain situations. Social awareness includes empathy, listening actively, and respecting group differences (**Figure 1**) [10, 11].

3. Assessment and interventions of life skills

In general practice, despite the fact that occupational therapists are more focused on rehabilitation and therapy rather than preventing strategies; in life skills training, this tendency decreases. For instance, the occupational therapist works with school aged adolescents in order to enhance their abilities to prevent them from drug, tobacco, and alcohol addiction. Further, occupational therapists provide life skills training for the immigrants that facilitate their coping, management, and employability skills. And of course, occupational therapy practitioners work with disadvantaged people like people with disabilities and drug users to rehabilitate them by improving their participation [13].

Life skills assessment can be done by observation, interviews, questionnaires, checklists, and standardized evaluations. Therapists are able to develop a checklist for certain person to follow the process. They can also apply questionnaires or checklists to screen life skills in a broad sense. Moreover, it is possible to employ a standardized test to define life skills in detail. The most commonly used standardized assessment instruments by occupational therapy practitioners are shown in **Table 1** [14–17].

Name of the instrument	Validation samples
Activities of Daily Living Situational Test (AST)	Alzheimer disease
Cognitive Performance Test (CPT)	Mild to moderate alzheimer disease
Direct Assessment of Functional Abilities (DAFA)	Demented participants
Direct Assessment of Functional Status (DAFS)	Alzheimer disease
Functional Performance Measure (FPM)	Alzheimer disease
Texas Functional Living Scale (TFLS)	Alzheimer disease
Bay Area Functional Performance Evaluation (BaFPE)	Psychiatric patients; Schizophrenia or depression patients
Kohlman Evaluation of Living Skills (KELS)	Designed for inpatient psychiatric unit, used with older adults
UCSD Performance-based Skills Assessment (UPSA)	Middle-aged schizophrenia patient
Independent Living Scales (ILS)	Independent and dependent adults; mentally retarded adults; TBI; dementia; and chronic psychiatric
Occupational Therapy Evaluation of Performance and Support (OTEPS)	Older adults referred for NP assessment upon admission to a geriatric psychiatry hospital. Sample includes; depression, anxiety, and probable dementia
Performance Test of Activities of Daily Living (PADL)	Consecutive inpatient admissions over age 65
St. George Hospital Memory Disorders Clinic Occupational Therapy Assessment Scale (OTAS)	Psychiatric disturbances, dementia
Activities of Daily Living Test (ADL-T)	Older healthy people
Everyday Problems Test (EPT)	Community-dwelling older healthy people
Observed Tasks of Daily Living (OTDL)	Educated older healthy people
Everyday Functioning Battery(EFB)	HIV+ individuals
Performance Assessment of Self-Care Skills (PASS)	Numerous populations
Beck Dressing Performance Scale (BDPS)	Cognitively impaired adults
Financial Capacity Index (FCI)	Alzheimer disease
Kitchen Task Assessment (KTA)	Alzheimer disease
Medication Management Ability Assessment (MMAA)	Schizophrenia and schizoaffective older than 45
Test of Grocery Shopping Skills (TOGSS)	Schizophrenia and schizoaffective
Time and Change Test (T&C)	Outpatients 75+ years, 36% demented
Drug Regimen Unassisted Grading Scale (DRUGS)	Older community dwelling people
Functional Ability to Take Medications (FATM)	Geriatric clinic inpatients and outpatients
Immersive Virtual Kitchen (IVK)	Traumatic brain injury
Rabideau Kitchen Evaluation Revised (RKE-R)	TBI men ages18–49

Name of the instrument	Validation samples
Medication Management Task (MMT)	HIV+ validation samples HIV+ adherence sample
Refined ADL Assessment Scale (RADL)	Cognitively impaired nursing home residents
Do-Eat	Developmental coordination disorder
School-Assessment of Motor and Process Skills (schoolAMPS)	Typically developing or attention-deficit hyperactivity disorder, learning disability or sensory integrative disorder
Functional Independence Measure for Children (WeeFIM)	Limb deficiency, Down's syndrome, spina bifida, cerebral palsy, extreme prematurity
Children's Assessment of Participation and Enjoyment (CAPE)	6-21 years old children with/without disabilities
School Function Assessment (SFA)	Elementary/ primary school children ages between 5 and 12, physical and/or sensory impairment
School Outcome Measure (SOM)	School aged children (3–18 years)
Children Helping Out: Responsibilities, Expectations, and Supports (CHORES)	6–11 years old children with/without disability
Assessment of LIFE-Habits for Children (LIFE-H)	5–13 years old children with disabilities
Canadian Occupational Performance Measure (COPM)	All ages and disabilities
Goal Attainment Scaling (GAS)	All ages and disabilities
Assessment of Functional Living Skills (AFLS)	2 years and up, developmental delays and autism

Table 1. The assessment tools that used commonly in life skills evaluation by occupational therapists.

When assessing life skills, it is important to note that occupational therapy approaches are individual and person centered. Each group and each person has specific characteristics in the mean of occupation. Therefore, the occupational therapy assessment of the life skills is provided individually by employing the practical reference models either for general praxis, such as Model of Human Occupation (MOHO) [18, 19], Person-Environment- Occupation Model (PEO) [20–22], and VdT Model of Creative Ability (MOCA) [23, 24] or the ones that particularly developed for this use, such as Occupational Therapy Life Skills Curriculum Model [13], Life Skills Training Approach [25], and etc.

MOHO provides a framework (or model) for occupational therapist to understand how to use daily activities therapeutically to support people's health. It seeks to explain how meaningful daily activities are motivated, patterned, and performed. MOHO focuses on the occupation in practice; the motivation for occupation; the patterning of occupational behavior/performance into routines and lifestyles; the nature of skilled performance; and the influence of the environment on occupational performance. It has assessments and intervention protocols, that are specific to itself, to support practitioner to understand the volition, habitation, roles, and performance capacity of the individuals. Life skills, in this model, are agent that both affect and are affected by the routines, roles, habits, and the capacity [18].

The fundamental belief of MOCA, which is an occupational therapy model, the motivation controls the action and the action is the manifestation or expression of motivation. According to Vona du Toit, humans develop a variety of skills in a sequential sequence as environmental/social/relationship/occupational demands change and influence them throughout the lifespan. That is why, action is examined by four skills of people. These are personal management, social ability, work ability, and use of free time. The role of the occupational therapist is to identify the client's current level of creative ability and how much independence s/he has at that level. This enables the therapist, team, client and/or carers to understand what the client is motivated for and the extent of his/her skills for doing things that s/he finds meaningful and is motivated toward. With this understanding, intervention can be offered to elicit motivation and participation in order to facilitate growth toward the next (higher) level of ability. In the case of a client with dementia, intervention is provided to maintain level of ability and prevent deterioration for as long as possible [26].

PEO model describes the interaction among person, environment, and occupation for clear understanding of occupational performance. The person component of this model is seen holistically as a combination of mind, body, and spiritual qualities. And also, each person has both learned and initiate skills in order to accomplish in occupational performance. The environment where the individual use their abilities to engage in occupation has four subscales: cultural, socioeconomic, institutional, physical, and social. Last but not the least, the occupation is a composite of activities and tasks that are necessary to function in life [20].

Occupational Therapy Life Skills Curriculum Model is created for promoting the nonpatient population via a unique, nontraditional occupational therapy role focusing on primary prevention, and community health and enhancement. This model includes a program, that is, named leisure skills/career development, for children of ages between 4 and 22. And the program divides the age bands to three: fantasy-exploration stage, tentative choice stage, and final realistic stage. Meantime, there are academic skills and leisure skills program for each of the stages both of them have specific subprograms [13].

After choosing the most appropriate approach for the patient and completing the evaluations, occupational therapists navigate the session to the intervention. The life skills training programs are created in order to increase one's participation in social, intellectual, creative, and physical activities. The life skills training programs can be administered as individually or modular. Programs such as social skills training, emotional skills training, and behavioral skills trainings can be considered as modular because, for example, social skills training generally contains social participation skills, interpersonal skills, assertiveness training, communication skills, etc. The individual trainings typically facilitate development of abilities in the three main component areas of daily living by developing daily organization and time management; personal health including sleep, medication management, healthy eating, and avoiding addictions; self-monitoring; stress management and relaxation techniques; leisure exploration and development; communication and relationships; managing public transport and mobility; conflict resolution skills; managing money; career exploration and planning; study, prevocational, and work readiness training; and vocational reintegration skills. The group trainings, generally, are provided after the need analysis of the group. In the life skills training for schizophrenics, for example, focus points of training are generally about interpersonal communication, nutrition, time management, etc., while the life skills training programs for homeless are about social action, individual justice, employment, money management, etc. [27–29].

4. Life skills in children and adolescents

Life skills trainings improve skills to create proficiency for human development and to indigenize appropriate behaviors that provide to deal with the difficulties of daily life in children and adolescents. Life skills also help children and adolescents to improve their psychosocial competence which is important to deal with challenges of daily life, promotion of health, and for well-being. Specially, where the health issues are associated with behaviors which cause inadequacy to cope with personal and social challenges powerfully, developing of psychosocial competence may be an important way to contribute well-being and health. Therefore, teaching of life skills to children and adolescents is one of the core elements to develop psychosocial competence [10].

Life skills training supports constructive behavior about health, relationships, and well-being. Optimally, it is critical to perform this training when the children and adolescents are at young age before adverse behaviors. Trainings of life skills are based on general life skills and their practice in connection with social and health issues. Methods and approaches such as cognitive-behavioral skills training techniques, didactic teaching methods, group discussion, brainstorming, and role play can be used in teaching of life skills [10, 27].

There are many evidence-based life skills programs which provide education about many issues, such as drug abuse prevention or preventing violence which are related with life skills. For example, the life skills training (LST) program which is a primary prevention program for adolescent drug abuse created positive behaviors about alcohol, tobacco, and other drug use. This program included drug resistance skills, self-management, and social skills. Methods which are used in this program were instruction, reinforcement, feedback, practice of the skill, and behavioral homework assignments [30, 31]. Another evidence-based program about life skills is coping skills training for youth with diabetes mellitus which was conducted by Grey and her colleagues. Role play about situations such as managing food choices, giving feedback, using of social problem-solving, and working with small groups are the methods which were used in this training. Results of this training showed that teenagers in the coping skills training program were likely able to cope with diabetes mellitus and other medical situations, and indicated less negative effect of diabetes on quality of life [32]. HIV prevention intervention which is done in Zimbabwe with adolescent female orphans is also an important research. In this intervention, HIV and health knowledge (e.g., condom use) and issues related to culture, gender, sexual, and physical violence were the topics in life skills curriculum of this research. According to the results of this study, participants earned personal hope and value, and effective communication skills [33].

The objective of the life skills education is to help children and adolescents to understand themselves, reach personal satisfaction, live life better, and achieve their goals. This education is essential for the personal and academic development of children and adolescents.

Therefore, considering of the certain strategies for life skills education may affect the impact of the education. These strategies are:

- Doing the education in schools because of the possibility to reach many children and adolescents and long- and short-term evaluation.
- Providing the education at young ages.
- Making the education part of the school curriculum.
- Using tested, evidence-based, well design life skills programs.
- Using an evaluation system for education.
- Determining objective of the education through need analyses.
- Inclusion of both knowledge and social attitudes and values.
- Improvement of all teachers, principals, other staff members about the topic of life skills education.
- Using methods such as role play, feedback about performance, practice of skills instead of just using didactic teaching.
- Starting with skills learning in nonthreatening situations and progressively moving on the practice of skills in high-risk situations.
- Creating the education with a multidisciplinary group such as professionals from schools, public health, and social services.

Apart from these strategies, conducting publicity campaigns to promote support and expectations of life skills education and publishing papers about education may increase the effect of life skills education [10, 34].

Mission of the school is to educate children and adolescents to be healthy, social skilled, responsible, and informed. With the school-based prevention and youth development programs, this mission is undergird [35]. Many teachers experience that many children in schools have poor social and communication skills because of computers and televisions [36]. Therefore, as we mentioned above, it is an important strategy to give life skills educations in schools. There are many life skills education programs for different age groups in many schools around the world. Some of them are: Promoting Alternative Thinking Strategies (PATHS); The School Mental Health Program (SMHP); The Smoking Prevention Program; The GOAL Program; UNESCO and Government of Ghana Life Skills Alcohol and Drug Prevention Program; Life Skills and Positive Prevention Programme; The Life Skills Training (LST) program; The Problem-Solving Program [10, 12, 27, 37–40]. For deeper explanation about the context of educations, you can find an example of school-based life skills education sessions about prevention of cigarette smoking in **Figure 2** [39].

Life skills are like physical skills in the way of learning methods, through modeling and practice. Many of the life skills learned in sport are quotable to other life areas. These skills may include: the abilities to show performance under pressure; communicate; meet challenges; set goals; solve problems; handle failure; work with a group; and receive feedback. Therefore,

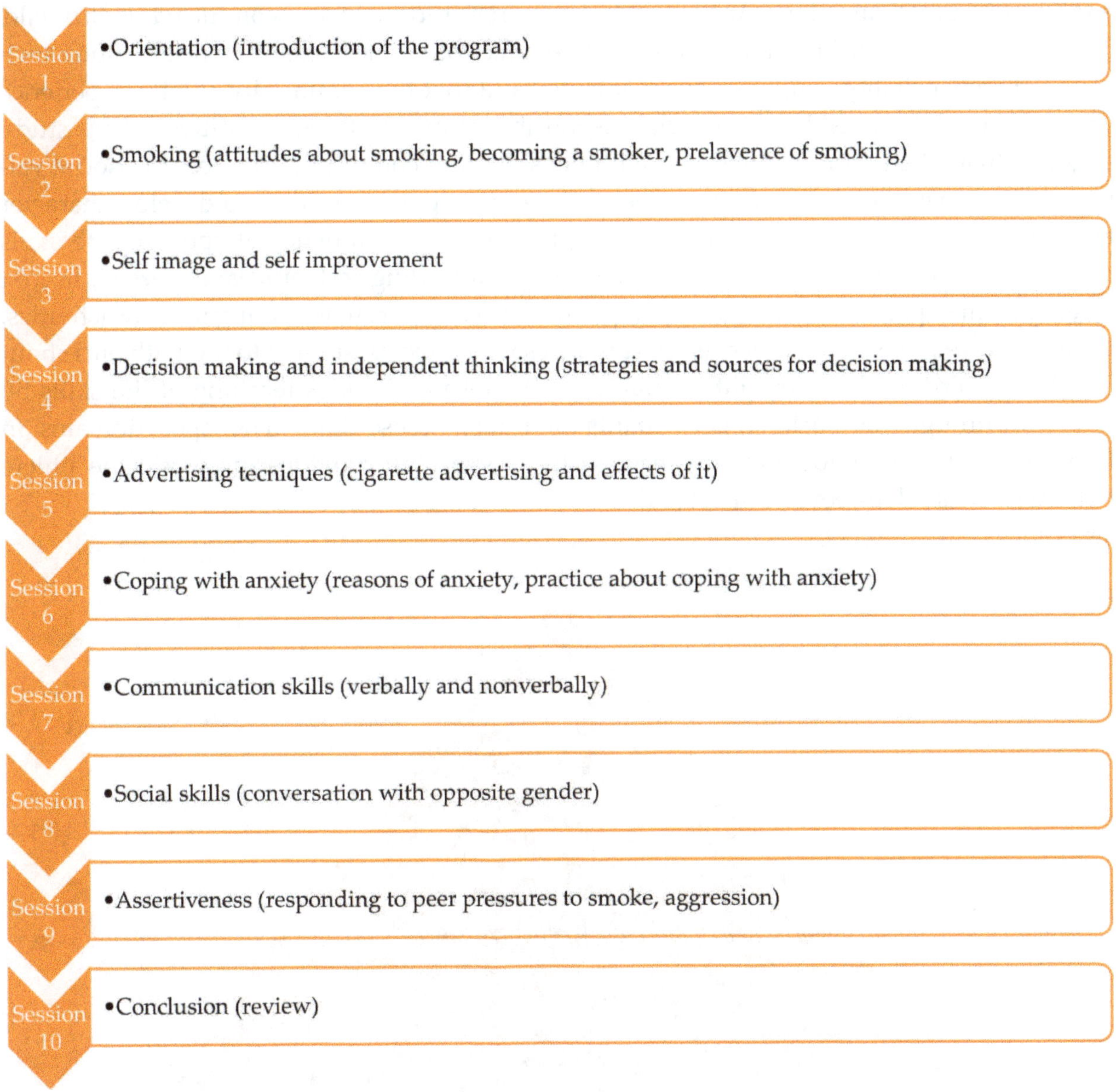
Session 1
•Orientation (introduction of the program)
Session 2
•Smoking (attitudes about smoking, becoming a smoker, prelavence of smoking)
Session 3
•Self image and self improvement
Session 4
•Decision making and independent thinking (strategies and sources for decision making)
Session 5
•Advertising tecniques (cigarette advertising and effects of it)
Session 6
•Coping with anxiety (reasons of anxiety, practice about coping with anxiety)
Session 7
•Communication skills (verbally and nonverbally)
Session 8
•Social skills (conversation with opposite gender)
Session 9
•Assertiveness (responding to peer pressures to smoke, aggression)
Session 10
•Conclusion (review)

Figure 2. School-based life skills education sessions about prevention of cigarette smoking [39].

sport participation which provides psychosocial development may contribute to life skills in children and adolescents [41]. Although there is not enough research focusing the effect of sports on life skills development, there is growing interest about the development of life skills through sport in children and adolescents and sport psychology. Many athletes have begun to understand the importance of using sport psychology strategies and techniques to improve their nonathletic life. One study which is about teaching life skills through sport, mentioned a program which calls Sports United to Promote Education and Recreation (SUPER). The objective of the program was to show participants the importance of physical and mental skills for sport and life and the existence of the effective student-athlete role models. In this program, topics such as similarities and differences of life skills and sport, being a good listener, speaking with the group were taught to the participants who are sport leaders. And these leaders taught students sport skills and life skills related with sport, coached the students to increase their sport performance [42]. Sport-based life skill education is also important on adolescents' prosocial values. According to a research study which is conducted by Brunelle, Sport-Based Life Skill Program had a positive effect on adolescents' prosocial values such as social responsibility, empathy, social interest, and that the community service experience affected the adolescents' levels of social responsibility and confidence positively. This study suggests that when sport is integrated with life skills and community services, prosocial values are improved in adolescent volunteers. Therefore, sport may serve to develop character and values when combined with life skills programs [43]. Influence of sport on life skills development occurs in different levels (**Figure 3**). According to Gould and Carson, in first level sport may prevent youth from getting into trouble and from involving in risky activities. In second level, role models such as sport coaches may affect positively to their athletes about life skills. Third level is more influential level. Because it includes teaching of life skills by coaches. Through this teaching, participants can transfer these skills to nonsport domains. In fourth level, the coach does not only teach skills for sport but provides and works the athlete to transfer these skills beyond sport [44].

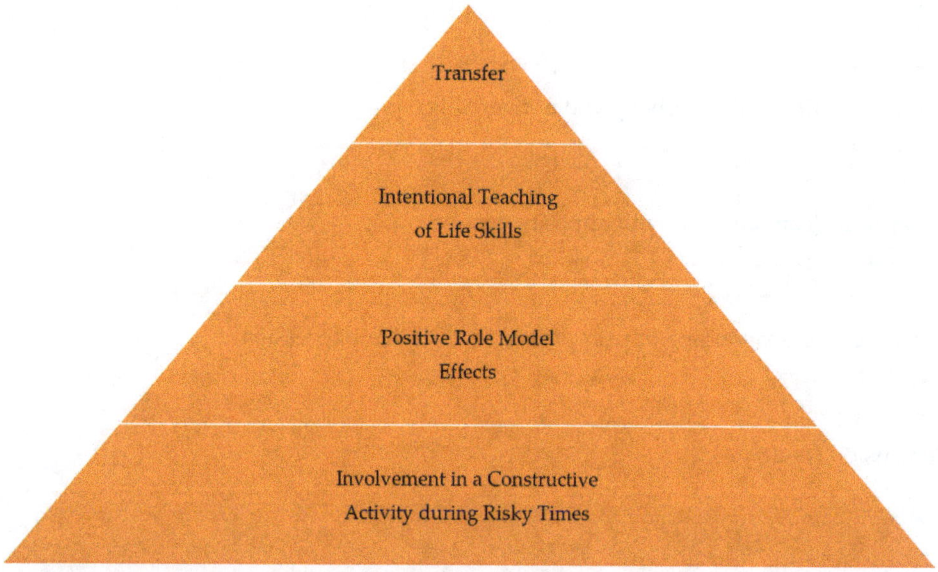

Figure 3. Levels of life skills development through sport [44].

5. Life skills for disadvantaged groups

Life skills programs enhance skills of vulnerable adolescent and young adult populations. These programs generally include a formal curriculum, along with a combination of group education, peer mentorship, one-to-one support, coaching, and experiential learning [45]. "Coaching" in which therapists guide people to examine their goals and identify changes to their performance [46], is one of these programs. It involves tailored, experience-based support in learning life skills and self-management strategies, and seeks to enhance people's self-efficacy and skill development by providing opportunities to learn new skills, make decisions, experience successes, and take calculated risks [47]. Life skills programs need to be intentionally designed. These programs offer experiential opportunities by providing new insights, self-realizations, and positive yet realistic views of the future to equip them with knowledge, skills, and confidence, and to motivate them to engage in new life directions [48].

Vulnerable children such as orphans, sexually exploited children, street children, and working children may need for life skills interventions. Although life skills play an important role in determining how children cope with difficult conditions, little is known about life skills interventions with vulnerable young people. Children with low socioeconomic backgrounds have a low self-concept and lack of self-efficacy and life skills. Their belief in their own abilities value is decreased due to the low attendance of school and the difficulties in school life [7, 49].

The term street children refers to a diverse group of young people dislocated from family, school, and community, who tend to work, congregate and/or live in inner city areas. Poverty in developing countries, associated with the collapse of rural economies and migration into overburdened urban environments, is the root cause of the street child phenomenon [50]. Life skills programs are necessary for health promotion and well-being for these groups. Life skills may include to identify health problems and the ways to prevent them, to analyze factors that impact growth and development from adolescence to adulthood, to describe the relationship between health and adolescent choices, to assess factors that influence emotional self-management and relationships with the environment [51].

Another disadvantaged group is individuals with addictions. It is supported by research that life skills training are the most effective approach in school-based drug prevention programs. The life skills training program for adolescent drug use focuses on the social and emotional factors that promote substance use. Separate curricula have been developed for students from different age groups as supportive interventions in schools. The program consists of three main components: drug resistance skills, personal self-management skills, and general social skills [52, 53].

Deaf individuals face many challenges during school years and during the transition to independent living. Research on the life skills in these individuals is very limited. Life skills training should be designed to meet the needs of deaf individuals. In a study, life skills training for vulnerable deaf adults includes money management and consumer awareness, food management, personal appearance and hygiene, health (e.g., knowing the symptoms and treatment of various illnesses), housing (e.g., knowledge of renters rights and obligations), housekeeping, educational planning, transportation, legal knowledge (rights when arrested, function of a lawyer), job seeking skills, job maintenance skills, knowledge of community resources, emergency and safety, interpersonal skills, pregnancy, parenting, and childcare [54].

People with schizophrenia are a disadvantaged group because of stigma. Negative labeling has an impact on public attitudes toward people with schizophrenia. Negative labeling has a strong negative effect on the way people react emotionally to someone with schizophrenia as a result of increasing the preference for social distance. Furthermore, people with schizophrenia have social withdrawal, employment problems, reduced social, or recreational activities. Life skills training for people with schizophrenia may include daily living activities, money management, communication and social skills, home management, community life skills, etc. [55–58].

Life skills training are also important for homeless people. Homeless individuals may experience problems with unemployment, loss of income, lack of social security, inadequate access to social support and health services, disability, substance abuse, or suicide attempts. Because life skills such as managing money, shopping, cooking, running a home, and maintaining social networks are essential for living independently. Some homeless people do not have all of these skills, because they never acquired them or lost them through extended periods of homelessness. The aim of the training is to promote self-sufficiency in homeless people. Life skills can be classified into three broad categories: (1) social skills (e.g., interpersonal skills, avoiding or dealing with neighbor disputes, developing self-confidence and social networks), (2) independent living skills (e.g., managing a household, budgeting, appointment keeping and contacting services, dealing with bills, and correspondence), and (3) core or basic skills (e.g., numeracy, literacy, and information technology). For example, a study is showed that homeless youth may need to personnel hygiene (body odor and sweating), oral health (including bad breath), oily skin and acne, unwanted or oily hair, feminine hygiene, piercing maintenance, budgeting and finance, and soft skills (motivation, self-awareness, and ability to work with others) [59, 60].

In the literature, there are different life skill training programs designed other disadvantaged groups such as criminals and refugees. Disadvantaged individuals face social, economic, and cultural challenges throughout their lives. A disadvantaged group may face multiple challenges. Some difficulties can be overcome or changed more easily than others. Because the difficulties that individuals experience and the ways in which they deal with them are different between the groups, life skills interventions may change from group to group. The ability to overcome difficulties in everyday life depends largely on the development of life skills. Life skills include skills that enable people to cope with their life, difficulties, and changes [61–63].

In summary, there is no definite classification of what psychosocial skills may be at the core of life skills, nor is there any clarity about the relationship of these skills to each other. However, it is seen that the skills defined as life skills are cognitive, emotional and behavioral, even though they are classified by different persons and institutions in different ways. These skills are vital to maintaining a productive and healthy lifestyle, having meaningful and satisfying roles, and promoting well-being. For this reason, it is quite natural that occupational therapy, which aims to promote functional independence of individuals in their daily life skills, includes life skills and related training programs.

Author details

Hatice Abaoğlu*, Özge Buket Cesim, Sinem Kars and Zeynep Çelik

*Address all correspondence to: haticeabaoglu@hacettepe.edu.tr

Faculty of Health Sciences, Occupational Therapy Department, Hacettepe University, Ankara, Turkey

References

[1] Chakra A. A life skills approach to adolescent development. International Journal of Home Science. 2016;**2**(1):234-238

[2] Miller EK. Occupational Therapists' Intervention Approaches in Secondary Transition Services for Students with Disabilities. [Doctoral dissertation]. Kentucky: Eastern Kentucky University; 2012.

[3] Chapparo C, Ranka J. Clinical reasoning in occupational therapy. In: Higgs J, Jones M, editors. Clinical reasoning in the health professions. Oxford: Butterworth Heinemann; 2000. p. 128-137.

[4] American Occupational Therapy Association. Occupational therapy practice framework: Domain and process. American Journal of Occupational Therapy. 2014;**68**(Suppl. 1):S1-S48

[5] Roberts M. Life skills. In: Creek J, Lougher L, editors. Occupational Therapy and Mental Health. 4th ed. London: Elsevier Ltd; 2008. pp. 359-381

[6] Mitchell L, Gunaratne E. Occupational therapists as life skills educators: Experiences at the gage transition to independent living program. Occupational Therapy Now. 2007;**9**(3):20

[7] World Health Organization. Partners in Life Skills Education. Geneva, Switzerland: World Health Organization, Department of Mental Health; 1999.

[8] UNICEF. Life skills-Based Education in South Asia, A Regional Overview Prepared For: The South Asia Life Skills-Based Education Forum. Paris: The United Nations Children's Fund (UNICEF); 2005.

[9] Hanbury C, Malti T. Monitoring and Evaluating Life Skills for Youth Development. Switzerland: Jacobs Foundations; 2011.

[10] Weisen RB, Orley J, Evans V, Jeff Lee T, Sprunger B, Pellaux D. Life Skills Education in Schools. Geneva, Switzerland: World Health Organization; 1994.

[11] World Health Organization. Preventing Violence by Developing Life Skills in Children and Adolescents. Geneva: World Health Organization; 2009.

[12] O'Hearn TC, Gatz M. Going for the goal: Improving youths' problem-solving skills through a school-based intervention. Journal of Community Psychology. 2002;**30**(3):281-303

[13] DeMars PA. An occupational therapy life skills curriculum model for a Native American tribe: A health promotion program based on ethnographic field research. American Journal of Occupational Therapy. 1992;**46**(8):727-736

[14] Moore DJ, Palmer BW, Patterson TL, Jeste DV. A review of performance-based measures of functional living skills. Journal of Psychiatric Research. 2007;**41**(1):97-118

[15] Linde B, Netten J, Otten E, Postema K, Geuze R, Schoemaker M. A systematic review of instruments for assessment of capacity in activities of daily living in children with developmental co-ordination disorder. Child: Care, Health and Development. 2015;**41**(1):23-34

[16] Sakzewski L, Boyd R, Ziviani J. Clinimetric properties of participation measures for 5-to 13-year-old children with cerebral palsy: A systematic review. Developmental Medicine & Child Neurology. 2007;**49**(3):232-240

[17] Partington JWP, Mueller MM. Assessment of Functional Living Skills (AFLS). [Internet]. 2012. Available from: http://www.wpspublish.com/store/p/2650/assessment-of-functional-living-skills-afls: WPS unlocking potential

[18] Kielhofner G, Forsyth K, Kramer J, Melton J, Dobson E. The Model of Human Occupation. Wellington: Queen Margaret College; 1988.

[19] Duncan E. The model of human occupation. British Journal of Occupational Therapy. 2010;**73**(11):497-498

[20] Law M, Cooper B, Strong S, Stewart D, Rigby P, Letts L. The person-environment-occupation model: A transactive approach to occupational performance. Canadian Journal of Occupational Therapy. 1996;**63**(1):9-23

[21] Hamera E, Brown CE. Developing a context-based performance measure for persons with schizophrenia: The test of grocery shopping skills. American Journal of Occupational Therapy. 2000;**54**(1):20-25

[22] Gol D, Jarus T. Effect of a social skills training group on everyday activities of children with attention-deficit-hyperactivity disorder. Developmental Medicine & Child Neurology. 2005;**47**(8):539-545

[23] Jansen M, Casteleijn D. Applying the model of creative ability to patients with diabetic foot problems. South African Journal of Occupational Therapy. 2009;**39**(3):26-32

[24] Williamson B. Creativity, the corporate curriculum and the future: A case study. Futures. 2001;**33**(6):541-555

[25] Wheeler SD, Lane SJ, McMahon BT. Community participation and life satisfaction following intensive, community-based rehabilitation using a life skills training approach. OTJR: Occupation, Participation and Health. 2007;**27**(1):13-22

[26] Sherwood W. An introduction to the Vona du Toit model of creative ability. Revista electrónica de terapia ocupacional Galicia, TOG. 2011;**14**:12

[27] Botvin GJ, Griffin KW. Life skills training: Empirical findings and future directions. Journal of Primary Prevention. 2004;**25**(2):211-232

[28] Mairs H, Bradshaw T. Life skills training in schizophrenia. British Journal of Occupational Therapy. 2004; **67**(5):217-224

[29] Arbesman M, Logsdon DW. Occupational therapy interventions for employment and education for adults with serious mental illness: A systematic review. American Journal of Occupational Therapy. 2011;**65**(3):238-246

[30] Botvin GJ. Preventing Adolescent Drug Abuse through Life Skills Training: Theory, Evidence of Effectiveness. In Crane J, editor. Social programs that work. New York, NY: Russell Sage Foundation; 1998. p. 225-257.

[31] Botvin GJ, Griffin KW, Paul E, Macaulay AP. Preventing tobacco and alcohol use among elementary school students through life skills training. Journal of Child & Adolescent Substance Abuse. 2003;**12**(4):1-17

[32] Grey M, Boland EA, Davidson M, Li J, Tamborlane WV. Coping skills training for youth with diabetes mellitus has long-lasting effects on metabolic control and quality of life. Journal of Pediatrics. 2000;**137**(1):107-113

[33] Dunbar MS, Maternowska MC, Kang MS, Laver SM, Mudekunye-Mahaka I, Padian NS. Findings from SHAZ!: A feasibility study of a microcredit and life-skills HIV prevention intervention to reduce risk among adolescent female orphans in Zimbabwe. Journal of Prevention and Intervention in the Community. 2010;**38**(2):147-161

[34] Singh H, Gera M. Strategies for development of life skills and global competencies. International Journal of Scientific Research. 2015;**4**(6):760-763

[35] Greenberg MT, Weissberg RP, O'Brien MU, Zins JE, Fredericks L, Resnik H, et al. Enhancing school-based prevention and youth development through coordinated social, emotional, and academic learning. The American Psychologist. 2003;**58(6-7)**:466-474

[36] Dwivedi KN, Harper P. Promoting the Emotional Well Being of Children and Adolescents and Preventing Their Mental Ill Health: A Handbook. London: Jessica Kingsley Publishers; 2004.

[37] Curtis C, Norgate R. An evaluation of the promoting alternative thinking strategies curriculum at key Stage 1. Educational Psychology in Practice. 2007;**23**(1):33-44

[38] Srikala B, Kishore Kumar K. Empowering adolescents with life skills education in schools — School mental health program: Does it work? Indian Journal of Psychiatry. 2010;**52**(4):344-349

[39] Botvin GJ, Eng A, Williams CL. Preventing the onset of cigarette smoking through life skills training. Preventive Medicine. 1980;**9**(1):135-143

[40] Alvarez J, Cotler S, Jason LA. Developing a problem-solving program in an elementary school setting. Education. 1984;**104**(3):281-286

[41] Papacharisis V, Goudas M, Danish SJ, Theodorakis Y. The effectiveness of teaching a life skills program in a sport context. Journal of Applied Sport Psychology. 2005;**17**(3):247-254

[42] Danish SJ, Nellen VC. New roles for sport psychologists: Teaching life skills through sport to at-risk youth. Quest. 1997;**49**(1):100-113

[43] Brunelle J, Danish SJ, Forneris T. The impact of a sport-based life skill program on adolescent prosocial values. Applied Developmental Science. 2007;**11**(1):43-55

[44] Gould D, Carson S. Life skills development through sport: current status and future directions. International Review of Sport and Exercise Psychology. 2008;**1**(1):58-78

[45] Kingsnorth S, Healy H, Macarthur C. Preparing for adulthood: A systematic review of life skill programs for youth with physical disabilities. Journal of Adolescent Health. 2007;**41**(4):323-332

[46] Graham F, Rodger S, Ziviani J. Effectiveness of occupational performance coaching in improving children's and mothers' performance and mothers' self-competence. The American Journal of Occupational Therapy. 2013;**67**:10-18

[47] Baldwin P, King G, Evans J, McDougall S, Tucker MA, Servais M. Solution-focused coaching in pediatric rehabilitation: An integrated model for practice. Physical & Occupational Therapy in Pediatrics. Epub ahead of print. 2013. DOI: 10.3109/01942638.2013.784718

[48] King G, Batorowicz B, Rigby P, McMain-Klein M, Thompson L, Pinto M. Development of a measure to assess youth self-reported experiences of activity settings (SEAS). International Journal of Disability, Development and Education. 2014;**61**(1):44-66

[49] Weidinger W. Promoting self-competences and life skills of children coming from vulnerable groups: Research-based development of an inclusive education program. The Fourth European Conference on Education. Official Conference Proceedings. Switzerland: Zurich University of Teacher Education; 2016.

[50] Richter LM. Street children: The nature and scope of the problem in southern Africa. Child Care Worker. 1988;**6**:11-14

[51] Swart-Kruger J, Richter LM. AIDS-related knowledge, attitudes and behaviour among South African street youth: Reflections on power, sexuality and the autonomous self. Social Science & Medicine. 1997;**45**(6):957-966

[52] Griffin KW, Botvin GJ. Evidence-based interventions for preventing substance use disorders in adolescents. Child and adolescent psychiatric clinics of North America. 2010;**19**(3):505-526.

[53] Bühler A, Schröder E, Silbereisen RK. The role of life skills promotion in substance abuse prevention: A mediation analysis. Health Education Research. 2008;**23**(4):621-632

[54] Mathews ES. Towards an independent future: Life skills training and vulnerable deaf adults. Irish Journal of Applied Social Studies. 2015;**15**(1):1

[55] Rüsch N, Angermeyer MC, Corrigan PW. Mental illness stigma: concepts, consequences, and initiatives to reduce stigma. European psychiatry. 2005;**20**(8):529-539

[56] Angermeyer MC, Matschinger H. The stigma of mental illness: Effects of labelling on public attitudes towards people with mental disorder. Acta Psychiatrica Scandinavica. 2003;**108**(4):304-309

[57] Tandon R, Jibson M. Negative symptoms of schizophrenia: How to treat them most effectively. Current Psychiatry Online. 2002;**1**(9):36-42

[58] Kopelowicz A, Liberman RP, Zarate R. Recent advances in social skills training for schizophrenia. Schizophrenia Bulletin. 2006;**32**(Suppl. 1):12-23

[59] Thomas Y, Gray M, McGinty S. A systematic review of occupational therapy interventions with homeless people. Occupational Therapy in Health Care. 2011;**25**(1):38-53

[60] Gopalan A, Reddy A, Roman B, Nkonde-Price C, Lee D, Fong HF, Rosenbaum L, Patel M. Developing a life skills curriculum for homeless youth. Philadelphia: Robert Wood Johnson Foundation; 2012.

[61] Mayer SE. What is a "Disadvantaged Group?" [Internet]. Minneapolis: Effective Communities Project; 2003 [Cited December 5, 2016]. Available from: http://www.effectivecommunities.com/pdfs/ECP_DisadvantagedGroup.pdf

[62] Yankey T, Biswas UN. Life skills training as an effective intervention strategy to reduce stress among Tibetan refugee adolescents. Journal of Refugee Studies. 2012;**25**(4):514-536

[63] Melton R, Pennell S. Staying out successfully: An evaluation of an in-custody life skills training program. San Diego, CA: San Diego Association of Governments; 1998.

2

Hearing Impairment in Professional Musicians and Industrial Workers — Profession-Specific Auditory Stimuli Used to Evoke Event-Related Brain Potentials and to Show Different Auditory Perception and Processing

Edeltraut Emmerich, Marcus Engelmann, Melanie Rohmann and Frank Richter

Abstract

Hearing impaired professional musicians or industrial workers often report that they were able to identify mistuned chords in a music piece or even slight changes in the noise of their machines (usually > 100 dB SPL) though they were handicapped in listening tasks in daily routine.

In order to assess central processing of acoustic stimuli, we analyzed auditory evoked potentials (AEP) and EEG spectra after stimulation with work-related auditory stimuli in healthy controls, in hearing impaired musicians or hearing impaired workers from the beverage industry. Stimuli were series of in-tune or mistuned synthetic piano chords or the original machine noise the workers heard in daily routine and the same noise with disturbing signals.

Professional musicians identified the mistuned stimuli and the AEP differed significantly. The workers recognized the disturb signals. In both groups the spectral analysis confirmed a frequency shift towards higher alpha frequencies and an altered spatial distribution of the EEG frequencies during presentation of the disturb signals.

We assume that professionalism causes learning of typical auditory stimuli that is important for auditory processing after hearing impairment. AEP component analysis and spectral analysis of the EEG are important tools to objectify this processing, in particular in hearing impaired employees.

Keywords: Auditory evoked potential, Mismatch negativity (MMN), Hearing impairment, Permanent threshold shift (PTS), Occupational disease

1. Introduction

The mismatch negativity component (MMN) of auditory evoked event-related potential can be elicited by deviant stimuli inserted into a follow-up of identical sounds [1]. See for review [2]. In the past, numerous studies had been performed in which changed attributes of the stimuli, such as decrement in duration [3], changes in frequency [4], or changed stimulus intensity [5], were used to differentiate between standard and deviant stimuli. MMN to musical stimuli has been investigated for a long time. It was shown that MMN was caused by a timbre change [6,7]. In a later study, it was shown [8] that comparison of MMN to omitted tones in a series of sine-wave tone pips could be used to differentiate between musicians and non-musicians. Violation of harmony rules elicited large MMN in the fronto-central cortex areas [9]. Slightly mistuned chords produced MMN in professional violinists, but not in non-musicians [10]. Similarly, larger and earlier MMN to rhythm variations were observed in jazz musicians than in non-musicians [11].

An earlier study of our group raised the issue that hearing-impaired professional musicians were able to play their instruments in the orchestras and to perform without problems when they were trained for years, regardless of their permanent threshold shift (PTS) [12]. Interestingly, those musicians reported on hearing problems when watching TV or if they wanted to have conversation in a noisy environment (party-noise effect). To our knowledge, there are only few studies about musicians dealing with the effects of occupational noise and central compensation after hearing damage. Therefore, we want to test whether differences exist in auditory event-related potentials (AEP) (amplitudes and latencies) and/or in MMN reflecting the sound processing while comparing normal hearing people and musicians (normal hearing and hearing impaired). The new aspect in our study is the use of typical musical stimuli, i.e., in-tune and mistuned chords. We assumed that professional musicians should be trained to these stimuli regardless whether they have normal hearing or not.

There is some evidence for the assumption that ongoing training of professional musicians would produce changes in the central processing of musical auditory signals since an earlier study did not find different neural generators for MMN while comparing musicians and non-musicians, but found typical differences in MMN between both groups after omitted tone pips [8]. From other data, it was supposed that ongoing professional training could result in a more accurate tuning of frequency-specific neurons in musicians [10]. Professional musicians are considered to be a model for cortical plasticity caused by ongoing musical training [13-17]. In a review [18], it was summarized that top-down and bottom-up plasticity exists in the auditory cortex, as well as in other somatosensory areas of the brain. This was supported by a recent study [19] that showed that the posterior medial cortex is involved in processing of melodic and harmonic information. If ongoing musical training participates in this process, it would be interesting to see whether a hearing deficit in trained professional musicians would interfere with, e.g., an improved tuning function or with the recognition of wrongly tuned sounds.

The present experiments investigated whether MMN could be detected in professional musicians, non-musicians, or industrial workers without formal musical training when typical musical stimuli (C-chords) were presented in the oddball-design. To get better information over the whole range of audibility, we applied the stimuli both in the mid-frequency and in the high-frequency range. We analyzed the amplitudes and latencies of the first positive and negative components of the AEP. We looked further for differences in the MMN between the three investigated groups. In another series of experiments, we tested with the same paradigm, whether MMN to mistuned high-frequency stimuli could still be observed in hearing-impaired professional musicians with a PTS in the high-frequency range between 3.000 Hz and 8.000 Hz. To evaluate to what extent the subjects were annoyed by the mistuned chords, we analyzed the EEG frequency activity in the interstimulus intervals and additionally looked for changes in heart frequency. To check, whether a long-lasting professional training might have induced a learning process for specific sounds, we repeated the EEG and heart frequency analysis in the group of hearing-impaired workers and presented them slightly disturbed machine noise they usually had heard in their daily working routine.

Hypotheses:

1. Ongoing professional training of musicians or of workers to listen to specific sounds either while performing music or watching machine sounds changes the central sound processing. These changes in AEP can be used to differentiate between untrained and trained persons.

2. The ongoing training to profession-specific sounds enables the trained person to recognize even slight deviations. The recognition is reflected by specific late components of the AEP, even when the person was not aware of the deviated stimulus.

3. The learned specific sounds could even be recognized when sound perception is disturbed by a permanent hearing impairment (PTS). External stimuli that were not trained would not be recognized even though they would be presented in the same sound intensity.

2. Materials and methods

2.1. Proband groups

Normal hearing and hearing-impaired non-musicians, aged 16 to 30 years

A group consisting of 16 members of the Medical Faculty of Jena (mean age 21.3 years) who had no hearing deficits, and who did not perform music regularly and never had formal training in music was categorized as non-musicians. The participants were all right-handed.

The hearing-impaired group (10 age-matched participants) had a hearing deficit (PTS) of about 20 dB SPL in the frequency range from 3.000 Hz to 8.000 Hz.

Normal hearing and hearing-impaired professional musicians, aged 28 to 68 years

In this part of the study participated 15 professional normal hearing musicians (mean age 41.4 years) who were employed at three German orchestras. The instrument groups were violins, trombones, oboes, bassoons, cellos, violas, and contrabasses. A second group of 10 professional musicians from the same three orchestras (mean age 48.1 years) had a hearing deficit (PTS) of more than 30 dB in frequencies larger 3 kHz. These 10 musicians played violins, contrabasses, bassoon, cello, trombones, and oboe.

Hearing-impaired industrial workers, aged 38 to 63 years

In this part of the study participated 20 industrial workers from a brewery who worked on bottle washing or bottle filling machines. Their hearing loss (PTS) of more than 20 dB SPL in the frequency range from 3.000 Hz to 8.000 Hz was officially recognized as an occupational disease. The workers were aged 38 to 63 years and had never had formal musical training or played any kind of music. All experiments were performed without hearing aids.

2.2. Study design

The study was approved by the local ethics committee of the University of Jena. All participants gave informed consent to this study and received monetary compensation for their participation. In a questionnaire, the participants were asked for their age; musical experiences, i.e., duration of employment in the orchestra or attending music school, instruments that are or were played, duration of training time per week, and the use of hearing protectors; occurrence of tinnitus; occurrence of ear, nose, and throat diseases; and hereditary ear diseases in the family. We also asked for noisy leisure time activities. The workers were asked similar questions with special respect for noise exposition per working shift. The hearing ability of the right and left ears in each participant was tested by means of a high frequency audiometer (Grahnert Präcitronic MA 22; Dresden, Germany, combined with a headphone HDA-200; Sennheiser, Hannover, Germany) and by measuring the otoacoustic emissions (DPOAE/TEOAE) (Madsen, Denmark). Details were given by our group in the literature [12].

To study the perception of auditory stimuli, we recorded MMN using the classical ac-EEG technique. Participants were seated comfortably with closed eyes. They listened to the stimuli that were presented via loudspeakers in the free field mode and were instructed only to listen relaxed and to avoid attention or any reaction to the stimuli to minimize artifacts caused by movements.

The ac-EEG was recorded from 32 electrodes (Figure 1) positioned according to the international 10/20 system over frontal, central, temporal and parietal brain areas of both hemispheres using the standardized Easy-Cap device (Easy Cap GmbH, Herrsching-Breitbrunn, Germany). A linked-mastoid electrode served as a reference. Impedance was maintained below 5 kOhm. An electrode at the forehead was used as a ground. The electrooculogram was recorded for rejection of artifacts (two electrodes above and below the eye, one electrode lateral to the eye).

The EEG was recorded with the Brain Products recording system (Brain Products GmbH, Gilching, Germany). The bandpass ranged from 0.1 Hz to 250 Hz. The amplified signals were digitized at a 5.000 Hz sample rate and analyzed off-line. The electrocardiogram was recorded for a beat-to-beat frequency analysis.

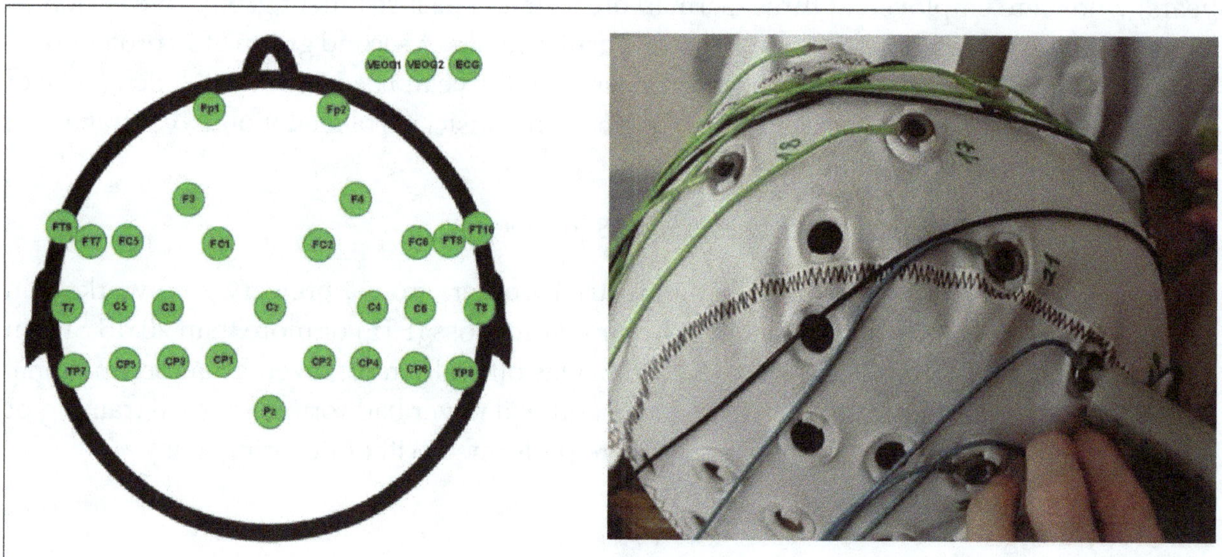

Figure 1. The left panel shows the typical electrode positions at the cap that were used in this study. Two additional reference electrodes were placed at the mastoids and as a ground electrode, the FPC position was used. To extract artifacts by eye movements, the VEOG was recorded with two electrodes. For analyzing the heart rate, the electrocardiogram in the Einthoven triangle was recorded (symbolized by the ECG marking). The right panel shows the Easy Cap device on the head while fixing the electrodes.

2.3. Auditory stimuli

Stimuli were pure C1-major chords, C3 chords, and respective mistuned chords in a classical oddball paradigm. The mistuned chords were generated by a synthesizer (variation +50 cent of the middle tone for the C-major chord, and variation +12 cent for the C3 chord) (Figure 2). A frequency and spectrogram analysis was performed to assure that the mistuned chords were in the same frequency range and had a similar intensity (integrating-averaging Sound Level Meter, type 118, class 1; Norsonic, Lierskog, Norway). Whereas the +50 cent variation was easy to differentiate from correct tunes, the +12 cent variation was difficult to discern for all non-trained listeners.

Stimuli were stored on a PC and presented in a free-field mode via the Presentation software (Presentation V9.12, NBS, Berkeley, CA) via two active loudspeakers as shown in Figure 3.

A recording session consisted of four trains per 200 single stimuli each. The participants listened with closed eyes to two trains of C1-major chords and to two trains of C3 chords. Parent and deviant stimuli were presented randomly in a 4:1 order and at randomized interstimulus intervals lasting from 2 to 6 seconds. We defined three different paradigms of stimulus occurrence: paradigm 1 had 150 normal and 50 mistuned C1-major chords, paradigm

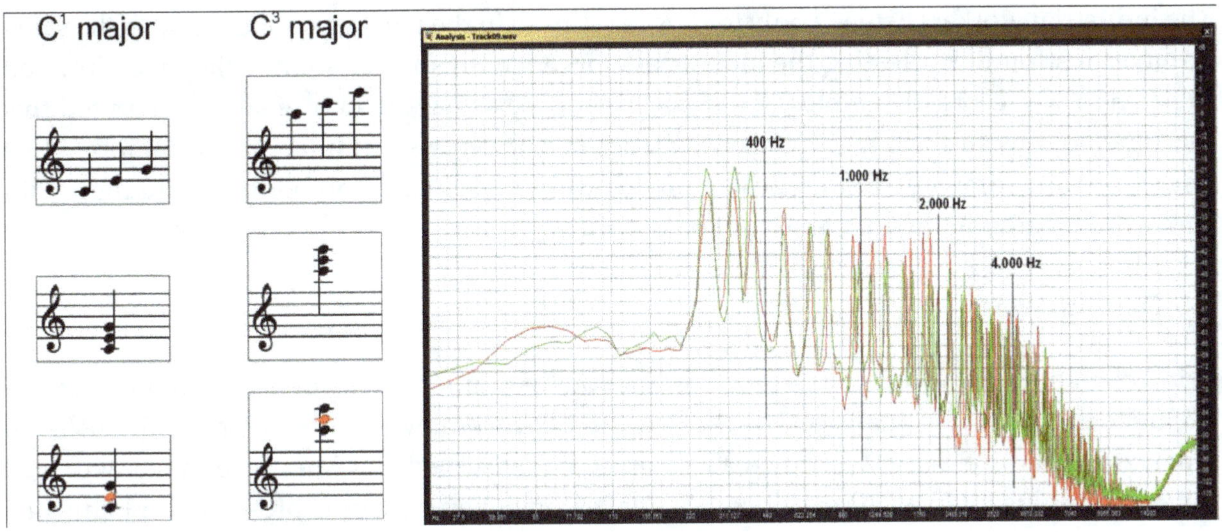

Figure 2. Design of the musical chords produced with a computer synthesizer. The C1 major (ca. 400 Hz) were the low frequency stimuli and the C3 major (ca. 1300 Hz) the high frequency stimuli. For mistuning, the middle tone E was modified (marked with red in the lower panels on the left side). The diagram on the right shows a screenshot with the intensities of both stimuli in a frequency spectrum. Note that there is no significant difference in intensity between the normal and mistuned stimuli.

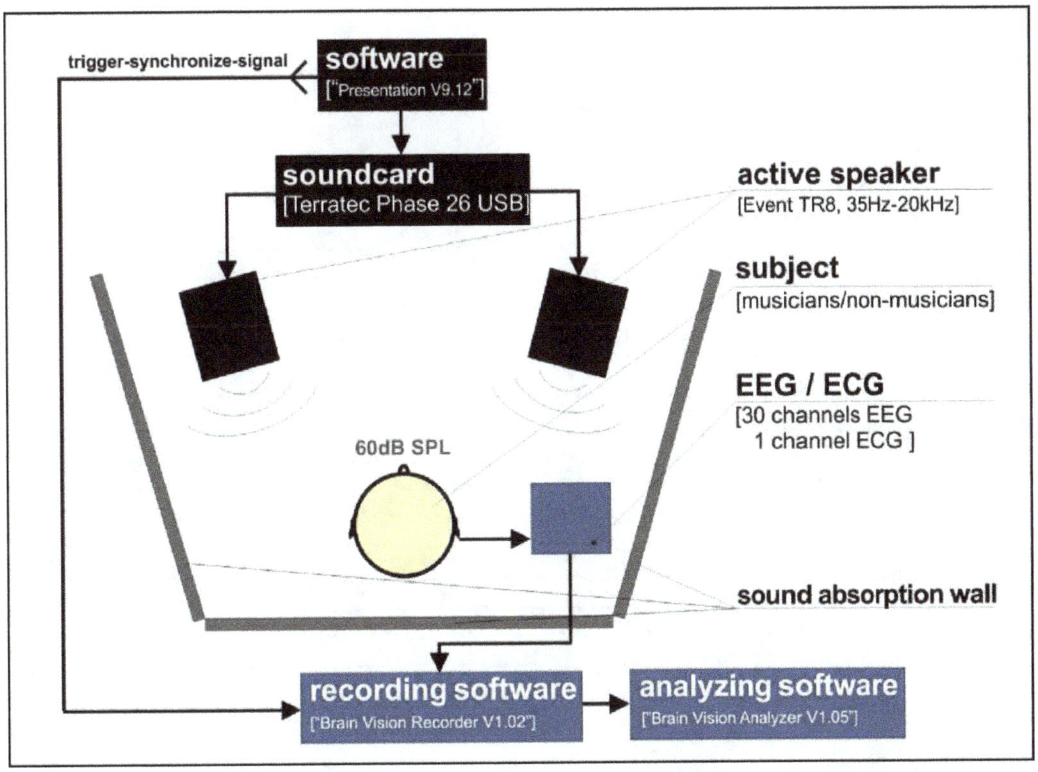

Figure 3. Schematic diagram of sound presentation and data recording setup in this study.

2 150 mistuned and 50 normal C1-major chords, and paradigm 3 150 normal and 50 mistuned C3-major chords. Non-musicians and professional musicians listened to all three paradigms. The stimulus intensity was set at 65 dB SPL.

The industrial workers listened only to musical stimuli in the paradigms 1 and 2 with the same number of stimuli. For testing the industrial workers with specific sounds they were trained to listen to we recorded samples of the machine noise as parent stimuli and interrupted this machine noise with short high-pitched whistles or with very short intervals of random white noise (deviant stimulus). Both types of stimuli were presented in an oddball paradigm with similar time intervals at an intensity of 65 dB SPL.

2.4. Data analysis

Trials contaminated with artifacts (e.g., contractions of mimic muscles or eye movements) were excluded from further analysis. The AEP in the EEG were evaluated using the BrainVision Analyzer 2 (Brain Products, Munich, Germany). We observed a 512 ms time range with a 50 ms pre-stimulus interval. A set of raw EEG data from all electrodes is presented in Figure 4.

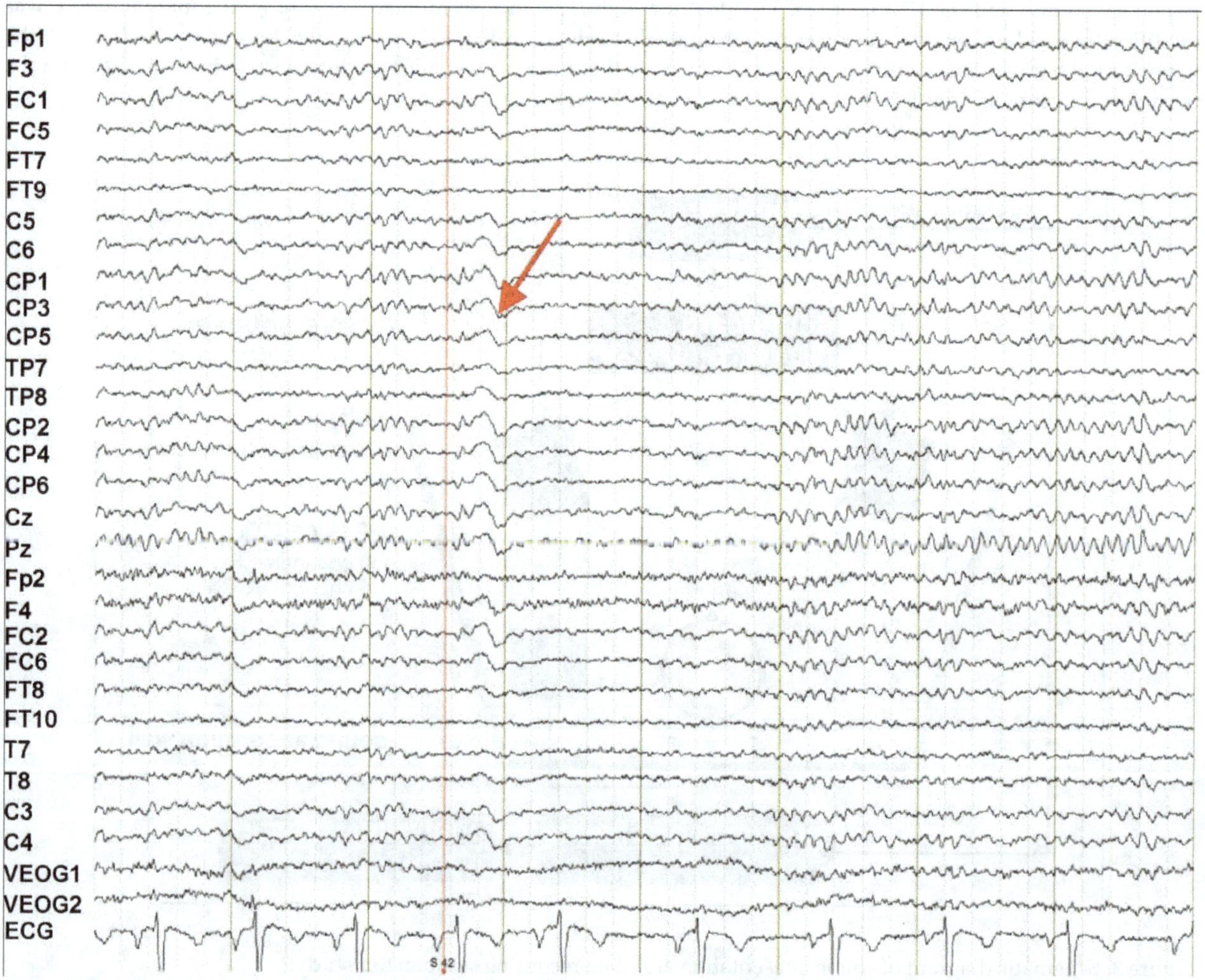

Figure 4. Specimen of an EEG recording, the recordings of EOG and of electrocardiogram with presentation of an auditory stimulus marked by the red dot and red line. The thin green lines indicate time intervals of 1 second. Note the desynchronization in the EEG beginning from the arrow for the next 1-2 seconds together with a longer lasting decrease in momentarily heart frequency.

According to widely accepted procedures [20-22], we analyzed the maximal amplitudes and latencies of the first negative component (N1), of the second positive component (P2), and we analyzed the area under the curve for the second negative component (N2) in the time range from 250-340 ms. The latter was done since not in all cases we could discern a typical or even a single peak for the component of the AEP. The MMN was measured as the difference curve between the AEP to deviant and parent chords in that time interval (Figure 5). Amplitudes and latencies were compared between parent and deviant stimuli by t-tests (student) and between the groups by one-way ANOVA as well. Separate tests were performed to determine whether the MMN-amplitudes differed for non-musicians and professional musicians as well as for normal hearing musicians and hearing-impaired musicians.

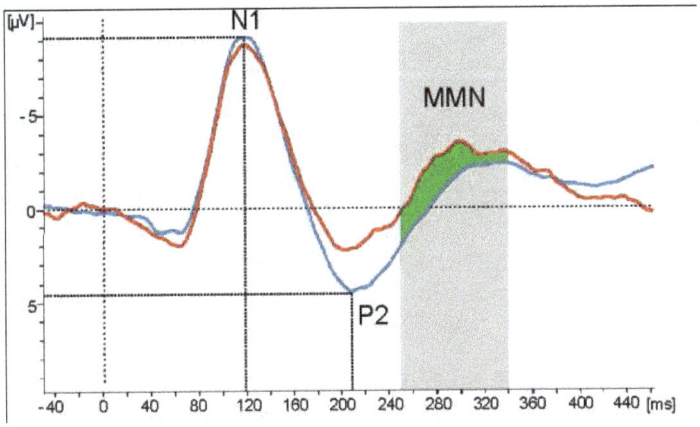

Figure 5. Specimen of a mean auditory evoked potential with labeling of the N1 and P2 components (amplitudes and latencies accentuated with dotted lines). The time interval in which we looked for the MMN is marked in grey, and the MMN is marked in green. The blue curve depicts the mean value to the frequently presented (parent) stimuli, the red one to the infrequently presented (deviant) stimuli.

To assess whether listening to mistuned chords had influence on momentary EEG-activity, we performed a Fast Fourier-Transformation (FFT) with the BrainVision Analyzer 2 in the interstimulus interval to see whether EEG-activity shifted to higher frequencies after mistuned chords. In addition, we analyzed the changes in mean heart rate (average of the heart rate during listening to in-tune music vs. mistuned tones) within the same time interval. A statistical comparison was made by means of the Wilcoxon matched pairs signed-ranks test. Statistical significance was set at 5%. Though we performed the analysis for all EEG electrodes, for better clarity we present here only data from the Cz electrodes.

3. Results

3.1. Amplitudes and latencies of N1 and P2 components of the AEP in normal hearing probands

As can be seen in Figure 6, our presented chords evoked stable and replicable AEP both in non-musicians and in professional musicians that differed only slightly between both groups.

In both groups the presentation of mistuned chords induced larger P2 components than the presentation of normal chords.

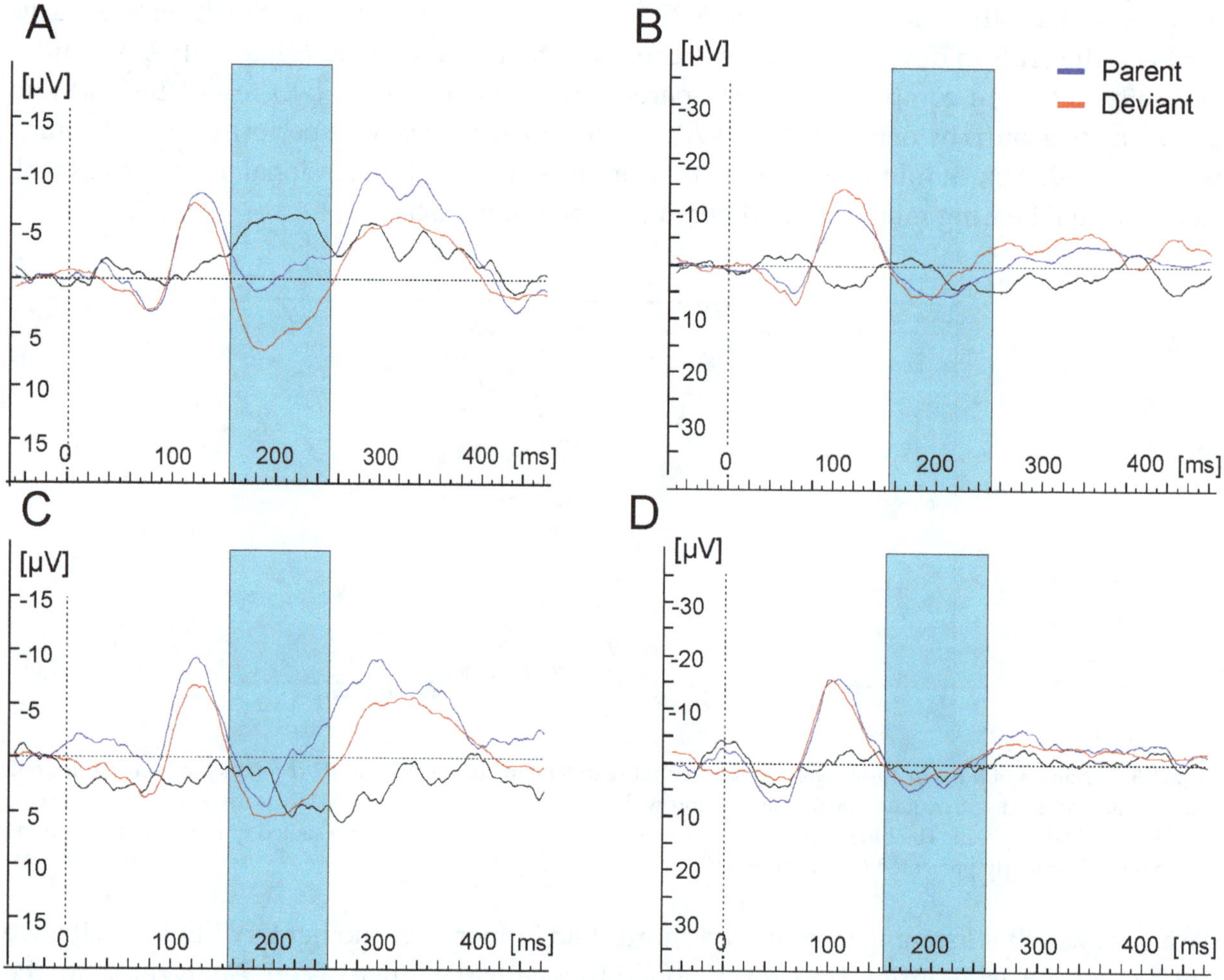

Figure 6. Mean values of AEP evoked by normal or mistuned stimuli in musicians (left diagrams) and in non-musicians (right diagrams). The bluish areas mark the time range in which we analyzed the differences between the AEP. The difference curves are shown in black. The blue lines represent AEP to frequently presented chords, the red lines AEP to the infrequently presented ones. For a better visibility the standard deviations of the curves are omitted. A and B show that normal chords occurred frequently (paradigm 1). C and D show that mistuned chords occurred frequently (paradigm 2). Note the small differences between normal tuned and mistuned chords in non-musicians in diagrams B and D.

The peak of the N1 component was seen at about 128 ms after the stimulus, the peak of the P2 component at about 224 ms after the stimulus. Mean N1 amplitudes amounted to about 7 µV, mean P2 amplitudes to 5 µV. A detailed comparison between the groups of musicians and non-musicians and the three paradigms is given in Figure 7. It should be noted that both C3-major chords resulted in markedly larger areas under the curve both for the N1 and for the P2 components in non-musicians and in musicians. However, the area under the curve of the P2 component was larger when C3-major chords were presented than when C1-major chords were presented.

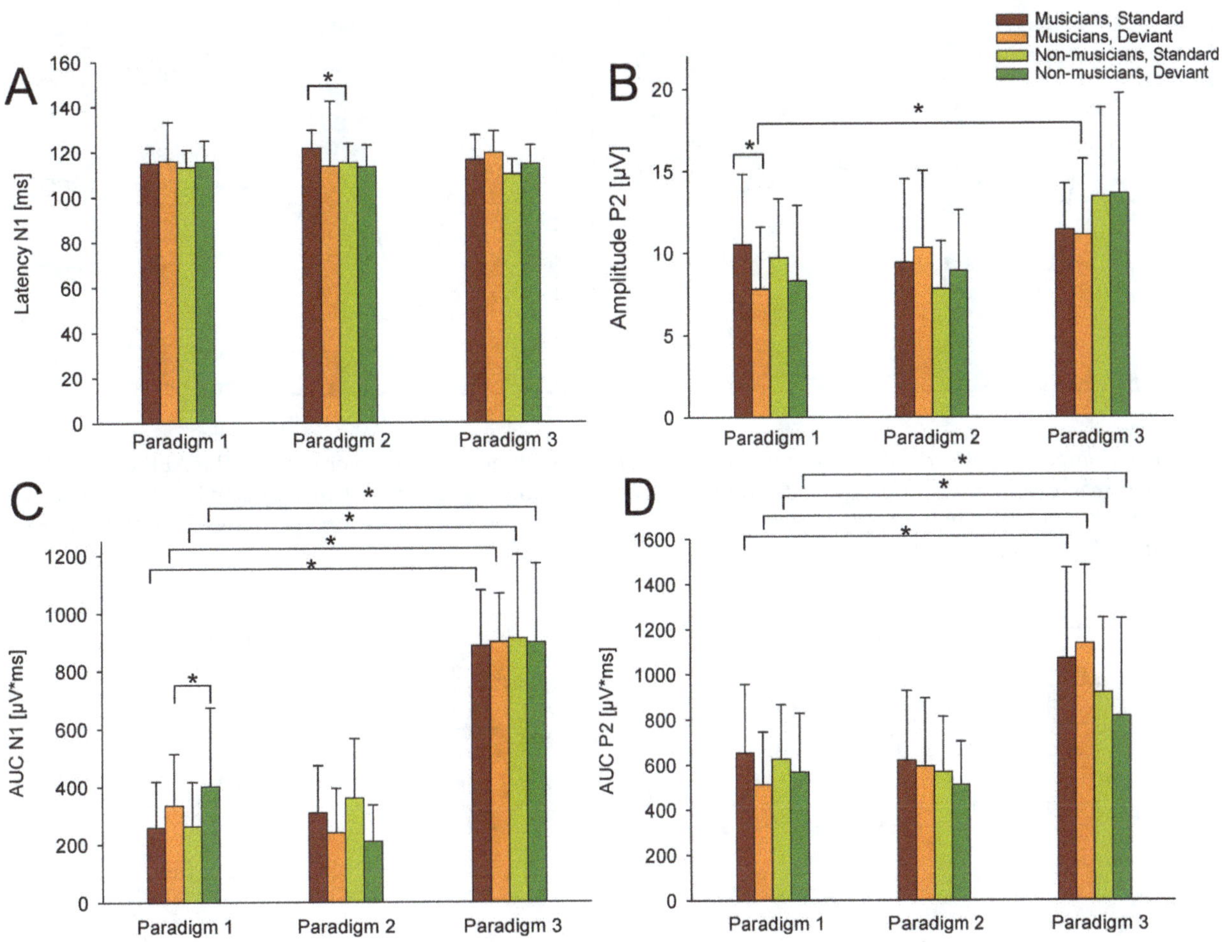

Figure 7. AEP components from normal hearing non-musicians and musicians. The bars give the mean values ± std. dev. The asterisks mark statistically significant differences ($p<0.05$). A) Latency times of the N1 component. B) Amplitudes of the P2 component. C) Areas under the curves of the N1 component. D) Areas under the curve of the P2 component.

Interestingly, the EEG activity differed markedly between both groups when the late components of the AEP were compared that were recorded from the Cz electrode and an activity map was computed by the brain vision software. Though the general pattern was alike, a general higher activity rate was seen in musicians over the temporo-occipital cortex and a lower activity in the vertex area of the brain (Figure 8).

3.2. Amplitudes and latencies of N1 and P2 components of the AEP in hearing-impaired probands

All professional musicians in this group had a hearing loss in the mid- and/or high-frequency range with a mean PTS up to 35 dB SPL. No significant differences were obtained when left and right ears were tested so a preferential side of hearing loss could be excluded. All hearing-impaired industrial workers suffered from hearing loss that was recognized as an occupational disease. The hearing deficit had a similar magnitude as in the hearing-impaired professional musicians and was also found at both ears with a slight but insignificant preference to the left ears (Figure 9).

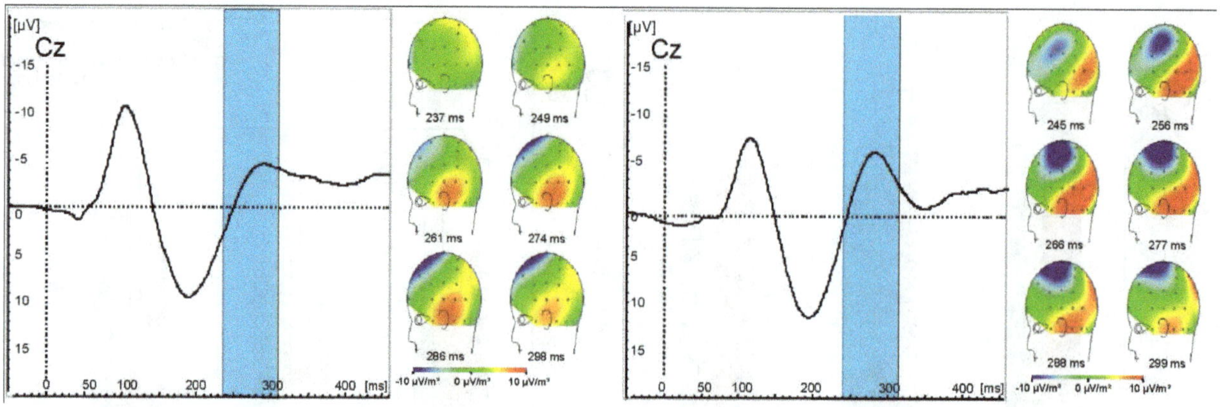

Figure 8. Comparison of cortical EEG activity after stimulation with normal C1-major chords. The AEP curves show the grand mean value from all participants and the activity maps the distribution of cortical activity at different moments after the stimulus in the time range marked in blue. A) Data from normal hearing non-musicians. B) Data from normal hearing musicians.

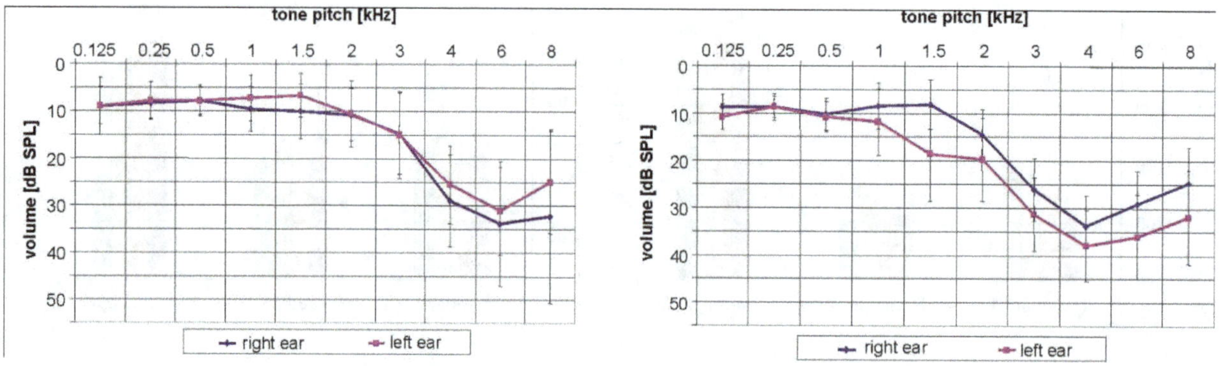

Figure 9. Mean values ± std. dev. of hearing loss in the left and right ears of the 10 hearing-impaired professional musicians (left) and of the 20 hearing-impaired industrial workers (right).

When tested with the auditory stimuli, the parameters of the AEP components differed from the data obtained in normal hearing musicians. The N1 peaks were found earlier (C1 chord 121 ms, C3 chord 109 ms after stimulus) and had larger amplitudes (C1 chord 11 µV, C3 chord 11 µV). The same was seen for the P2 peaks (latency for C1 chords 213 ms, for C3 chords 202 ms; amplitude for C1 chords 5 µV, for C3 chords 8 µV). The latter difference was even significant between C1 chords and C3 chords in this group.

For both stimulus types (normal or mistuned), neither amplitudes nor latencies of the N1 component showed significant differences between non-musicians, normal hearing or hearing-impaired musicians. Responses to parent or deviant stimuli did not differ, regardless whether in-tune or mistuned chords were given as parent stimuli. Similarly, no significant difference existed when comparing the N1 components to the mid-frequency (C1; paradigm 1) or to high-frequency (C3; paradigm 3) stimulation when the chords were mistuned by either 50 cent or by 12 cent.

The workers were first presented the same auditory stimuli as the other participants in this study, i.e., C1-major chords. When analyzing the AEP, we found later N1 amplitudes (peak

134 ms after stimulus) when the paradigm 1 was used, and same latencies as in non-musicians, when the paradigm 2 was used (N1 peak 128 ms after stimulus). The N1 amplitudes ranged from 10 to 12 μV and differed only slightly from those we obtained in non-musicians (Figure 10A and 10B). A similar result was seen when we analyzed the P2 components of the AEP. In this group, the latencies ranged from 228 to 237 ms after stimulus in paradigm 1 and from 218 to 226 ms in paradigm 2 that was later than in musicians, but in the same range as in non-musicians. The P2 amplitudes ranged from 7 to 11 μV and did not differ significantly to the other participants. Both musicians and industrial workers had larger P2 areas under the curve either when the mistuned stimuli were presented rarely in the paradigms 1 (Figure 10C) or often in the paradigms 2 (Figure 10D).

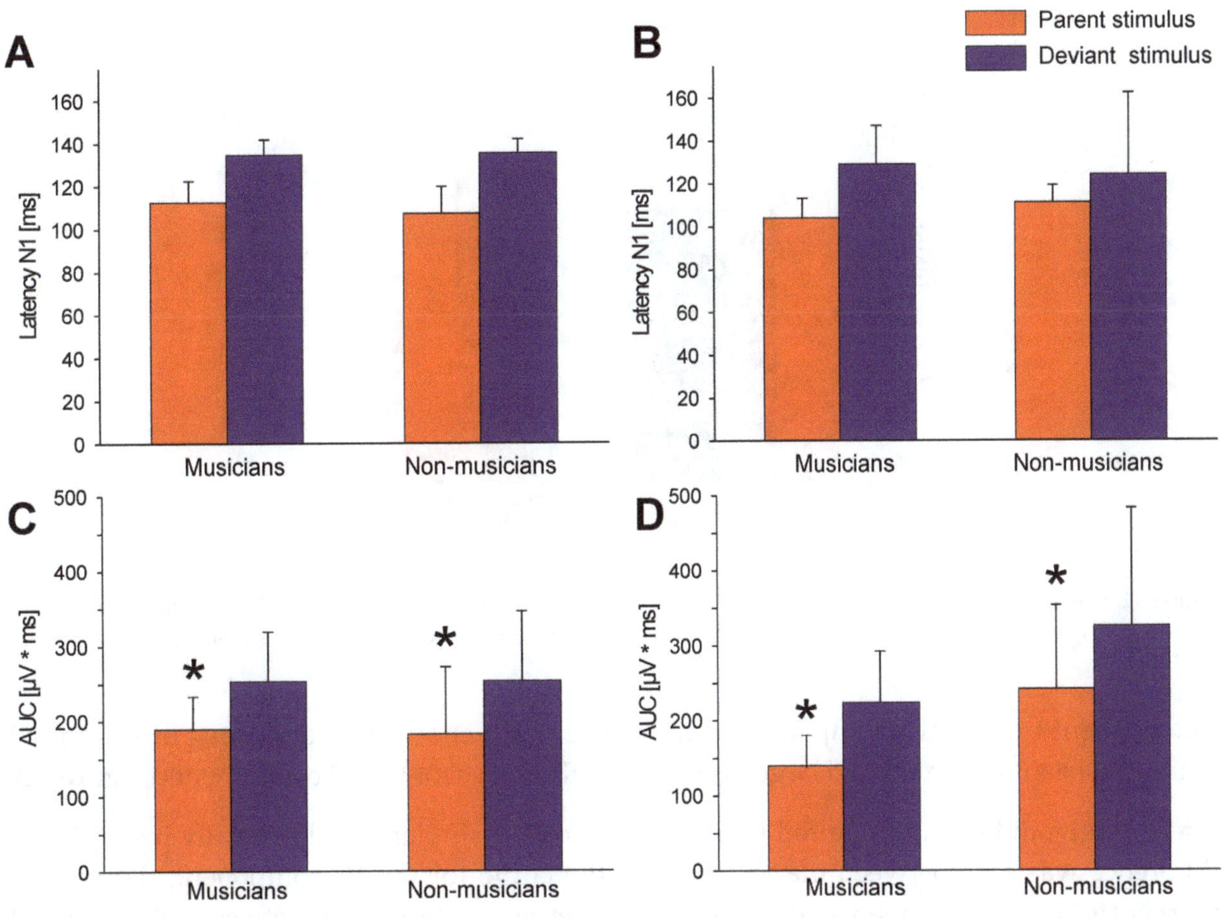

Figure 10. Comparison of amplitudes of the N1 components and of the areas under the curve for the P2 components of the AEP in hearing-impaired musicians and in hearing-impaired industrial workers. Data are presented as mean values ± std. dev. The asterisk marks statistically significant differences ($p<0.05$). A) N1 latencies in paradigm 1. B) N1 latencies in paradigm 2. C) P2 areas under the curve in paradigm 1. D) P2 areas under the curve in paradigm 2.

In a second part of the study, the workers had to listen to machine noise that was either unchanged (parent stimulus) or interrupted/disturbed by short high-pitched whistles. This type of stimulation did not evoke typical AEP, but was used to look for activity changes in the EEG (see below).

3.3. Comparison of the MMN

When interviewed after the series both normal hearing and hearing-impaired musicians complained about the mistuned chords. They told us that they were annoyed at the mistuned chords, but hearing-impaired non-musicians and hearing-impaired industrial workers had not perceived the small differences between the stimuli.

Hearing-impaired musicians were still able to distinguish between in-tune and mistuned chords in both the C1 and in the C3 chords regardless of the degree of mistuning. Their areas under the curve for the MMN were significantly larger when the C1 chords were presented and mistuned stimuli occurred rarely (paradigm 1), which is shown in Figure 11.

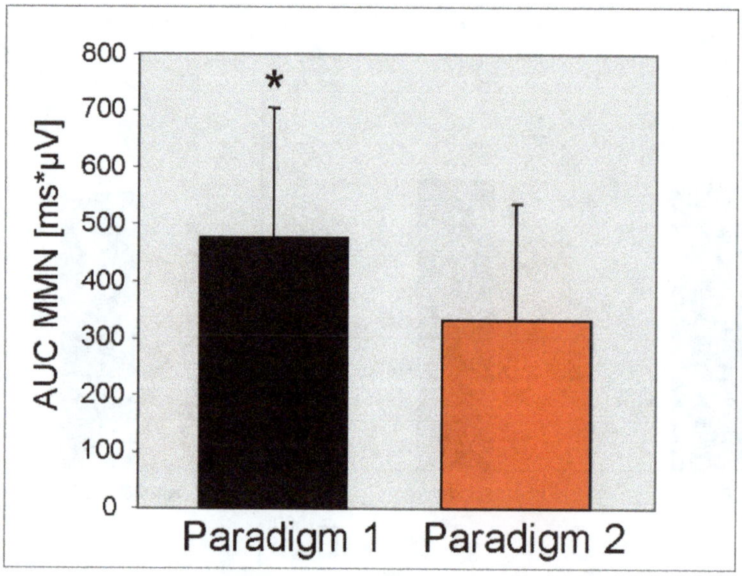

Figure 11. Comparison of areas under the curve for the stimulation with C1 chords in paradigm 1 (black bar) and in paradigm 2 (red bar). Data are presented as mean values ± std. dev. The asterisk marks a significant difference ($p<0.05$).

Independent from hearing impairment, rarely occurring chords (either normal or mistuned) in the musicians group evoked larger areas under the curve for the P2 components (Figure 12).

Interestingly, in hearing-impaired industrial workers, a similar but statistically insignificant difference was seen between the areas under the curve for the P2 component, though the workers told in the interview that they did not observe any differences between the presented chords. This difference was seen both when the mistuned stimulus was presented rarely or often (Figure 13).

The investigation of the MMN curves (AEP to deviant minus AEP to standard stimuli) confirmed differences between non-musicians and both groups of musicians. In normal hearing musicians, the MMN was found in the time range from 180-250 ms after stimulus and a similar, but even longer lasting MMN (up to 300 ms after stimulus), was seen in hearing-impaired musicians. The MMN curves after high-frequency stimulation (C3 chords), however, allowed a clear differentiation between professional musicians and non-musicians. Non-

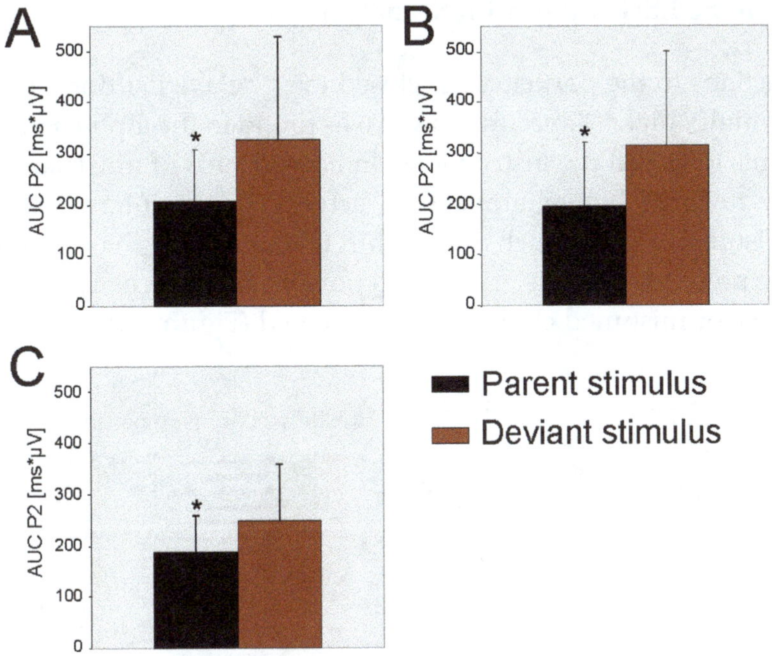

Figure 12. Comparison of the areas under the curve for the P2 components of the AEP in hearing-impaired professional musicians. Data are presented as mean values ± std. dev. The asterisks mark significant differences ($p<0.05$). Black bars show responses to the parent stimuli, the brown bars show the responses to the deviant stimuli. A) C1 chord, paradigm 1. B) C1chord, paradigm 2. C) C3 chord, paradigm 3.

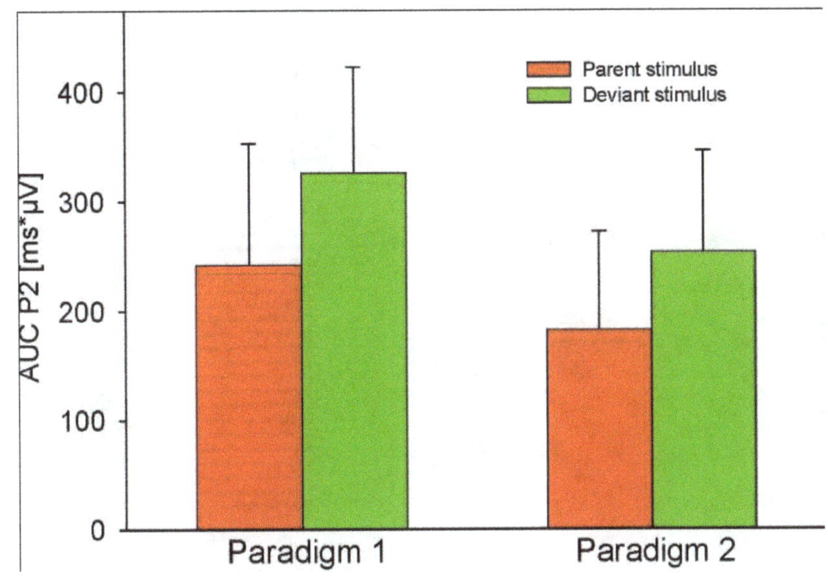

Figure 13. Areas under the curve for the P2 component recorded in hearing-impaired workers. Data are presented as mean values ± std. dev. The red bars show responses to parent stimuli, the green ones to deviant stimuli. A) Presentation in paradigm 1 (mistuned stimuli occur rarely). B) Presentation in paradigm 2 (normal stimuli occur rarely).

musicians had no typical MMN in the observed time range. In normal hearing musicians, this MMN occurred in the range of 250-340 ms after stimulus and a small, but clearly discernable MMN was also found in hearing-impaired musicians. In the latter group, however, the MMN started earlier (220-230 ms after stimulus).

3.4. FFT analysis of the EEG and heart rate analysis

Due to the instructions to the participants (closed eyes, relaxed sitting position, no directed attention to the stimuli), highest spectral power was found in the alpha band, thus confirming that the participants followed the instructions. In both groups of musicians, we found a shift in power density towards higher alpha EEG activity in the interstimulus intervals after presentation of mistuned chords. Such a large shift failed to occur in non-musicians, when the same stimuli were presented. In this group EEG power spectra density was the same, regardless whether in-tune or mistuned chords were presented (Figure 14).

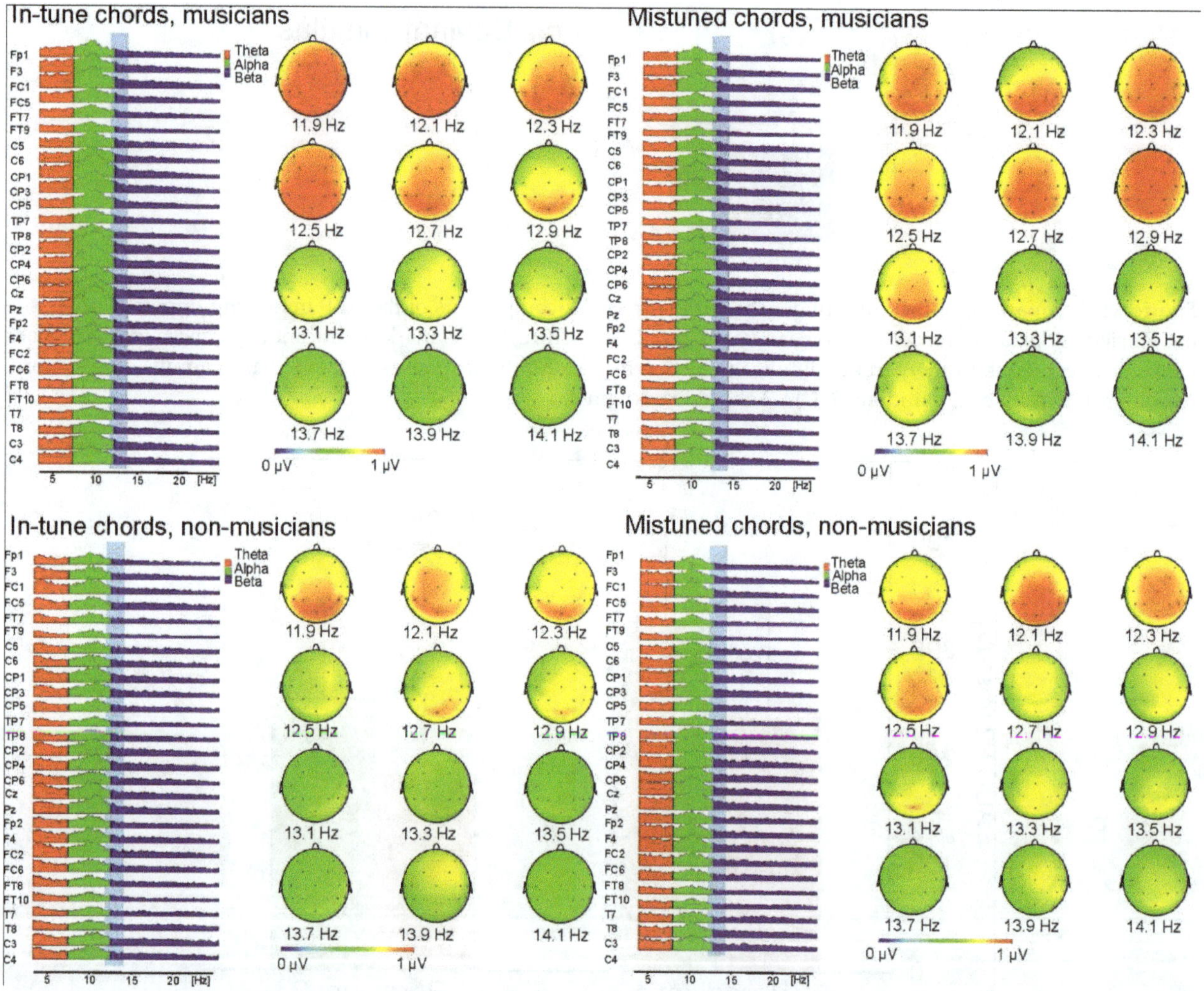

Figure 14. FFT-analysis of the EEG shown as diagrams of regional spectral EEG power and as frequency split maps for musicians (top) and non-musicians (bottom). The light blue bar in the power spectra marks the frequency range that is further analyzed in the frequency split maps. Note the activity shifts towards higher alpha frequencies in musicians when mistuned stimuli were presented. Such a shift failed to occur in non-musicians.

In the same groups we analyzed the heart rates and found a significant increase in mean heart rate in musicians after listening to mistuned chords compared to the resting situation, but no significant differences when comparing resting situation vs. hearing of in-tune chords (resting situation 69.6±12.4 beats per minute, 70.2±12.4 beats per minute after in-tune chords, 71.4±11.5

beats per minute after mistuned chords; n=15; Wilcoxon matched pairs signed-ranks test, p=0.0353). The mean heart frequency, however, did not change in non-musicians (resting situation 60,7±8.1 beats per minute, 60.5±7.5 beats per minute after in-tune chords, 60.8±8.7 beats per minute after mistuned chords; n=10).

Hearing-impaired industrial workers always negated to have noticed the mistuned stimuli, though we had recorded typical MMN to the rare stimulus. In order to present a profession-specific sound to this group, we had used short sequences of the unchanged machine noise and the same noise with high-pitched whistles that sounded like very short pips.

As expected from the pre-trial interviews where the hearing-impaired workers claimed that they easily could discern even one broken bottle in the machine sound, the workers confirmed after the trials that they had heard the rarely occurring disturbed noise samples. In the EEG, the occurrence of these rare stimuli caused a desynchronization lasting for 5-6 seconds (Figure 15).

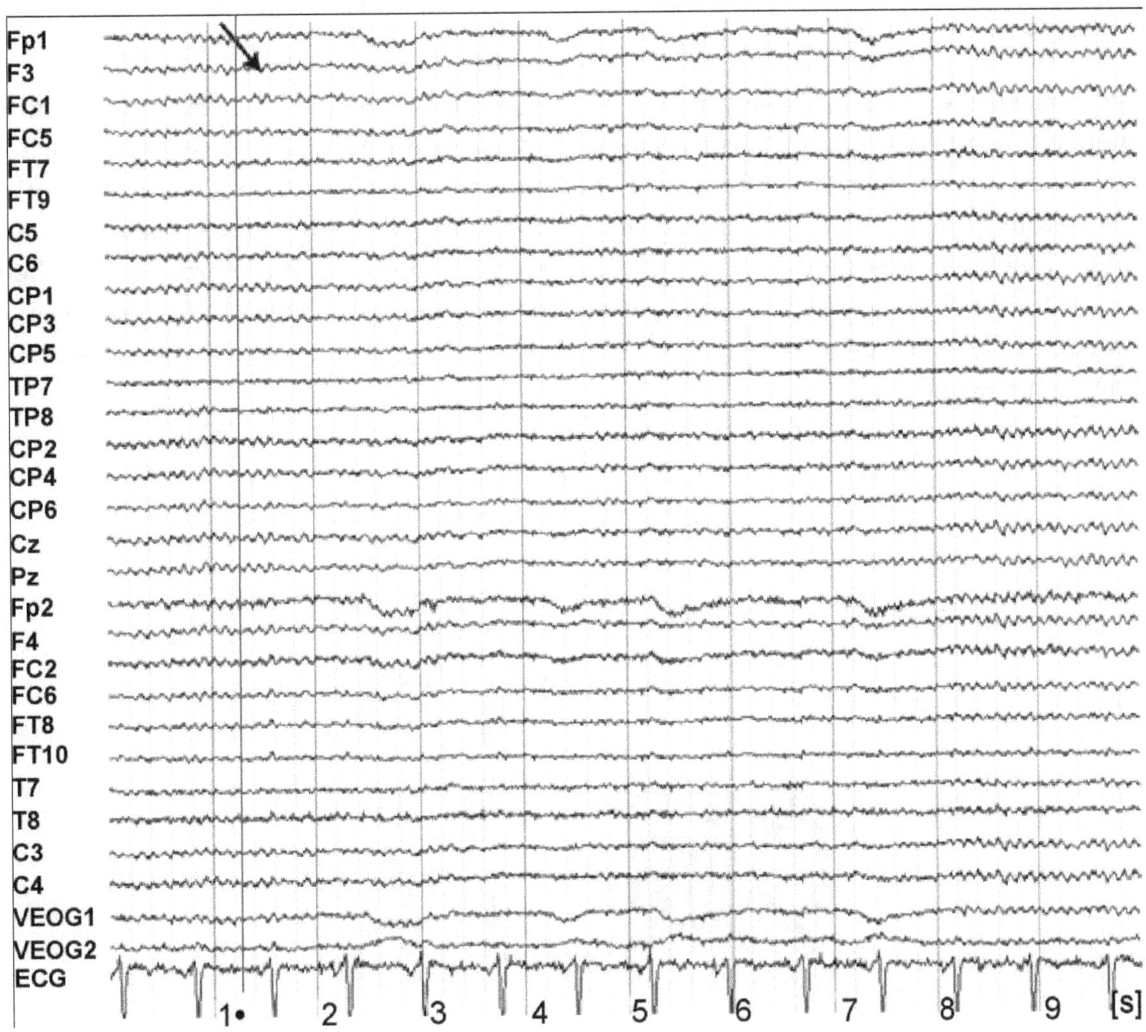

Figure 15. Sample EEG recording from one hearing-impaired industrial worker. The black dot at the bottom marks the presentation of the disturbed machine noise; the onset of the desynchronization in the EEG is marked by an arrow.

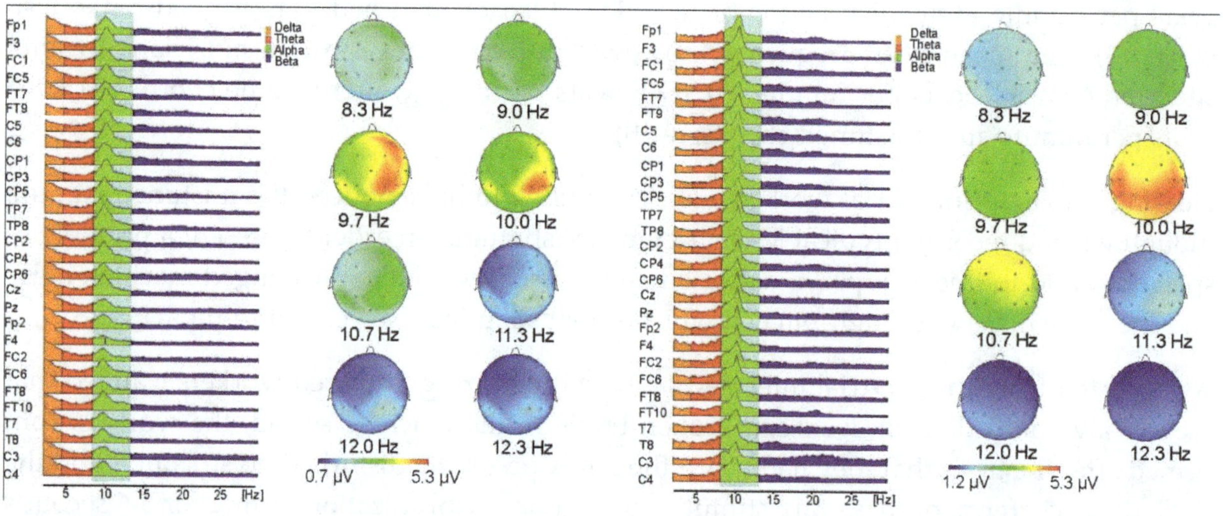

Figure 16. FFT-analysis of the EEG shown as diagrams of regional spectral EEG power and as frequency split maps for normal undisturbed machine noise was presented (left panel), and when the machine noise was disturbed by short pips (right panel). The light blue bar in the power spectra marks the frequency range that is further analyzed in the frequency split maps.

We performed the same FFT-analysis of the EEG in the workers and revealed a shift in the frequency towards higher alpha bands when the disturbed noise was presented (Figure 16). During undisturbed noise the EEG activity had its maximum at 9.7 Hz and was preferentially distributed in the right hemisphere, and only a small area of this hemisphere showed a 10.0 Hz EEG. When we presented the disturbed noise, in a larger area of the brain at both hemispheres a 10.0 Hz EEG and in the frontal parts of the cortex even a 10.7 Hz EEG were observed. The mean EEG frequency increased from 9.2±0.6 Hz during undisturbed noise to 9.4±0.6 Hz during disturbed noise.

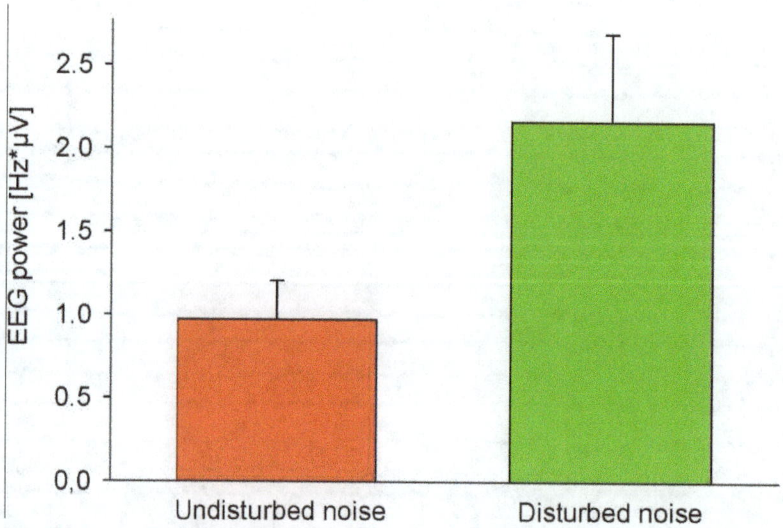

Figure 17. Mean values of EEG power spectra ± std. dev. in hearing-impaired industrial workers when typical machine noise was presented. The red bar shows the data during undisturbed noise; the green one shows the data during disturbed noise.

In addition, we analyzed the power spectra in the frequency range from 12 to 14 Hz at the Cz electrode and found significantly higher regional EEG spectral power in hearing-impaired industrial workers when disturbed machine noise was presented (Figure 17).

4. Discussion

For the first time in this study, profession-specific stimuli were used to assess the effects of hearing deficits in professional musicians and in industrial workers. Here we have shown that parameters of AEP and MMN to mistuned chords differ between musicians and non-musicians, as well as between normal hearing and hearing-impaired musicians, and that components of the AEP and the MMN can be used to differentiate between the three investigated groups. FFT analysis of the EEG in the interstimulus intervals confirmed that mistuned chords caused a state of higher EEG activity only in musicians, regardless of their hearing loss. Another evidence was the occurrence of heart rate changes only in musicians. Therefore we conclude that both perception and processing of musical signals differ between musicians and non-musicians. In hearing-impaired workers, the disturbed machine noise caused a state of higher EEG activity as well.

It is known that complex stimuli such as complex derived words can produce MMN [23]. The stimuli we used were chosen from the typical occupational environment of the professional musician, i.e., musical chords. Complex musical sounds are used to produce MMN, e.g., to compare timbre processing in harmonically rich sounds versus single sinusoidal tones [24]. We had expected that musicians with ongoing musical training over several years have learned to hear and to evaluate these stimuli with their professional memory. Marked differences between tuned and mistuned chords should be recognized easily by musicians, but also by non-musicians. Smaller differences, however, when stimuli were presented in the high-frequency range should be recognized only by musicians. To our knowledge, such a study had not been done before in hearing-impaired musicians.

Intense musical training resulted in an increase in area of primary and secondary auditory cortices [25-27]. In line with this finding, fMRI investigations in musicians revealed a co-activation of both auditory and sensomotor areas in the cortex, thus showing that musical training changes the connectivity and probably also the processing strategies in the brain of musicians [28-30]. Long-term musical training enhances the short-term memory for auditory stimuli and eased behavioral tasks, e.g., detection of deviant tones in a series of auditory stimuli [31].

Our results confirmed the efficacy of comparison of event-related potentials to differentiate between trained musicians and non-musicians [32,33]. The effect of training to induce neural plasticity in the auditory system has been shown in musical conductors compared to non-musicians in a spatial detection task [34], in a pitch detection task [35] or in MMN evoked by variations of complex tone patterns, where long-term musical training modulated the encoding of wrong tones in the right hemisphere of musicians [36]. This is an ongoing process starting in pre-adolescence, since musically trained children had larger MMN to slightly mistuned tones compared to age-matched, non-trained children already at the age of 11, thus confirming that musical training indeed could be responsible for the larger negativity [37]. The cortical plasticity can even be improved, if not only auditory but also somatosensory tasks should be solved, e.g., learning to judge whether music was correctly played versus learning to play an instrument [38]. Interestingly, in hearing-impaired musicians we found clearly distinguishable MMNs, as well as changes in EEG power spectra after presentation of mistuned chords. Even when the stimulus was in the frequency range that was affected by the hearing disability (C3 paradigm), the professional musicians were able to differentiate between in-tune and mistuned chords. However, the normal hearing untrained non-musicians were only able to differentiate to heavily mistuned (50 cent) stimuli, but the hearing impaired did not. The results of interviews confirmed that the mistuned stimuli were recognized both by normal hearing and by hearing-impaired musicians and caused a state of unhappiness.

We could prove this when we tested the hearing-impaired workers with chord stimuli. The workers had similar hearing deficits in a similar frequency range as the hearing professional musicians. The musicians easily recognized the mistuned stimuli and commented on their occurrence in the interviews after the trials, but the workers who never before had heard those stimuli did not. The early AEP components (N1 amplitudes and latencies) did not indicate different processing of the mistuned chords by the workers. The late AEP components (P2 area under the curve and MMN), however, indicated that the mistuned stimuli were sensed and processed differently, even if the person was not aware of this stimulus [39]. Unfortunately, we could not test this phenomenon reversely with the professional musicians, since they refused stimulation with machine noise. We suppose that such unfamiliar stimuli would be difficult to discern by the musicians.

To explain the ability of hearing-impaired musicians to differentiate between "right" and "wrong" tunes several considerations are necessary. We can exclude a significantly varied loudness of the tuned versus the mistuned stimuli. In the group of hearing-impaired musicians, audiological investigations provided evidence for a diminished peripheral input. This impairment might explain the delayed and smaller amplitude of the P2 component as well as the smaller areas under the curve for the N2 component and the smaller resulting MMNs than in normal hearing musicians. Interestingly, the AEP had a similar amplitude and time shape both after stimulation with the high-frequent C3 paradigm and with the mid-frequent C1-major chords, thus confirming that the hearing damage should have affected a larger part of the cochlea. In agreement with a previous study [8], we had instructed the participants to sit relaxed and not to pay attention to the chords. Therefore, we conclude that we were able to record a non-attentional, automatic processing of musical signals. Musicians that were trained to those signals should process this information more effectively [8]. In line with this, musicians were less dependent on the salience of an acoustical environment, but in non-musicians salience had a stronger impact on the processing of complex tone patterns [36]. Assuming that musical training had already caused this effect before hearing impairment started, it is likely that the diminished input could be processed in professional musicians with still higher efficacy than in untrained non-musicians. Another statement in the literature [10] gives support to our interpretation: musical training should result in a more accurate tuning of the frequency-specific neurons in musicians compared to non-musicians. There is indication for a better top-down modulation of auditory processing in trained musicians for both musical sounds and speech [40]. We suppose, therefore, that a better tuning function of the neurons would result in more accurate processing of the rest of a signal when the input is diminished by cochlear damage. In line with this, we found in hearing-impaired musicians significant earlier N1 and P2 components than in hearing-impaired industrial workers when musician-specific chords were used as stimuli.

We conclude that our observed smaller MMNs to mistuned chords in hearing-impaired professional musicians reflect central compensation mechanisms that are able to improve the processing of profession-specific signals, i.e., musical chords. This compensation does not take place in situations of normal life (i.e., without ongoing formal training), e.g., watching TV, using a headphone or cellular phone, or in situations with a loud background that disturbs the incoming signals. In these situations, hearing-impaired musicians complain about the hearing deficit though they are able to play their instruments correctly.

The musicians investigated in our study were interested in learning about hearing damage and the proper use of hearing protectors. Nevertheless, the acceptance of hearing protectors (custom-built ear plugs for specific instruments) among musicians in classical orchestras is very small; more than 90% dislike such devices. Another number has been observed among rock musicians - there is a rate of nearly 50% who accept such hearing protectors [41,42]. Hearing loss among professional musicians in Germany has so far not been accepted as an occupational disease though sound intensities exceed the limits allowed for a working shift in many orchestras [12,43]. The lack of rules to prevent hearing loss in professional classical musicians and the ongoing dispute whether sound exposure during rehearsals or performances is high enough to induce hearing loss hinders the discussion to foster the use of hearing protection in that profession [44-48].

In conclusion, our data indicate that a differentiation between non-musicians and musicians is possible by analyzing AEP components or the MMN when profession-specific stimuli are used. The MMN was still present in hearing-impaired professional musicians, although they had a hearing deficit in the frequency range of the musical stimuli. Probably, the intense musical training has enhanced the processing structures and/or efficacy to evaluate the musical stimulus. A similar result was seen in the workers: ongoing professional training enabled the detection of disturbed machine noise though this group was unable to detect differences in non-trained musical sounds.

To answer the hypotheses postulated at the beginning:

1. Musical chords are a suitable stimulus to evoke stable and replicable AEP both in musicians and in people who are not trained to musical stimuli. AEP evoked by those stimuli can be used to differentiate between trained and untrained persons. Especially the late components of the AEP differ and depend on the learned stimulus. Ongoing professional training to specific sounds is a learning process that is reflected in different sound processing and in the late components of the AEP.

2. After ongoing training to profession-specific sounds, a person is able to notice even small differences of a stimulus, even though the stimulus is presented in a frequency range with impaired hearing function. This phenomenon should be noted when hearing thresholds are measured. A PTS does not always represent an inability to perform a specific (learned) hearing task.

3. The occurrence of differences in the stimuli that is reflected in different parameters of the AEP does not imply an awareness of perception of the stimulus. This is important when foreign stimuli are used and the proband is asked for recognition of different stimuli.

Nomenclature and Abbreviations

AEP; Auditory evoked potential

ANOVA; Analysis of variance

DPOAE; Distortion product otoacoustic emissions

EEG; Electroencephalogram

FFT; Fast Fourier transformation

MMN; Mismatch Negativity

PTS; Permanent threshold shift

TEOAE; Transient-evoked otoacoustic emissions

VEOG; Vertical electrooculogram

Acknowledgements

The study has been supported by a grant of the Berufsgenossenschaft Nahrungsmittel und Gaststätten (Employer's Liability Insurance Association) and by the Kompetenzzentrum für Interdisziplinäre Prävention (KIP) of the Friedrich Schiller University Jena.

Author details

Edeltraut Emmerich, Marcus Engelmann, Melanie Rohmann and Frank Richter*

Institute of Physiology I/Neurophysiology, University Hospital Jena - Friedrich Schiller University, Jena, Germany

References

[1] Näätänen R, Gaillard AWK, Mäntysalo S. Early selective-attention effect on evoked potential reinterpreted. Acta Psychologica. 1978;42:313-329.

[2] Näätänen R, Paavilainen P, Rinne T, Alho K. The mismatch negativity (MMN) in basic research of central auditory processing: A review. Clinical Neurophysiology. 2007;118(12):2544-2590.

[3] Näätänen R, Paavilainen P, Reinikainen K. Do event-related potentials to infrequent decrements in duration of auditory stimuli demonstrate a memory trace in man? Neuroscience Letters. 1989;107(1-3):347-352.

[4] Hari R, Hämäläinen M, Ilmoniemi R, Kaukoranta E, Reinikainen K, Salminen J, Alho K, Näätänen R, Sams M. Responses of the primary auditory cortex to pitch changes in a sequence of tone pips: Neuromagnetic recordings in man. Neuroscience Letters. 1984;50(1-3):127-132.

[5] Näätänen R, Paavilainen P, Alho K, Reinikainen K, Sams M. The mismatch negativity to intensity changes in an auditory stimulus sequence. Electroencephalography & Clinical Neurophysiology. 1987;Suppl. 40:125-131.

[6] Tervaniemi M, Winkler I, Näätänen R. Pre-attentive categorization of sounds by timbre as revealed by event-related potentials. Neuroreport. 1997;8(11):2571-2574.

[7] Rahne T, Plontke SK, Wagner L. Mismatch negativity (MMN) reflects timbre discrimination thresholds in normal-hearing listeners and cochlear implant users. Brain Research. 2014;1586:143-151.

[8] Rüsseler J, Altenmüller E, Nager W, Kohlmetz C, Münte TF. Event-related brain potentials to sound omissions differ in musicians and non-musicians. Neuroscience Letters. 2001;308(1):33-36.

[9] Leino S, Brattico E, Tervaniemi M, Vuust P. Representation of harmony rules in the human brain: Further evidence from event-related potentials. Brain Research. 2007;1142:169-177.

[10] Koelsch S, Schröger E, Tervaniemi M. Superior pre-attentive auditory processing in musicians. Neuroreport. 1999;10(6):1309-1313.

[11] Vuust P, Pallesen KJ, Bailey C, van Zuijen TL, Gjedde A, Roepstorff A, Østergaard L. To musicians, the message is in the meter pre-attentive neuronal responses to incongruent rhythm are left-lateralized in musicians. Neuroimage. 2005;24(2):560-564.

[12] Emmerich E, Rudel L, Richter F. Is the audiologic status of professional musicians a reflection of the noise exposure in classical orchestral music? European Archives of Otorhinolaryngology. 2008;265(7):753-758.

[13] Bormann V, Sust CA, Heinecke-Schmidt R, Fuder G, Lazarus H., editors. Schwerhörigkeit und Sprachkommunikation am Arbeitsplatz. Schriftenreihe der

Bundesanstalt für Arbeitsschutz und Arbeitsmedizin - Fb 1041. Dortmund: Wirtschaftsverlag NW; 2005.

[14] Gentsch G. Differenzierung reiner und verstimmter Akkorde bei hörgeschädigten Berufsmusikern: Eine Analyse akustisch evozierter Potentiale. MD thesis. University Hospital Jena - Friedrich Schiller University; 2010.

[15] Rohmann M. Analyse von akustisch evozierten Potentialen nach reinen und verstimmten Akkorden bei hörgesunden Musikern und Nichtmusikern. MD thesis. University Hospital Jena - Friedrich Schiller University; 2012.

[16] Münte TF, Altenmüller E, Jäncke L. The musician's brain as a model of neuroplasticity. Nature Reviews Neuroscience. 2002;3(6):473-478.

[17] Parbery-Clark A, Anderson S, Kraus N. Musicians change their tune: How hearing loss alters the neural code. Hearing Research. 2013;302:121-131.

[18] Kral A, Eggermont JJ. What's to lose and what's to learn: Development under auditory deprivation, cochlear implants and limits of cortical plasticity. Brain Research Reviews. 2007;56(1):259-269.

[19] Spada D, Verga L, Iadanza A, Tettamanti M, Perani D. The auditory scene: An fMRI study on melody and accompaniment in professional pianists. Neuroimage. 2014;102:764-775.

[20] Koelsch S, Gunter TC, Wittfoth M, Sammler D. Interaction between syntax processing in language and in music: An ERP Study. Journal of Cognitive Neuroscience. 2005;17(10):1565-1577.

[21] Sussman ES, Gumenyuk V. Organization of sequential sounds in auditory memory. Neuroreport. 2005;16(13):1519-1523.

[22] Tata MS, Ward LM. Early phase of spatial mismatch negativity is localized to a posterior "where" auditory pathway. Experimental Brain Research. 2005;167(3): 481-486.

[23] Hanna J, Pulvermuller F. Neurophysiological evidence for whole form retrieval of complex derived words: A mismatch negativity study. Frontiers in Human Neuroscience. 2014;8:886.

[24] Christman, CA, Lachmann T, Berti S. Earlier timbre processing of instrumental tones compared to equally complex spectrally rotated sounds as revealed by the mismatch negativity. Neuroscience Letters. 2014;581:115-119.

[25] Altenmüller E. Brain electrical correlates of cerebral music processing in the human. European Archives of Psychiatry and Neurological Sciences. 1986;235(6):342-354.

[26] Ragert P, Schmidt A, Altenmüller E, Dinse HR. Superior tactile performance and learning in professional pianists: Evidence for meta-plasticity in musicians. European Journal of Neuroscience. 2004;19(2):473-478.

[27] Koelsch S. Brain correlates of music-evoked emotions. Nature Reviews Neuroscience. 2014;15(3):170-180.

[28] Gaser C, Schlaug G. Brain structures differ between musicians and non-musicians. The Journal of Neuroscience. 2003;23(27):9240-9245.

[29] Lotze M, Scheler G, Tan HR, Braun C, Birbaumer N, The musician's brain: Functional imaging of amateurs and professionals during performance and imagery. Neuroimage. 2003;20(3):1817-1829.

[30] Schlaug G, Norton A, Overy K, Winner E. Effects of music training on the child's brain and cognitive development. Annals of the New York Academy of Sciences. 2005;1060:219-230.

[31] Boh B, Herholz SC, Lappe C, Pantev C. Processing of complex auditory patterns in musicians and nonmusicians. PLoS One. 2011;6(7):e21458.

[32] Münte TF, Nager W, Beiss T, Schroeder C, Altenmüller E. Specialization of the specialized: Electrophysiological investigations in professional musicians. Annals of the New York Academy of Sciences. 2003;999:131-139.

[33] Paraskevopoulos E, Kuchenbuch A, Herholz SC, Pantev C. Statistical learning effects in musicians and non-musicians: An MEG study. Neuropsychologia. 2012;50(2): 341-349.

[34] Münte TF, Kohlmetz C, Nager W, Altenmüller E. Neuroperception. Superior auditory spatial tuning in conductors. Nature. 2001;409(6820):580.

[35] Münte TF, Nager W, Rosenthal O, Johannes S, Altenmüller E. Attention to pitch in musicians and non-musicians: An event-related brain potential study. In: Nakada T. (ed.) Integrated Human Brain Science. Amsterdam: Elsevier; 2000. p. 389-398.

[36] Kuchenbuch A, Paraskevopoulos E, Herholz SC, Pantev C. Effects of musical training and event probabilities on encoding of complex tone patterns. BMC Neuroscience. 2013;14:51.

[37] Putkinen V, Tervaniemi M, Saarkivi K, de Vent N, Huotilainen M. Investigating the effects of musical training on functional brain development with a novel Melodic MMN paradigm. Neurobiology of Learning and Memory. 2014;110:8-15.

[38] Pantev C, Lappe C, Herholz SC, Trainor L. Auditory-somatosensory integration and cortical plasticity in musical training. Annals of the New York Academy of Sciences. 2009;1169:143-150.

[39] Engelmann M. Untersuchungen von Komponenten akustisch evozierter Potentiale an schwerhörigen Industriearbeitern. MD thesis. University Hospital Jena - Friedrich Schiller University; 2012.

[40] Tervaniemi M, Kruck S, De Baene W, Schroger E, Alter K.Friederici AD. Top-down modulation of auditory processing: Effects of sound context, musical expertise and attentional focus. European Journal of Neuroscience. 2009;30(8):1636-1642.

[41] Axelsson A, Eliasson A, Israelsson B. Hearing in pop/rock musicians: A follow-up study. Ear and Hearing. 1995;16(3):245-253.

[42] Schmuziger N, Patscheke J, Probst R. Hearing in nonprofessional pop/rock musicians. Ear and Hearing. 2006;27(4):321-330.

[43] Emmerich E, Richter F, Hagner H, Giessler F, Gehrlein S, Dieroff HG. Effects of discotheque music on audiometric results and central acoustic evoked neuromagnetic responses. International Tinnitus Journal. 2002;8(1):13-19.

[44] Toppila E, Koskinen H, Pyykkö I. Hearing loss among classical-orchestra musicians. Noise & Health. 2011;13(50):45-50.

[45] O'Brien I, Driscoll T, Ackermann B. Hearing conservation and noise management practices in professional orchestras. Journal of Occupational and Environmental Hygiene. 2012; 9(10):602-608.

[46] Schmidt JH, Pedersen ER, Paarup HM, Christensen-Dalsgaard J, Andersen T, Poulsen T, Bælum J. Hearing loss in relation to sound exposure of professional symphony orchestra musicians. Ear and Hearing. 2014;35(4):448-60.

[47] Schink T, Kreutz G, Busch V, Pigeot I, Ahrens W. Incidence and relative risk of hearing disorders in professional musicians. Occupational & Environmental Medicine. 2014;71(7):472-476.

[48] Raymond DM 3rd, Romeo JH, Kumke KV. A pilot study of occupational injury and illness experienced by classical musicians. Workplace Health & Safety. 2012;60(1): 19-24.

3

Measurement of Participation: The Role Checklist Version 3 - Satisfaction and Performance

Patricia J. Scott, Kelsey McKinney, Jeff Perron,
Emily Ruff and Jessica Smiley

Abstract

Participation in society is an area of interest to both clinicians and population researchers. Measurement of participation is therefore important, yet differences in definition, in terms of both content and scope, have made general agreement on one instrument tool elusive. What is recognized is the need for a theoretically based tool that captures both the insider and the outsider perspective. The outsider perspective, inclusive of the generally held views of a society, supports the utility for aggregating population data, whereas the insider perspective provides the internally held views of an individual needed for client-centered treatment planning. The Role Checklist Version 3 modifies one of the most commonly used assessment tools in occupational therapy practice, has good preliminary psychometric properties, and is theoretically consistent with both the ICF and the Model of Human Occupation. The Model of Human Occupation is the most widely used theoretical model in occupational therapy. This chapter provides an overview of the theoretical development, empirical testing, and implications for use of this participation measure by occupational therapists along with implications for population researchers.

Keywords: role checklist, measurement, participation, Model of Human Occupation, occupational therapy

1. Introduction

Humans interact with each other in consistent and scripted ways. *This interaction is known as participation and takes the form of roles*. These roles have specific meaning both to the person performing: the insider, and to those around them: the outsiders. A person's identity and sense of competency are tied inextricably to this role participation. Role participation is both persistent and changes over time, as people go through both planned and unplanned life transitions. Clinically, a person's role participation becomes the focus of the occupational therapist when disability-related limitations affect a person's capacity to participate in desired and meaningful roles.

Occupational therapists aim to assure that persons with disabilities have the motivation, opportunities, and capacity to overcome disability-related limitations and participate in social life. The International Classification of Health, Disability and Function (ICF) seeks to establish uniform definitions worldwide [1]. The American Occupational Therapy Association includes the ICF definition of participation in their practice framework [2] (see Box 1). The ICF is a classification system that "conceptualizes a person's level of functioning as a dynamic interaction between her or his health conditions, environment, and personal factors" [1]. Haglund et al. [3] found that the ICF classification aides occupational therapists in their practice; however, it alone does not encompass all that is needed for good practice. Therefore, it was found to be important to discover a tool consistent with the ICF that also is grounded in the theory of occupational therapy.

The ICF defines participation as "involvement in life situation" different than it defines activities which are "the execution of a task or action by an individual" [1] (p. 10). Despite the difference in definition, the ICF places both activities and participation together in one chapter and specifies four ways for ICF users to distinguish between the two. This ambiguity has resulted in an entire thread of literature as rehabilitation researchers seek to identify ways to approach measurement of participation. For if there is no agreement around the definition and scope, how can there be agreement on how to measure? This difficulty does not, however, make the task any less important.

BOX 1.

"Achieving health, well-being, and participation in

life through engagement in occupation is the overarching

statement that describes the domain and process of occupational

therapy in its fullest sense."

"Participation—"involvement in a life situation" (WHO, 2001, p. 10). Participation naturally occurs when clients are actively involved in carrying out occupations or daily life activities they find purposeful and meaningful. More specific outcomes of occupational therapy intervention are multidimensional and support the end result of participation."

AOTA Occupational Therapy Framework

(March/April 2014, Volume 68 Supplement 1, p. S4)

The Model of Human Occupation (MOHO) is the theoretical approach used most commonly commonly worldwide [4–6]. Developed by Kielhofner [7] and colleagues, Kielhofner's vision for MOHO is to support practice that is occupation focused, client centered, holistic, evidence based, and complementary to practice based on other occupational therapy models and interdisciplinary theories [8]. In this chapter, therefore we use the approach of differentiating between activities and participation by using the theory of MOHO to provide a framework that explains how participation in occupation is achieved.

Occupational performance (1976-2002)

- Perceived incumbency
- Values

Occupational participation (2002-present)

- Occupational performance
- Satisfaction with performance

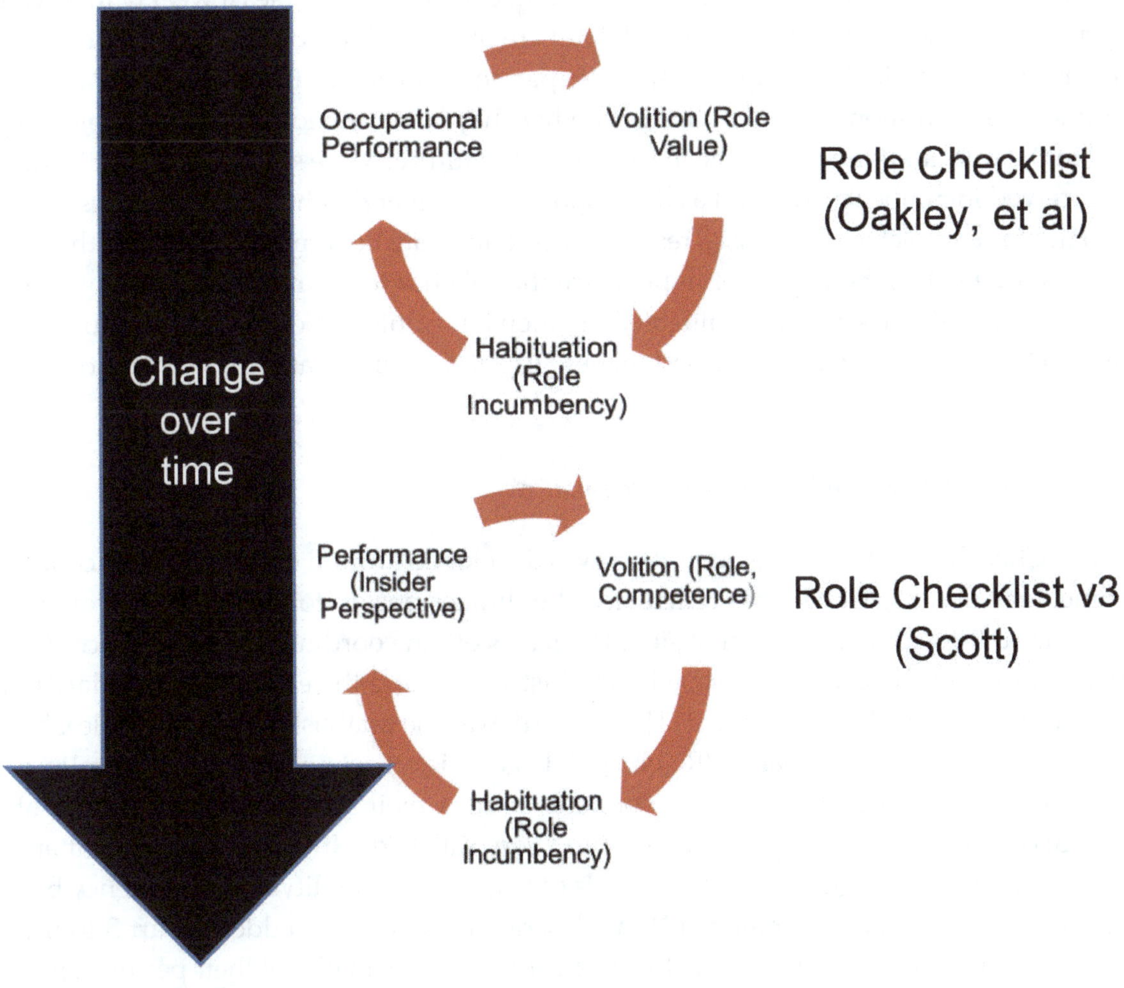

Figure 1. Underlying concepts and their influence on Role Checklist revisions.

The Role Checklist, theoretically grounded in MOHO, was developed by Frances Oakley in 1981 to capture occupational performance by measuring role incumbency and value [8]. However, over time the concepts of MOHO have evolved. In 2002, Kielhofner introduced the dimensions of doing [7]. Scott responded to this new concept by revisiting the Role Checklist, and began the process of revising the Role Checklist (see **Figure 1**). The latest MOHO text, the 5th edition, places the Role Checklist Version 3: Participation and Satisfaction (RCv3) among measures of occupational participation [8]. This chapter describes the process of revision and establishment of the psychometric properties needed to prepare the RCv3 as a cross-culturally valid measure of participation.

1.1. Role Checklist revisions: history and timelines

The Role Checklist, developed in 1981, is a short, two-part assessment tool that captures a person's perceived incumbency and role value in relation to the following 10 roles: student, worker, volunteer, caregiver, home maintainer, friend, family member, religious participant, hobbyist/amateur, and participant in organizations. Each role is provided with a brief definition followed by examples. The definitions contained a criterion of at least weekly involvement as occupational therapists who employ MOHO are interested in how these roles do or do not structure the respondent's occupational participation. For each of these 10 roles, Part 1 of the assessments asks respondents to indicate whether they have previously held the role, are currently in the role, and/or expect to be in the role in the future. More specifically, Part 1 is assessing perceived incumbency, defined as the respondent's belief that he or she occupies a role [9]. Once Part 1 is completed, Part 2 asks respondents to indicate how much they value the role. To determine role value, the degree of importance the role has to the respondent, he or she must rank each of the 10 roles as "very valuable," "somewhat valuable," or "not at all valuable." The Role Checklist is available now in 20 languages [10], and available at http://www.cade.uic.edu/moho.

1.1.1. *Role Checklist Version 2: quality of performance*

The Role Checklist, as it was created in 1981, was developed around current MOHO concepts of the time. However, as MOHO has articulated the dimensions of doing, revisions were needed to respond to these changes. In a first step, Patricia Scott, in coordination with Frances Oakley, responded to both clinical experience with the instrument and the established standards in the field of measurement of participation [11]. The result was the establishment of the Role Checklist Version 2: quality of performance (RCv2:QP). This revision retains the same 10 roles as the original Role Checklist and prompts respondents to rank their satisfaction with quality of performance on a scale from "very dissatisfied" to "very satisfied." In a 2014 study, Scott and colleagues found the RCv2:QP to have high levels of test-retest reliability and consistency between paper and electronic administration [12]. As described above, Scott added a Part 3 to the Role Checklist to enable respondents to rate their perception of the quality of their performance. This addition made the Role Checklist more sensitive to change and added a component to enable the "insider view," an important aspect of the person's self-assessment of adequacy or acceptability. Part 3 brought the Role Checklist closer to meeting the criteria for measures of participation [11].

1.1.2. Role Checklist Version 3: performance and satisfaction

While creating a scoring system, Scott recognized a need for a reflection of desired participation. Scoring had been elusive in the past, in great part due to the lack of accepted standards for patterns of role participation. With the client at the focal center, and role incumbency being an internalized concept, occupational therapists do not endorse the adoption of a universal standard for desired roles. The focus on individualizing contextual performance is based on current role satisfaction and the desirability of delaying engagement (or not) in desired future roles. This effort led to the reconceptualization of Part 3 and synthesis into a one-page document. This version is named Role Checklist Version 3: Satisfaction and Performance.

This one-page assessment tool is written as follows. Each role is first defined; the definitions have remained the same for the roles of student, worker, caregiver, and home maintainer. However, the time specifications for volunteer, friend, family member, hobbyist, and participant in organizations have changed from a weekly basis to "on a regular basis." Lastly, to identify as a religious participant, involvement is no longer required to be "at least once a week," and instead has no time frame. To complete the assessment, for each role, the respondent is asked to indicate if he or she is currently performing the role. If the respondent indicates "Yes" to currently performing the given role, he or she then is prompted to indicate his or her level of satisfaction with their role performance. If the respondent indicates "No" to currently performing the given role, he or she is then asked to indicate his or her interest in role participation in the future by selecting "I would like to do this NOW," "I would like to do this IN THE FUTURE," or "I am NOT INTERESTED in doing this."

This new, revised assessment tool is no longer concerned with past role incumbency or role value. Instead, the RCv3 elicits information that allows clinicians to provide a client-centered plan of care and monitor client progress, and researches a measure to collect outcome data on an individual or population level.

1.2. Connection to international audiences

In a 2014 publication, Scott [13] presented the case for the Role Checklist Version 2: Quality of Performance as valid measure consistent with the ICF definition of participation. Her work drew the attention of International colleagues who joined Scott and formed the International Role Alliance for the study of Participation (IRAP) in October 2013.

The International Role Alliance for the Study of Participation (IRAP) maintains the mission to promote participation in society for all persons with disabling conditions. Specifically, this group seeks to establish the revised Role Checklist as a cross-culturally valid method of measuring participation, actual participation, and desired future participation, contextualized by the value and satisfaction a person associates with that participation. IRAP core members are academic clinical scholars from universities in Switzerland (German), Sweden, Japan, USA, UK, and Norway. Each has completed translations and contributed data to establish the initial psychometric properties of the Role Checklist Version 2: Quality of Performance. Initial investigations of the utility of the tool and its clinical applicability took place in Sweden and in Norway.

Among one of the first agendas of this group was to establish valid cross-cultural guidelines for translation. These guidelines would, to quote Dr. Lena Haglund from Sweden, a founding IRAP member, "place a fence around the translation process to keep the MOHO concepts in." These guidelines have been tested for feasibility and implementation. Collaborators from Iceland and China have completed valid translations of the RCv3, and Spanish and Norwegian translations are in progress. Now the translation guidelines are shown to produce culturally equivalent versions, more than a dozen collaborators are on board to complete further translations.

IRAP members work through a worldwide network of occupational therapists who provide services to persons with disabilities across the globe. This network is enabled on two fronts: first, the MOHO Clearing House, which is the source for a dozen measurements, instruments in 20 languages and second, the World Federation of Occupational Therapy with 77 member organizations, which represent over 350,000 occupational therapists internationally.

2. Concepts of concern: ICF and MOHO levels of doing

In this section, it is useful to better understand the differences between activities and participation or, as understood in MOHO, occupational participation and occupational performance [3]. In Section 1, we offered the definitions from the ICF of activities and participation. They are worth repeating here:

> *Participation: "involvement in life situation"*
> *Activities which is "the execution of a task or action by an individual"*
>
> *(WHO* [1], *p. 10)*

Occupational therapists are inherently attuned to and concerned with the things people do and how they do them. Doing is described in MOHO at three levels: occupational skill, occupational performance, and occupational participation. Kielhofner [7] refers to this hierarchy as the "dimensions of doing." Occupational skill can be simply described as purposeful actions needed to carry out a task. They are the motor skills, process skills, and communication and interaction skills that come together to make up occupational performance [14]. Occupational performance is the act of utilizing these skills to carry out a task. These acts of occupational performance comprise occupational participation; however, there is more to participation than performance alone [15]. Kielhofner [14] explains that participation is composed of occupations that are, "part of one's sociocultural context and that are desired and/or necessary to one's well-being." They are linked to a sense of belonging, value, and meaning [15]. This is the dimension of doing in which roles reside. These levels of doing can be best understood through examples. The ability to push, grasp, and categorize would be considered occupational skill. Occupational performance would include such activities as vacuuming, scrubbing a kitchen counter, or sorting laundry. Partaking in and identifying with the role of home maintainer would be considered as occupational participation.

Occupational role participation is more than partaking in an activity [15]. Kielhofner [7] explained that it "refers to engaging in work, play, or activities of daily living that are part of one's sociocultural context and that are desired and/or necessary to one's well-being" (p. 101). Dijkers [15] notes that there are many aspects of participation, including, but not limited to frequency of activities, value and meaning, responsibility, autonomy, reciprocity, location, and the company of others. Driving a car is an activity performed by many throughout the course of a day; however, it is not always perceived the same way. A teenage boy, whom may not value his education and finds the daily commute to school quite cumbersome, may view it as nothing more than a daily task. However, later that day he may take that same route during his work hours as a pizza delivery boy. He finds the task of driving to be a necessary aspect of his valued occupation of work. Even further, the addition of friends as passengers on the way to a Friday night football game can be considered engagement in social participation. The line between participation and common performance lies within the individual's perception. Bonsaksen and colleagues analyzed over 7000 role examples and associated them with these levels of doing.

3. Reliability and validity psychometrics of RCv3

Although several studies have supported the psychometric properties of the Role Checklist, it has not yet achieved the level of psychometric evidence to be included among other MOHO assessments. **Table 1** charts the history of studies of different versions of the Role Checklist. It is

Properties verified	Title	Authors	Year	Comments
The Role Checklist				
Reliability	The Role Checklist: Development and empirical assessment of reliability	Oakley, F., Kielhofner, G., Barris, R., & Reichler, R. K.	1986	Construct
Cross-cultural validity & reliability	Spanish Translation of the Role Checklist	Colón, H., & Haertlein, C.	2002	No application to RCv3
Cross-cultural validity & test-retest reliability	Cross-Cultural Reproducibility of the Brazilian Portuguese Version of the Role Checklist for Persons With Chronic Obstructive Pulmonary Disease	Cordeiro, J. R., Camelier, A., Oakley, F., & Jardim, J. R.	2007	No application to RCv3
The Role Checklist Version 2: Quality of Performance				
Electronic administration & test-retest reliability	The Role Checklist Version 2: Quality of Performance: Reliability and validation of electronic administration	Scott PJ, McFadden, R, Yates, K, Baker, S. & McSoley, S.	2014	Supports electronic administration & test-test reliability
Feasibility	Using the Role Checklist Version 2: Quality of Performance in the Occupational Therapy Process in a Psychiatric Hospital	Aslaksen, M., Scott, P., Haglund, L., Ellingham, B., & Bonsaksen, T.	2014	Informs responsiveness and utility

Properties verified	Title	Authors	Year	Comments
Construct validity with ICF	Measuring participation outcomes following life-saving medical interventions: The Role Checklist Version 2: Quality of Performance	Scott, P.J.	2014	Same roles are used in all versions
Construct validity with MOHO levels of doing	Does the Role Checklist Measure Occupational Participation?	Bonsaksen, T., Meidert, U., Schuman, D., Kvarsnes, H., Haglund, L., Prior, S., Forsyth, K., Yamada, T. & Scott, P.J.	2015	Role examples reflect mixed classification into occupational performance and occupational participation
Concurrent validity	Establishing Concurrent Validity of the Role Checklist version 2 with the OCAIRS in Post Liver transplant patients	Scott, PJ, Cacich D., Fulk, M., Michel, K., & Whiffen, K	2016	Both assessments measure the construct of participation
Content validity	Measuring Participation According to the ICF With the Modified Role Checklist	Meidert, U., Bonsaksen, T., & Scott, P.	n.d.	97% of role examples classified as consistent with ICF construct of participation
Role Checklist Version 3: Performance and Satisfaction				
Cross-cultural validity	Translation Guidelines for the revised Role Checklist	Van Antwerp, L., Haglund, L., Fenger, K., & Scott, P.	2016	Translation guidelines are feasible
Discriminate validity	Measurement of Participation: The Role Checklist Version 3.	Scott, P., & Latham, K.	n.d.	Discriminates between persons identifying disability-related limitations and those without.

Table 1. Psychometric properties of the various versions of the Role Checklist.

important to note that caution must be used in the assignment of psychometric properties found for one version to another. The only consistent feature across all three versions is the 10 roles. The Role Checklist, original and versions 2 and 3, have excellent validity and cross-cultural reproducibility; however, there is still a need for feasibility, utility, and reliability testing of the RCv3.

3.1. Feasibility

In 2014, Aslasken and colleagues [16] completed a pilot study to verify subject feasibility and to illustrate how an occupational therapist used the translated RCv2: QP to direct a clinical intervention. Aslaksen reported on the feedback from four Swedish therapists and one case report from Norway. The therapists each reported that a revised tool would be helpful if it were (1) provided on a single page layout, (2) had opportunity for comments, and (3) gathered information for each role one at a time [16]. The respondent who took the RCv2: QP reported frustration with the definitions provided for each role. Despite feeling as though he identified with select roles, he did not qualify as a participant in such roles according to the provided definitions [16]. In creating the RCv3, Scott took note of these recommendations and included changes addressing several of these concerns. The new RCv3 presents on a single page and prompts answers for each role one at a time. In addition, the time specifications used to define volunteer, friend, family member, hobbyist, participant in organizations, and religious participant have changed. As Aslasken's study did, this study aims to show subject feasibility, among other psychometric properties, through employing therapist and client thought on the updates when compared to the original Role Checklist, developed in 1981 by Fran Oakley.

3.2. Utility

Utility is being the degree to which the treatment outcome is positively influenced by an assessment, in this case, the RCv3. Hayes et al. [17] provide a functional approach to evaluating an assessment's quality. The authors justify that treatment utility is not a matter of cost-benefit ratio, but instead it is the "demonstration of a particular type of benefit" ([17], p. 964). Nelson-Gray [18] provided examples of typical treatment utility questions: "(a) Does treatment selection that is based on a particular assessment result in a more successful client outcome? And (b) Does supplying outcome data to therapists result in a more successful outcome?" These are the questions Aslasken et al. [16] provides only a partial answer to—these two questions remain largely unanswered for the RCv3.

3.3. Test-retest reliability

Establishing reliability is crucial to substantiate an assessment. Kerlinger [19] supported this notion when stating, "concern for reliability comes from the necessity for dependability in measurement" (p. 442). There are three definitions of reliability [19]. The first is characterized by the question of accuracy and stability. Does this instrument truly measure the outcome measure it sets out to find? The second looks to inquire the instrument's error of measurement. This refers to its precision; how far it is from "hitting the bullseye" [20]. The third focuses on the stability, dependability, and predictability through multiple administrations. The first definition, hitting the mark, is appropriate for the RCv3. The 10 roles listed in the Role Checklist, all versions, are mutually independent, that is, no scaling is possible. For example, being in the role of a home maintainer is not necessarily associated with being a friend, any more than being a volunteer is associated with being a religious participant. Therefore, it is not surprising that the test-retest reliability performed on the 1981 version is associated with that performed in 2014 on the RCv2:QP.

3.4. Flexible administration

Previous studies have found that assessments administered electronically are consistent with paper and pencil administrations [21]. Using electronic means to administer the assessment allows for flexibility versus being limited to paper and pencil format. Because technology is advancing and becoming more prevalent in our society, clients benefit from having the option of taking an assessment in an electronic format. The RCv3 can be administered as a self-report, completed on a variety of electronic devices such as a smartphone, a tablet, or a laptop, or as an interview with the answers being submitted by the therapist. Studies have shown that clients often feel more at ease when taking surveys online versus on paper due to feeling less concerned with societal norms and how others might perceive them especially when it comes to personal and sensitive topics such as role incumbency and satisfaction [21, 22]. Additionally, using electronic means to gather data eliminates human error when transferring data into a database for analysis and is time and cost-effective [22, 23].

Although using electronic means to implement an assessment has many benefits, there are some shortcomings as well. Based on a study conducted by Gwaltney et al. [21], there are two reasons why administering an assessment electronically may not be equivalent to paper and pencil administration. First, the assessment tool presents itself different on paper versus electronically. Aspects such as letter size, spacing, or how many items per screen can vary between the two and ultimately alter the way a client would respond. Second, some clients may not feel comfortable using a computer or other electronic devise such as an iPad or a smartphone. This is especially true for the older population in which paper and pencil are most familiar. For these reasons, it is important to have an administrator around to address confusion or questions the client might have, as well as aid clients who may have a cognitive impairment, low vision, physical challenges, or lack of experience using technology.

3.5. Summary

As seen in **Table 1**, the RCv3 has established validity and cross-cultural standards; however, there is currently an obvious need for feasibility, utility, and replication of reliability. Establishing test-retest reliability for the RCV3 will improve the psychometrics that assessment tools needed to be considered a valid standardized instrument for occupational therapists to confidently use in treatment planning, goal progression, and outcome measurement. Verifying the RCv3 as a psychometric tool with feasibility and treatment utility through therapist perceptions, as well as replicating reliability will validate revisions to the assessment tool.

4. Use as a population-based measure

Thus far, we have addressed the use of the RCv3 as a client-centered measure of participation theoretically grounded in MOHO. It also has implications for a population-based population measure of interest to policy makers, as well as health and disability scholars.

In the 2011 World Report on Disability, the World Health Organization claims that improvement within a person's social participation may be made when the health-care professional addresses barriers, which hinder their everyday activities (WHO [24], p. 4). These barriers must be identified through reliable measures, which measure participation. The CRPD, Convention on the Rights of Person's with Disabilities, specifies that there is a need and an obligation for development of assessments, which promote participation (WHO [24], p. 11). Recommendation 8 describes the need to develop methodologies for data collection on persons with disabilities, which are tested cross-culturally and applied consistently.

5. Chapter summary

There are currently no general appropriate assessments, which may be reliably scored among health-care professionals on a multidisciplinary team, are cross-culturally consistent, and are both cost-effective and efficient. We have presented the Role Checklist Version 3: Quality and Performance as a way to fill this void. In this chapter, we have defined participation as defined by international standards, the ICF, and theoretically according to the most widely used model in occupational therapy, MOHO. We have substantiated conceptual consistency with the ICF participation domains. In addition, cross-cultural translational guidelines have been developed and internationally established as both feasible and valid [25]. Therefore, the revised Role Checklist that meets criteria for a balanced measure of participation [26] is conceptually consistent with the ICF [13], has cross-culturally valid translation guidelines [25], construct validity as a MOHO-based measure of participation [27] and concurrent validity with an established measure of participation [12].

Author details

Patricia J. Scott*, Kelsey McKinney, Jeff Perron, Emily Ruff and Jessica Smiley

*Address all correspondence to: scottp@iu.edu

Indiana University, Indianapolis, IN, USA

References

[1] WHO. International Classification of Functioning, Disability and Health. Geneva: World Health Organization; 2001

[2] American Occupational Therapy Association. Occupational therapy practice framework: Domain and process. American Journal of Occupational Therapy. 2008;**62**:625-683

[3] Haglund L, Henriksson C. Concepts in occupational therapy in relation to the ICF. Occupational Therapy International. 2003;**10**(4):253-268

[4] Haglund L, Ekbladh E, Thorell L-H, Hallberg IR. Practice models in Swedish psychiatric occupational therapy. Scandinavian Journal of Occupational Therapy. 2000;7(3):107-113

[5] Law M, McCoLL MA. Knowledge and use of theory among occupational therapists: A Canadian survey. Canadian Journal of Occupational Therapy. 1989;**56**(4):198-204

[6] Lee SW, Taylor R, Kielhofner G. Choice, knowledge, and utilization of a practice theory: A national study of occupational therapists who use the Model of Human Occupation. Occupational Therapy in Health Care. 2009;**23**(1):60-71

[7] Kielhofner G. Model of Human Occupation: Theory and Application. 3rd ed. Baltimore: Lippincott Williams & Wilkins; 2002

[8] Taylor R, editor. Kielhofner's Model of Human Occupation: Theory and Application. 5th ed. Philadelphia: Wolters Kluwer Health. New Jersey; 2017

[9] Oakley F, Kielhofner G, Barris R, Reichler R. The Role Checklist: Development and empirical assessment of reliability. Occupational Therapy Journal of Research. 1986;**6**(3):158-170

[10] Hemphill-Pearson B, editor. Assessments in Occupational Therapy Mental Health: An Integrative Approach. 2nd ed. Slack INC; 2008

[11] Brown M, Dijkers MPJM, Gordon WA, Ashman T, Charatz H, Cheng Z. Participation objective, participation subjective: A measure of participation combining outsider and insider perspectives. The Journal of Head Trauma Rehabilitation. 2004;**19**(6):459-481

[12] Scott PJ, McFadden R, Yates K, Baker S, McSoley S. The Role Checklist V2: QP: Establishment of reliability and validation of electronic administration. British Journal of Occupational Therapy. 2014;**77**(2):96-102

[13] Scott PJ. Measuring participation outcomes following life-saving medical interventions: The Role Checklist Version 2: Quality of performance. Disability and Rehabilitation. 2014;**36**(13):1108-1112

[14] Kielhofner G. Model of Human Occupation: Theory and Application. 4th ed. Baltimore: Lippincott Williams & Wilkins; 2008

[15] Dijkers MP. Issues in the conceptualization and measurement of participation: An overview. Archives of Physical Medicine and Rehabilitation. 2010;**91**(Suppl 9):S5–S16. DOI: 10.1016/j.apmr.2009.10.036

[16] Aslaksen M, Scott P, Haglund L, Ellingham B, Bonsaksen T. The Role Checklist Version 2: Quality of performance in the occupational therapy process in a mental health setting. Ergoterapeuten. 2014;**4**:38-45

[17] Hayes SC, Nelson RO, Jarrett RB. The treatment utility of assessment: A functional approach to evaluating assessment quality. American Psychologist. 1987;**42**(11):963

[18] Nelson-Gray RO. Treatment utility of psychological assessment. Psychological Assessment. 2003;**15**(4):521

[19] Kerlinger FN. Foundations of Behavioral Research (New York: Holt, Rinehart, and Winston, 1964). Health Behavior and Health Education: Theory, Research and Practice. 4th ed. San Francisco: Jossey Bass; 2008. pp. 26-27

[20] Riegelman RK. Studying a Study and Testing a Test: How to Read the Medical Evidence. Baltimore: Lippincott Williams & Wilkins; 2005

[21] Gwaltney CJ, Shields AL, Shiffman S. Equivalence of electronic and paper-and-pencil administration of patient-reported outcome measures: A meta-analytic review. Value in Health. 2008;**11**(2):322-333. DOI: http://dx.doi.org/10.1111/j.1524-4733.2007.00231.x

[22] Kiesler S, Sproull LS. Response effects in the electronic survey. Public Opinion Quarterly. 1986;**50**(3):402-413

[23] Weber BA, Yarandi H, Rowe MA, Weber JP. A comparison study: Paper-based versus web-based data collection and management. Applied Nursing Research. 2005;**18**(3):182-185

[24] WHO. United Nations World Report on Disability: Summary 2011. World Health Organization. 2011. Retrieved from: http://www.refworld.org/docid/50854a322.html

[25] Van Antwerp L, Crabtree JL, Scott PJ. Translation guidelines for the Role Checklist Version 2: Quality of performance. In: Feasibility study in Iceland and China: American Occupational Therapy Association 96th Annual Conference and Expo; April 7-10; Chicago; 2016

[26] Brown M, Dijkers MPJM, Gordon WA, Ashman T, Charatz H, Cheng Z. Participation objective, participation subjective: A measure of participation combining outsider and insider perspectives. The Journal of Head Trauma Rehabilitation. 2004;**19**(6):459-481

[27] Bonsaksen T, Meidert U, Schuman D, Kvarsnes H, Haglund L, Prior S, et al. Does the Role Checklist measure occupational participation? The Open Journal of Occupational Therapy. 2015;**3**(3):2

4

Psychomotor Therapy for Patients with Severe Mental Health Disorders

Michel Probst

Abstract

Psychomotor therapy is defined as a method of treatment based on a holistic view of the human being that is derived from the unity of body and mind. Assessments (observation and/or evaluation) are essential to achieving concrete psychosocial objectives methodically. Psychomotor therapy uses movement, body awareness and a wide range of movement activities to optimize movement behaviour as well as the cognitive, affective and relational aspects of psychomotor functioning (i.e. the relationships between physical movements and cognitive and social-affective aspects). Consequently, the approach to this type of therapy integrates the physical, cognitive and emotional aspects of functioning in relation to the capacity of being and acting in a psychosocial context in order to achieve clearly defined goals in consultation with the patients. Psychomotor therapy framework consists of three different approaches: a health-related approach, a psychosocial approach and a psychotherapeutic approach, which can be embedded in several psychotherapeutic approaches. Through the implementation of both systematically planned evaluations and individually targeted interventions in group, the psychomotor therapist strives to broaden the general action competences and specific skills and to stimulate a positive self-image and personal well-being in balanced social relationships. Today, there is sufficient evidence that psychomotor therapy has a major contribution to both well-being and mental health of patients with severe psychiatric problems. In Flemish psychiatric hospitals, psychomotor therapy is imbedded in different treatment programmes. In this chapter, the theory behind this approach and some practical examples will be provided.

Keywords: body image, physical activity, mental health disorders, psychiatry, psychotherapeutic accent, movement therapy, psychomotor therapy

1. Introduction

In Belgium [1], the Netherlands [2] and Germany [3], psychomotor therapy has been well integrated into psychiatry care since 1965. Psychomotor therapy is defined as a method of treatment that systematically uses a wide variety of physical activities as cornerstones of its approach. It is considered a supplement to and a support for residential psychiatric treatment [4]. Psychomotor therapy attempts to achieve positive therapeutic results regarding the psychiatric problems of the patient (depression, anxiety, schizophrenia, autism, eating disorders, etc.) by systematically using adapted body experiences and physical activities, movement, sensory awareness and sport-derived activities. In this sense, psychomotor therapy is more than just "doing exercise" or "performing recreation activities". The foundation of psychomotor therapy is based on the well-accepted relationship between mental health and physical activity [5, 6]. It is imbedded in different multidisciplinary psychotherapeutic treatment programmes (behavioural, cognitive, or psychodynamic therapy) for different diagnosis-related patient settings [4]. Psychomotor therapy (see **Figure 1**) stimulates and integrates motor, cognitive and affective competences as inherent aspects of human behaviour, thereby enabling a person to act autonomously within his own psychosocial context [7]. Psychomotor therapy focuses on the somatic effects of physical activity (at the morphological, muscular, cardiorespiratory, metabolic, and motor levels) and on the physio-psychological effects as the core of the treatment. The experiences during PMT and the responses that arise from these experiences function as a dynamic source of change [1, 4]. Psychomotor therapy is mostly a group therapy based on the ideas of Yalom [8]. It has no real side effects, and its safety rules are transparent.

This chapter clarifies the background, history and clinical implementation of psychomotor therapy for patients with severe mental health disorders in psychiatry.

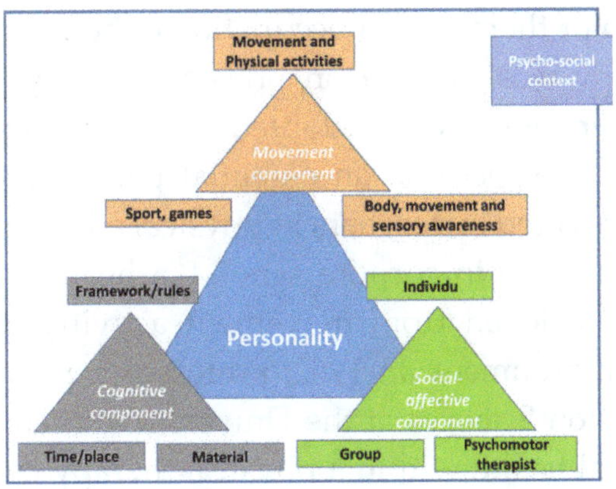

Figure 1. Psychomotor therapy: motor, cognitive and social-affective components.

2. From occupation to psychomotor therapy: a historical perspective

The French Revolution was a milestone in the treatment of patients with psychiatric problems. Pinel (France, 1745–1826) and his contemporaries Esquirol (France, 1772–1840), Tuke

(England, 1745–1813), Greisinger (Germany, 1817–1868), Chiarugi (Italy, 1759–1820), Riedel (Czech Republic, 1803–1870), Rush (USA, 1745–1813) and Guislain (Belgium, 1797–1860) transferred the ideas of the French Revolution to the treatment of patients with psychiatric disorders [9]. A repressive approach (i.e. detention, chaining of patients) was replaced with a more humane and moral treatment that consisted of daily rounds by the medical doctor and different daily activities (housekeeping activities, gardening, working in a vegetable garden, and others). Later, other milestones were important in the development of treatments for patients with severe mental health disorders: The Great World War (1914–1918), the development of neuroleptics (1952), the influence of philosophers and phenomenologists on (mental) health care (Kierkegaard, Husserl, Heidegger, Merleau-Ponty and Sartre) and the development of different types of psychotherapy and adjunctive or complementary therapies.

The book "Aktive Krankenbehandlung in der Irrenanstalt" [10], by Simon (1867–1947), a German psychiatrist, led to new ideas concerning more active treatments for patients with mental illnesses. The approach aimed to address and stimulate the healthy part of the personality of each patient.

Albert Day (1812–1894) developed an institution in New York to treat alcohol addiction. This gymnasium featured appropriate fitness equipment for its time [11, 12]. Shepherd Ivory Franz (1874–1933) [13] studied the effects upon the retardation in conditions of depression. In the United States, Meyer (1866–1950) [14] reported the positive effects of daily activities on mental health. He underlined the unity between body and mind and the effect of exercise on the balance between thinking, doing and being. He was convinced of the effects of activity as a type of therapy and of the advantages in social life for patients with mental illness. Movement activities for psychiatric patients were derived from the so-called active therapies (called "occupational therapy" in some countries) that were organized in psychiatric hospitals [1].

Until 1960, occupational therapy and psychomotor therapy were based on the same ideas [15]. In Belgium, psychomotor therapy and occupational therapy developed as two different tracks. Psychomotor therapy was focused on physical activity [1]. In the Flemish part of Belgium, Simon's and Meyer's ideas were adopted by several psychiatrists after the Second World War. Movement therapy became an essential part of mental healthcare treatment services and was initially provided by teachers in physical education settings. The philosophy of this approach was "mens sana in corpore sano" ["a healthy mind in a healthy body"]. Gradually, the attention broadened from movement activities themselves to how people move in relation to their environment. In 1962, Professor De Nayer, dean of the Faculty of Kinesiology and Rehabilitation Sciences at the University of Leuven, introduced courses on movement therapy in mental health within a physical therapy curriculum. At that time, this idea was very innovative. Professors Pierloot [16] and Van Coppenolle [17] developed the theoretical and practical content. Both were influenced by Simon and Meyer who, together with Van Roozendaal (1922–1996) [18], were the trendsetters in the use of movement activities in psychiatry. At the end of the 1960s, the term "movement therapy" was replaced by "psychomotor therapy". Psychomotor therapy focused on the interactions between the body in motion and the mind, especially from a behavioural perspective. Methods derived from more physical therapy- and body-oriented approaches, such as relaxation and sensory- and body awareness, became an integral part of therapy [1, 4].

3. Definition of psychomotor therapy

Psychomotor therapy was defined as a method or treatment that uses corporality and movement as a driver of its approach and in which the clinician tries—after having performed a methodical psychomotor examination and in consultation with the patient—to realize clearly formulated goals that are relevant to the patient's problems [19]. This definition refers more to the structure than the content of the psychomotor therapy. Psychomotor therapy in mental health is person-centred and aimed at children, adolescents, adults and elderly individuals with common and severe, acute and chronic mental health problems. Psychomotor therapists provide health promotion, preventive health care, treatment and rehabilitation for individuals and groups, mostly in inpatient treatment. They create a therapeutic relationship to provide assessment and services specifically to the complexity of mental health within a supportive environment, applying a bio-psychosocial model. The core of psychomotor therapy is to optimize well-being and empower the individual by promoting physical activity, exercise, movement awareness and functional movement, bringing together physical and mental aspects. Psychomotor therapists play a key role in an integrated multidisciplinary team and in an interprofessional care. Psychomotor therapy in psychiatry is based on the available scientific and best clinical evidence [20].

The main purpose of psychomotor therapy is to demonstrate how goal-directed movement situations can have a positive psychological effect, not only physical skills but also cognitive, perceptual, affective and behaviour. The moving body in all its aspects is the cornerstone of the psychomotor approach. This characteristic distinguishes psychomotor therapy from other approaches in psychiatry. Movements that represent real-life situations provide the patient good structure and the opportunity to create a realistic image of his/her own capabilities and boundaries. The commitment requires discipline, responsibility and perseverance. In the first stage of therapy, mostly individualized treatment is offered depending on the problems the patient presents. At a later stage, more group and interactive activities are proposed [1]. Through the implementation of both systematically planned evaluations and individually targeted interventions, psychomotor therapy stimulates and integrates motor, cognitive and affective competences as inherent aspects of human behaviour, thereby enabling a person to act autonomously within his/her own psychosocial context. The goal is to stimulate a positive self-image and personal well-being in balanced social relationships. Psychomotor therapy is used in individual and in group sessions, mostly in inpatient settings. The theoretical foundation of psychomotor therapy came from various disciplines, such as medicine (neurology, psychiatry), psychology (clinical and exercise), pedagogy, sociology, kinesiology and exercise physiology.

4. Some clinical guidelines for optimizing psychomotor therapy

On the one hand, physical activity is currently well accepted in the treatment of patients with mental health problems. On the other hand, data indicate that patients with mental illness have higher levels of social anxiety in physical activity situations compared with healthy control subjects [21]. Consequently, psychomotor therapists should consider social anxiety when trying to improve the outcomes of patients with mental illness and their adherence to physical activity interventions. Prescribing "sport" activities for patients with severe mental illness without any clarification is therefore counterproductive for the majority of these patients. Most of these patients think they are not skilful enough to fulfil expectations or are afraid of criticism from peers; therefore, they will find many excuses for not attending these activities. Most people are convinced that physical activity is healthy for people with mental illness. This is not always the case, however, as illustrated in the following example of Ellen. This story is an eye-opener.

4.1. Example: Ellen, a 31-year-old patient with borderline personality

Swimming can be an aspect of psychomotor therapy. Swimming is a basic activity, but on an individual level, swimming can have other meanings. The therapist must keep in mind that what obvious is to them is not so obvious to the patient.

A 31-year-old female with borderline personality with eating disorder features was invited to attend a weekly swimming session at the hospital's swimming hall. The treatment was a group approach based on Linehan [22]. The patient had a negative attitude towards the swimming sessions. She discussed the problem with her therapist. She had difficulties sharing and expressing her feelings. The psychomotor therapist encouraged her to try to attend the session and to write about her experience.

"The whole day, I felt anxious about the fact that I have to go to the swimming session and that I wouldn't fit in my swimsuit anymore. It would definitely be too small, and I too fat. I imagined a fat, bulging body. The warm weather made me uncomfortable. Sweating gave me the feeling of being too fat and too indolent, which made the thought of putting on my swimsuit quite hard. The other group members were really enthusiastic. This was unimaginable for me. I could not, and still cannot, comprehend that they like to put on their bikini and have fun in the swimming pool. When I put on my swimsuit, it was larger than the last time. I saw that my belly wasn't sticking out. I felt quite good about my body. The water was less cold than I remembered from the last time. My skin felt soft in the water. I felt a very big contrast between the other group members and me as they moved freely through the water. Some even dared to sit on the edge of the swimming pool. I would have wanted to swim a lap, but I literally felt restricted. It was as if I wasn't able to swim. I didn't even know how to start, although I know that I'm a good swimmer. I had the tendency to constantly contract my muscles. When my muscles were tensed, my body felt so much better, less mushy. After a while, I asked to take a shower. The therapist gave me permission. It was very difficult for me to get out of the swimming pool. Everyone would now be able to see me. I didn't even dare to take a shower. In my fitting room, I really felt…anxious, close to despair. Drying myself and putting on my clothes was very hard for me. I cried, I felt the urge to harm myself, to cut and to ruin myself. I wanted to feel sick and weak by drinking something. However, I didn't do it. Mostly, I felt very and extremely tired".

5. The different dimensions in psychomotor therapy

As indicated in Section 1, psychomotor therapy is more than just physical activity. In psychomotor therapy, physical activities are used in relation to psychological dimensions. **Table 1** provides an overview of the different dimensions and the more concrete action points and clarifications used during the sessions. It is clear that the classification presented in **Table 1** is artificial. There is indeed a connection among thoughts, mood, behaviour, physical reactions and the environment (life experiences = outside the person). The advantage of such a table is that it clarifies what is meant by the situation and the psychomotor, cognitive, affective, behaviour and symbolic dimension. Different situations can lead to different thoughts, moods, behaviours, and physical reactions.

A seesaw was built with benches and mattresses, as presented in **Figure 2**. *The exercise was successful if the group could keep the seesaw in balance with all participants for at least 5 min. Even a small movement could dramatically affect the balance.*

Psychomotor dimension: In addition to the essential skills (balance and the perception of body tonus by the patients), the patient realizes that the physical skills are not the only ones necessary to achieve a

Dimension	Feature
Psychomotor dimension	Physical sensations (heart rate, sweating, dizziness, shortness of breath, blushing, stomach distress, muscle tension, trembling, headaches, restlessness, fatigue irritability, pain, energy and fatigue). Body, movement and sensory awareness; physical fitness; psychomotor skills (manual skills, eye hand coordination, balance, posture, lateralization, time place orientation…).
Cognitive dimension	Including communication aspects. Issues: What are the person's thoughts and beliefs before, during and after the activity? Are the thoughts accurate? Is the person worried about what might occur? Does the person ruminate about the past? Does the person show thoughts of being in danger, narrow attention, and impulsivity? How are the person's planning and organizational skills? How does the person communicate verbally and non-verbally?
Affective dimension	Including the relational dimension and the emotional distress. What are the person's feelings before, during and after the situation? How are the person's relationships with peers and the therapist? How does the person cope with feelings such as sadness, anger, surprise, disgust, shame, hopelessness, being overwhelmed, numbness …? How is the person's self-esteem, self-image, and attitude? How is his/her level of tolerance or frustration? Who takes the lead? Who follows? Who dares to voice his own opinions?
Behavioural dimension	What is the behaviour of the subject in the given situation? What does the person choose to do or not to do? How does the person overcome the problem; what are his/her problem-solving skills? What type of strategy is used in the given situation? Does the patient use avoidance or checking behaviours, rituals, repetitive behaviour or specific habits (for instance tapping feet, biting fingernails)? Does the patient want to escape the exercise? What is his/her social behaviour like? How does the person function in team efforts? Is he able to achieve the task?
Symbolic dimension	There is a link between the proposed exercise within the therapy and with the outside world (outside the therapy, within society). The proposed exercise contains a life message. The exercise evokes conscious or unconscious events from the past.

Table 1. The different dimensions in psychomotor therapy.

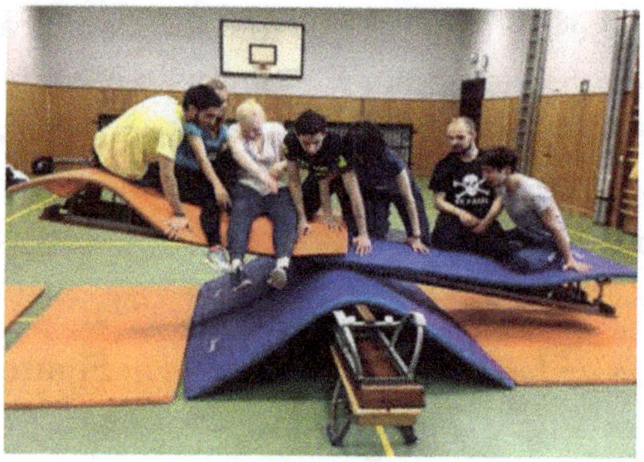

Figure 2. The seesaw: a group activity in psychomotor therapy.

goal. Other group members intrude into their comfort zone, and the patients are confronted with body contact. For some patients, this is a stress situation. How can they cope with this stress?

Cognitive and communication dimension: What are the thoughts involved in solving the problem? Who presents a substantial proposal for addressing the challenge? How is the communication among the group? Are the basic rules of communication respected? How is the group members' attention and concentration?

Affective and relational dimension: Which emotions come up with this exercise? Are the participants able to feel what the others are experiencing and anticipate their actions? Do they realize that personality and reactions may affect the way the person acts during this exercise? This exercise also led to the visible election of a leader who would be at the centre, giving instructions to the rest of the group. How does he/she lead the group? Which members are passive, and which are active? In this exercise, the value of teamwork is emphasized. How are the social interactions? What is the role of each individual in the group?

Behaviour dimension: What is the role of the patient (active or passive) throughout the task?

Symbolic dimension: Patients are always seeking balance in their life. People with eating disorders will see a weight scale but will soon realize that weight is not important in this exercise. The experiences during psychomotor therapy and the responses that arise from these experiences function as dynamic powers or change.

6. Observation and evaluation in psychomotor therapy

The need for treatment at a psychiatric hospital does not arise from physical or motor deficits but from psychological problems. Psychomotor therapists must therefore focus not only on physical goals but also on relevant psychological goals.

Within psychomotor therapy, observation is an important source of information that cannot always be obtained through tests or other measurement instruments. Even in group therapy, each individual reacts in a specific way. Observation can be helpful for establishing goals and a tailored treatment. **Table 2** provides an inventory of the important general mental health functions to observe individual along with some specific features and descriptions. These functions include the first impression, cognitive functions, affective functions and the conative functions [23]. Motor functions can be assessed using tests such as the Bruininks

Functions	Features	Description
First impressions	Appearance	Self-neglect, excessive self-care, differences between biological and calendar age; over- or underweight; piercings, tattoos, injections, self-harming, amputations
	Contact	Eye contact, looking away, looking around; handshake; non interactiveness; non reactivity
	Posture	Postural slumping, body immobility
	Complaints	Inconsistency between the symptoms and the presentation of the complaints
Cognitive functions	Awareness	Somnolent, soporific, semi-comatose, stupor, narrowed/constricted consciousness
	Attention	Cannot attract or maintain his/her attention
	Concentration	
	Orientation	To time, place and person
	Memory	Imprinting, short- and long-term memory
	Intellectual functions	Assessment skills, intelligence, awareness of illness, abstraction ability, executive functions
	Experience	Illusions, hallucinations, derealization, depersonalization
	Concrete thinking	Slowed thinking, rapid thinking, longwinded thinking, incoherence, …
	Substantive thinking	Poverty of thought, preoccupation, obsession, rumination, delusions
Affective functions	Mood	Gloomy, anhedonic, apathetic, anxious, dysphoric, euphoric
	Affect	Incongruent, flat, unstable, exaggerated, dramatic
	Somatic affective characteristics	Muscle tension, flushing, tachycardia, shortness of breath, sweating and clammy hands
	Vital signs	Sleep disorder, fatigue, loss of appetite, loss of body weight and loss of libido
	Suicidality	
Conative functions	Psychomotor	Mimicking, expression: immutable, excessively slow, absent; facial immobility
	Motivation and behaviour	Loss of decorum, inactivity, loss of initiative, lethargy, avolition, impulsive actions and behaviour, compulsive behaviour, motor agitation

Table 2. Observation of an individual patient with psychiatric disorders (adapted from Hengeveld and Schudel [23]).

Motor Ability Test [24] for gross and fine motor skills, the six-minute walk test [25–28] for measuring functional exercise capacity: alternative Leger test [29] or the Spartacus test [30].

6.1. The Louvain observation scales for objectives in psychomotor therapy

The development of the Louvain Observation Scales for Objectives in Psychomotor Therapy (LOFOPT) followed the "Bewegingsonderzoek" of Van Roozendaal [31], which became obsolete due to the time investment required. The LOFOPT was based on the premise that the observation method should offer direct and relevant information about psychosocial aspects of functioning. These observational scales offer direct indications for goals in psychomotor therapy. The disturbed characteristics of the personality in movement situations are directly related to goals. The LOFOPT observation consists of nine categories of goals that are important to psychiatric patients: improving emotional relationships, self-confidence, activity, relaxation, movement control, focus on the situation, movement expressivity, verbal communication, and social regulation ability (see **Table 3**). The LOFOPT can be considered objective and reliable [32].

Observation categories	Description
Emotional relationship	The extent to which the patient can make contacts that are emotional (i.e. experiencing a connection with fellow patients and the therapist with a certain degree of emotionally).
Self-confidence	The extent to which the patient moves independently from others, without underrating him/herself and in a non-anxious way
Activity	The extent to which the patient actively participates in movement situations
Relaxation	The extent to which the patient carries out or observes movement tasks without excessive muscle tension or nervousness
Movement control	The extent to which the patient moves calmly can control his own body and paces his efforts
Focussing attention on the situation	The extent to which the patient can give account of the situation and remain adjusted to it (concentration and task tension)
Movement expressivity	The extent to which the patient does or does not express something in his/her movements, posture and facial expressions
Verbal communication	The extent to which the patient can make verbal contact with others in a meaningful way according to the situation
Social regulation ability	The extent to which the patient is able to observe predetermined agreements and rules of behaviour during the session

Table 3. The Louvain Observation Scales for Objectives in Psychomotor Therapy: observation categories for group activities [31].

Different questionnaires related to (physical) self-concept and body image are used within psychomotor therapy: the self-description questionnaire by Marsh and O'Neill [33], the physical self-description questionnaire by Marsh et al. [34], the Body Attitude Test [35, 36], physical self-perception profile [37], and the physical self-inventory [38]. Other questionnaires are IPAQ [39] and SIMPAQ [40] and the psychomotor therapy satisfaction questionnaire by Vandensande and Probst [41].

7. The scope of psychomotor therapy

Depending on the problem analysis and the related psychomotor therapy goals, the competence of the patient, and the psychological frame of reference, the psychomotor therapist will be able to choose a more health-related approach, a psychosocial approach or a psychotherapeutic physiotherapy method (see **Figure 3**). Concrete activities are offered to motivate patients to act, interact, learn, experience, and express.

7.1. Health-related approach

The physical health-related approach aims to improve global physical health and is focused on the somatic functional status of the patient. Studies have shown that people with mental health problems are more susceptible to inactivity and are at risk of a sedentary lifestyle. In addition, the use of psychotropic drugs can result in the development of metabolic syndrome, obesity, osteoporosis and cardiovascular disease. The health-related approach is consistent with the recent recommendations of the World Health Organization (WHO) regarding the relationship between "physical inactivity" and poor health, which represents a serious threat to quality of life [42]. Clinical practice shows the importance of tailoring physical activity to each person's individual abilities to influence quality of life [43–46]. The challenge is to motivate people to remain active throughout their daily lives. People who do not continue exercising lose independence and will not maximize their potential in life. The American College of Sport Sciences offers guidelines for physical activity. It is the task of the psychomotor therapist to integrate and adapt these guidelines to the context of the person with mental health problems [47].

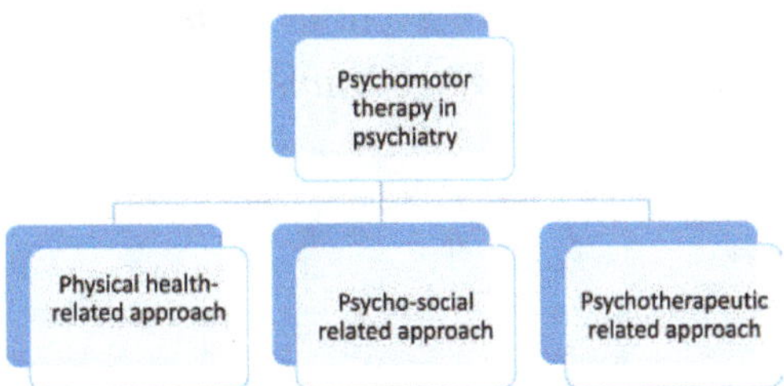

Figure 3. The scope of psychomotor therapy.

7.2. Psychosocial-oriented and psychophysiological approaches

The psychosocial-oriented approach emphasizes the acquisition of mental and physical skills related to the moving body and to support people's ability to function independently in society. The activities focus on learning, acquiring and maintaining psychomotor, sensorimotor, perceptual, cognitive, social and emotional proficiencies. More concretely, the following aspects are highlighted: paying attention, interacting with materials, recognizing stimuli, suppressing passivity, altering behaviour, performing goal-oriented work, enhancing attention to others, improving social proficiency, learning to collaborate, learning to cope with emotionality, learning to accept responsibilities, and being able to put oneself in someone else's place. Other elementary proficiencies are stressed, such as relaxation education, relaxation skills, stress management, breathing techniques, psychomotor and sensory skills and cognitive, expressive and social skills. Through exercises, patients acquire a broader perspective and can experience their own abilities. Moreover, education regarding the basic rules of communication is also integrated [4]. The psychophysiological approach focuses on the use of physical activity to influence mental health problems, such as depression and anxiety [48–54]. In the literature, the benefits of physical activity for mental health are well accepted. Physical activity has a positive influence on mental well-being, self-esteem, mood, and executive functioning. These effects can halt the downward spiral leading to dejection. Well-balanced and regularly executed endurance activities (walking, biking, jogging, swimming), power training (fitness training) and mindfulness-derived exercises augment physical and mental resilience improve the quality of sleep; enhance self-confidence, energy level, endurance level and relaxation; and in general, decrease physical complaints. Some examples will illustrate this approach.

7.2.1. Calculator

The goal of this exercise consists of tapping all the numbered cards located in the large square (calculator) by hand, in order and in the shortest possible time span.

The cards are numbered from 1 to 30 but are scattered randomly throughout the square. Only one player may be in the calculator at any time. A subsequent player can therefore only enter the machine when the other player leaves the square. The cards may not be moved. The time starts when the first player passes the start line. The stop time is at the time at which the last player returns to behind the start line. The level of difficulty can be increased by changing the rules, for instance, to tapping the cards from 30 to 1 or tapping every other card in order (1,3,5,7…). The activity can be adapted for elderly patients by allowing them to tap the cards with a foot or by placing the cards on tables or chairs. It is not necessary to include a competition between two teams. This situation focuses on coping with stress and on cognitive and social skills.

7.2.2. The Duplo game

The group is divided into subgroups of three patients each. The therapist and each group receive the same number of different coloured Duplo blocks. Each subgroup designates a "go-between" and two builders. The therapist constructs a model using the different Duplo blocks and places the model so that the builders cannot see it. The group must then reproduce the model following specific rules.

The go-between is the only person who is allowed to look at the hidden model made by the therapist. The go-between from the group has to perform a circuit to be able to see that figure. After circling and checking the figure, he can come back and answer the questions of the other two members, who will ask yes/no questions and construct the figure. The winner is the group that builds the figure first. In this exercise, patients have to cope with frustration. Communication is very important, as is memorization. It is very important from a symbolic point of view that the "go-between" who checks the figure is very sure of what he/she is doing.

7.3. Psychotherapeutic-oriented approach

The psychotherapeutic-oriented physiotherapy approach uses the motor domain as a gateway for ameliorating social-affective functioning. Using movement activities with a psychotherapeutic accent, the psychomotor therapist creates a setting that favours the initiation and development of processes designed to help patients gain better insight into their own functioning. During these activities, patients are invited to venture outside their comfort zones, think outside the box, experience new things, become more in touch with their inner self and cope with many emotions (depressive feelings, fear, guilt, anger, stress, feelings of unease, estrangement and dissatisfaction) and negative thoughts (intrusion, obsession, morbid preoccupations and worrying). Moreover, they will confront their behaviours (i.e. impulses, lack of abilities) or cognitive symptoms (i.e. derealisation, lack of concentration). Throughout psychomotor therapy interventions, an alternative perspective of experiences can be proposed. Becoming aware that an alternative may exist will trigger new emotions and experiences, and a discrepancy between reality and the patient's perception of their reality will emerge. Consequently, it is important to note that it is not the physical activity itself but the patient's experiences and inner perception that play the central role. Different issues are elaborated during psychomotor therapy, such as being aware of one's body and movement, expressing and regulating emotions, augmenting tolerance for frustration, refraining from impulsive behaviour, improving orientation to reality, improving social interaction, learning to define limits, strengthening self-confidence, improving body perception and self-perception, dealing with fear of failure, developing self-reflection, exploring one's actual emotional and social life and providing better insight into one's conscious through inter and intrapsychic conflicts. The careful guidance and encouragement of the psychomotor therapist and the opportunity to experience feelings in a safe environment allow the patient to develop behaviours that he/she would not have developed otherwise. The underlying problems are not necessarily resolved, but the therapist tries to improve the patient's management of problems. The patient shares his/her behaviour, feelings, and thoughts, initially with the therapist and eventually with peers. More emphasis is placed on experiences and how reactions to these experiences function as a dynamic source of power. Some examples of psychomotor therapy activities clearly illustrate the underlying message of the psychotherapeutic approach.

7.3.1. Blind squares

Blindfolded participants look for two ropes in a defined area. With these two ropes, they need to make two perfect squares, a small one in the middle of a large one. The entire length of the rope should be used. The ends of each rope are tied together. Self-confidence, communication, problem solving, orientation and concentration are the main aspects in this exercise.

7.3.2. The carpets

One person is invited to stay on a carpet. The carpet measures 70 cm by 70 cm. The top and the underside of the carpet are different colours. In this exercise, a person must turn over the carpet without touching the floor. If the person succeeds, he/she invites a second (third, fourth, fifth…) person to join him and turn the carpet back. The level of difficulty increases as the number of people on the mat increases. This is a great exercise to improve participants' balance and test their problem-solving skills. In dialogue, the participants should find the appropriate strategy for turning over the carpets. This exercise also requires leadership, coordination and co-operation skills to succeed. Closeness, bodily contact and touch are difficult issues for people with mental health problems such as eating disorders, post-traumatic stress disorders, and personality disorders to cope with. Patients will feel others invading their comfort zone. This exercise imitates real-life situations, such as rush hours on the bus, train or tube. Patients can become aware of their own thoughts, feelings, and behaviours while at the same time searching for new strategies to cope with this uncomfortable situation.

7.3.3. The window with 16 sections

The therapist designs a frame with 16 sections. Different letters lay in all but one of the sections. Using these letters, four group members must make a sentence following the rules of a sliding window. The person and the letters can only move horizontally or vertically. Letters and people cannot move diagonally.

An alternative form of this activity could be to place a person in all but one of the sections, with the goal of moving the youngest person to the beginning of the framework and the oldest to the end.

This exercise requires problem solving, communication skills, and attention.

7.3.4. Push and pull activity, a dance experience within psychomotor therapy

Patients are asked to be aware of the concepts "push" and "pull". During a warm-up, they can experience the meaning of "push" and "pull" separately in practice. Afterwards, the participants are asked to form to equal groups (in terms of both the number of members and strength) for a tug-of-war. The next step is to experience the push and pull concept during a two-minute music sequence. The participants are able to move freely during the activity and can choose whether to come in contact with other group members. The last step is to push and pull for 15 min along with music, starting from an as small a space as possible for the patient to feel safe. The patients are invited to increase the tempo in the room by touching, pushing and pulling. Again, they can decide whether other group members are allowed in their comfort zone.

These activities require self-esteem for the patient to use the whole space of the room or only the borders, to move without the concerns about the others, and to move in three dimensions. Attracting and rejecting or pushing away; greeting, meeting and then leaving; and coming together versus separating are well-known strategies for double messages and are congruent with eating and not eating, exerting control and not exerting control, tensing and relaxing, daring and not daring, and jumping and not jumping.

8. Psychomotor therapy interventions examples in psychiatry: depression, schizophrenia, personality disorders and eating disorders

8.1. Psychomotor therapy intervention for patients with depression

Table 4 shows the most important goals of psychomotor therapy for patients with depression. The approach focuses on providing regular successful experiences through realistic and individualized goals using mastery experiences [64] and group dynamism [8] as a mean to develop adequate coping strategies. Training effects are important but not necessary to improve the patient's physical self-concept. Therefore, the psychomotor therapist should focus on strategies for improving physical self-concept [4, 37, 55–57].

8.2. Psychomotor therapy for patients with schizophrenia

In addition to the basic goal of maintaining good physical condition, the psychomotor therapist will offer a wide range of movement activities to expand skills and structure their behaviour. Based on recent research, the evidence-based psychomotor programme consists of (a) a stress-reduction programme, (b) a movement activation programme and (c) a psychosocial therapy programme [58]. *The stress-reduction programme* consists of (1) progressive muscle relaxation, (2) yoga/tai chi therapy [65], (3) aqua therapy and (4) stress management training. This programme provides patients self-maintenance coping skills that help reduce psychological distress and improve subjective well-being [66]. In the *movement activation programme* (e.g. "start to walk" sessions, psychoeducation sessions regarding lifestyle, physical activity and fitness sessions), health-related issues (the metabolic abnormalities associated with atypical antipsychotics; sedentary lifestyle) should be of special interest. The self-determination theory [67] is an appropriated approach to motivate patients to move [68]. The psychosocial therapy programme focuses on a group setting and group involvement. In the group, patients will experience during the different group processes of co-operation, compromise, confrontation and conformity during movement sessions. Clinical observations confirm the conclusion of Faulkner and Biddle [69] that exercise can be a coping mechanism for positive symptoms, such as auditory hallucinations (see **Table 4**).

8.3. Psychomotor therapy in a clinical psychotherapy setting for patients with personality disorders

Twemlow et al. [70] suggest the use of movement in physically oriented therapies combined with psychodynamic psychotherapy. In psychomotor therapy, those ideas are applied for individuals with personality and behaviour disorders. In this setting, physical work in

Psychomotor therapy for patients with depression [55–57] • *Improving objective and subjective fitness: stimulating health-related physical fitness and improving general physical condition by running, swimming, cycling, (Nordic) walking* • *Reducing feelings of anxiety and tension* • *Providing experiences of success; improving self-image* • *Psychoeducation and coaching concerning physical fitness and personal well-being and teaching patients to actively search for solutions* • *Assisting people with lower verbal skills* ***Psychomotor therapy for patients with psychosis and schizophrenia*** [46, 58, 59] • *Improving poor physical health (cardiovascular fitness) caused by a low level of physical activity and a sedentary lifestyle* • *Increasing the level of "activity", "attention", "initiative", "communication" and "social contact" by offering a stress-reduction programme, a movement activation programme and a psychosocial therapy programme* ***Psychomotor therapy for patients with eating disorders*** [60–62, 36] • *Rebuilding a realistic self-image using posture exercises, massage, mirror exercises, breathing exercises, and sensory, movement and body awareness exercises* • *Curbing hyperactivity, impulses, and tensions using relaxation, yoga, tai chi and other physical activities* • *Developing social skills using problem-solving exercises* • *Psych-education concerning the body and physical activity. Coaching concerning physical fitness and personal well-being* ***Psychomotor therapy for patients with personality disorders*** **[63]** • *Re-tooling the person's experiences under the guidance of a healthy role model. Movement is used as a therapeutic tool for stimulating the part of the mind that requires specific training and skills. The process of mentalization during movement sessions is a crucial therapeutic force*

Table 4. Goals in psychomotor therapy for patients with depression, psychoses, eating disorders and personality disorders.

psychomotor therapy and psychological work in psychotherapy are combined. Psychomotor therapy is viewed as an important complementary approach to psychodynamic therapies. Individuals are allowed to re-tool their experiences under the guidance of a healthy role model [63]. Psychomotor therapy (see **Table 4**) aims to perceive and interpret the patients' behaviour in terms of intentional mental states, such as needs, desires, feelings, beliefs, goals, purposes, and reasons [71]. The different activities are used to experiment with and to learn how to address emotions [4].

8.4. Psychomotor therapy in a cognitive behavioural setting for patients with eating disorders

The cornerstones of psychomotor therapy for patients with eating disorders are the patient's specific relationship with his/her body (unfamiliarity with their own body, body dissatisfaction and social anxiety) and the drive for exercise, expressed as restlessness or hyperactivity in anorexia and bulimia nervosa or passivity (physical inactivity and a sedentary life style) in binge eating disorder [35]. The therapy focuses on the patient's impression (physical self-concept), expression (the emotional self-concept) and communication (social self-concept) using postural awareness exercises; breathing exercises; relaxation exercises; sensory, body and movement awareness; massage; mirror exercises; physical activity; yoga; tai chi; self-confrontation techniques; psychoeducation; guided imagery exercises; dance and expression; and problem-solving exercises in a group [17, 35, 60–62, 72] (see **Table 4**).

9. Conclusion

Psychomotor therapy in the field of psychiatry is a relatively recent and evolving domain. Depending on the patient's request for assistance, competence or therapeutic possibilities and his/her goals and psychological frame of reference, the psychomotor therapist can choose either a more health-related, a more psychosocial or a more psychotherapeutic approach. The therapist has access to a wide variety of activities. The emphasis is to activate patients, to offer them new experiences, and to stimulate them to express their feelings. The psychomotor therapist needs to have good motivation skills as well as creativity and adaptation skills. Because psychomotor therapy encompasses more than just movement, good communication skills are also important. The focus lays on improving the patient's actions and interaction with peers, learning new skills, behavioural change, new experiences and expression of emotions.

After a phase of clinical observations and explanations, the use of psychomotor therapy in psychiatry is now in a phase of testing the effectiveness of psychomotor interventions in different populations and settings. Many factors will influence clinical practice: the evidence, the skills of the patient and the therapist, the enthusiasm of the therapist's message the marketing, the referral systems, the health service systems and of course the economic situation. Compared with the health-related approach, the efficacy of the psychosocial and psychotherapeutic approaches of psychomotor therapy is hard to prove due to the scientific need to control for large numbers of variables. However, qualitative studies concerning patient satisfaction showed that the adjunctive approach is very helpful for many patients [73]. Future research must analyze which patients benefit the most from this approach.

The psychomotor therapist will face various challenges. Interdisciplinary and transdisciplinary are the future of mental health care. Under these approaches, professionals will reach out to other mental health caregivers who use the same methods as the core of their approach. Hopefully, this will open doors for a more intensive interchange of ideas, and the gap between the different adjunctive therapies that developed in the 1960s will begin to close.

In the future, therapists will need to obtain informed consent for each treatment. Each therapist will need to prove that his/her methods have value for the patient and provide information about what, why, where, when and how he/she will proceed and what the possible outcomes are. The move from inpatient treatment (residential therapy) to community treatment is another important challenge.

In Anglo-Saxon countries, psychomotor therapy as such is not well known as in Flanders, The Netherlands, and Germany. This approach is an evolving domain within psychiatry and can be seen as an adjunct bio-psychosocial treatment, in accordance with internationally accepted models. In Flanders, psychomotor therapy is taught at the university level and integrated in the dominant health care system [4].

Inviting people with mental health problems to participate in psychomotor therapy is not about finding a direct solution; rather, it is about starting a dialogue with the person with mental health problems.

Author details

Michel Probst

Address all correspondence to: michel.probst@kuleuven.be

Department of Rehabilitation Sciences, KU Leuven, Belgium

References

[1] Probst M, Bosscher RJ, editors. Ontwikkelingen in de Psychomotorische Therapie [Developments in Psychomotor Therapy]. Zeist: Cure & Care Publishers; 2001

[2] de Lange, editor. Psychomotorische therapie. Lichaams- en bewegingsgerichte interventies in de ggz [Psychomotor Therapy: Body and Movement Oriented Interventions in Mental Health Care]. Amsterdam: Uitgeverij Boom; 2010

[3] Hölter G. Bewegungstherapie bei psychischen Erkrankungen: Grundlagen und Anwendung [Movement Therapy in Mental Disorders]. Köln: Deutscher Ärzteverlag; 2011

[4] Probst M, Knapen J, Poot G, Vancampfort D. Psychomotor therapy and psychiatry: What is in a name? The Open Complementary Medicine Journal. 2010;**2**:105-113. DOI: 10.2174/1876391X010020010105

[5] Faulkner G, Carless D. Physical activity in the process of psychiatric rehabilitation: Theoretical and methodological issues. Psychiatric Rehabilitation Journal. 2006;**29**:258-266. DOI: 10.2975/29.2006.258.266

[6] Swarbrick M. A wellness approach. Psychiatric Rehabilitation Journal. 2006;**29**:311. DOI:10.2975/29.2006.311.314

[7] Simons J. Inleiding in de psychomotorische therapie [Introduction in Psychomotor Therapy]. Antwerpen: Garant; 2014

[8] Yalom ID. The Theory and Practice of Group Psychotherapy. 5th ed. New York: Guilford; 2005

[9] Probst M, Carraro A. Physical Activity and Mental Health; A Practice-Oriented Approach. Milan: Edi Ermes; 2014. ISBN: 978887051386-8,978887051387-5

[10] Simon H. Aktivere Krankenbehandlung in der Irrenanstalt. 2nd ed. Berlin: W. de Gruyter; 1929

[11] Day A. Superintendent's report to the board of trustees of the New York State Inebriate Asylum. New York; 1867

[12] Bonwill CEH. The New York State Inebriate Asylum at Binghamton. Harper's Weekly, A Journal of Civilization. 1869;**13**:828

[13] Franz SI, Hamilton GV. The effects of exercise upon the retardation in conditions of depression. American Journal of Insanity. 1905;**17:**239-256

[14] Meyer A. The philosophy of occupation therapy. American Journal of Occupational Therapy. 1977;**1:**1-10

[15] Creek J, Lougher L, Van Bruggen H. Occupational Therapy and Mental Health. 4th ed. London: Churchill Livingstone Title; 2011

[16] Pierloot R. Algemene grondslagen van de bewegingstherapie in de psychiatrie [Fundamentals in Movement Therapy in Psychiatry]. Leuven: Fonteyn; 1968

[17] VanCoppenolle H. Algemene grondslagen van psychomotorische therapie voor psychisch gestoorden [Cornerstones of Psychomotor Therapies in Mental Health]. Leuven: Acco; 1978

[18] Van Roozendaal NP. Grundlagen der Bewegungstherapie in der psychiatrischen Anstalt [Cornerstones for movement therapy in psychiatry]. Folia Psychiatrica, Neurologica et Neurochirugica Neerlandica. 1954;**57**:356-366

[19] Knapen J, Vancoppenolle. Een poging tot opstellen van een verkorte vorm van het bewegingsonderzoek van N.P. Van Roozendaal. Vlaams Tijdschrift voor Psychomotorische Therapie. 1978;**3**:83-93

[20] Probst M, Skjaerven LH, Parker A, Gyllensten AL, IJntema R, Catalán-Matamoros D. Do you support this definition of physiotherapy in mental health? In: 6th International Conference on Physiotherapy in Psychiatry and Mental Health; Madrid: Fisioterapia; 2016;**38**:49

[21] De Herdt A, Knapen J, Vancampfort D, De Hert M, Brunner E, Probst M. Social anxiety in physical activity participation in patients with mental illness: A cross-sectional multicenter study. Depression and Anxiety. 2013;**30:**757-762. DOI:10.1002/da.22059

[22] Linehan MM. Cognitive-Behavioral Treatment of Borderline Personality Disorder. 5th ed. New York: Guilford Publications; 1993

[23] Hengeveld MW, Shudel WJ. Het psychiatrisch onderzoek. 3e ed. Utrecht: Uitgeverij de Tijdstroom; 2003

[24] Bruininks BD, Bruininks RH. Occupational and Physical Therapy: Bruininks Motor Ability Test. Bloomington NM: Pearson, Ontario; 2012

[25] Engright P. The six-minute walk test. Respiratory Care. 2003;**48:**783-785

[26] Brooks D, Solway S. ATS statement on six-minute walk test. American Journal of Respiratory and Critical Care Medicine. 2003;**167:**1287-1287. DOI:10.1164/ajrccm.167.9.950

[27] Troosters T, Gosselink R, Decramer M. Six minute walking distance in healthy elderly subjects. European Respiratory Journal. 2009;**14:**270-274. DOI:10.1034/j.1399-3003.1999.14b06.x

[28] Vancampfort D, Rosenbaum S, Schurch F, Ward P, Richards J, Mugisha J, Probst M, Stubbs B. Cardiorespiratory fitness in severe mental illness: A systematic review and meta-analysis. Sports Medicine. 2010. DOI: 10.1007/s40279-016-0574-1

[29] Léger A, Mercier D, Gadoury C, Lambert J. The multistage 20 meter shuttle run test for aerobic fitness. Journal of Sports Sciences. 1988;**6:**93-101

[30] Rey O, Rossi D, Nicol C, Mercier C, Vallier J, Maïano C. Évaluation indirecte de la capacité aérobie d'adolescents obèses: Intérêt d'un test de course à pied intermittent court, progressif et maximal. Science & Sports. 2013;**28:**e133–e139

[31] Simons J. Psychomotor observation in psychiatry. Construction and evaluation of an objective directed observation method [doctoral dissertation]. Leuven: KU Leuven; 1987

[32] Van Coppenolle H, Simons J, Pierloot R, Probst M, Knapen J. The Louvain observation scales for objectives in psychomotor therapy. Adapted Physical Activity Quarterly. 1989;**6:**145-153. DOI:10.1123/apaq.6.2.145

[33] Marsh HW, O'Neill R. Self-description questionnaire III: The construct validity of multidimensional self-concept ratings by late adolescents. Journal of Educational Measurement. 1984;**21:**1745-3984. DOI:10.1111/j.1745-3984.1984.tb00227.x

[34] Marsh HW, Martin AJ, Jackson S. Introducing a short version of the physical self-description questionnaire: New strategies, short-form evaluative criteria, and applications of factor analyses. Journal of Sport and Exercise Psychology. 2010;**32:**438-482. DOI:10.1123/jsep.32.4.438

[35] Probst M, Van Coppenolle H, Vandereycken W. The Body Attitude Test for patients with an eating disorder: Psychometric characteristics of a new questionnaire. Eating Disorders. 1995;**3:**133-144. DOI: 10.1080/10640269508249156

[36] Probst M, Pieters G, Vanderlinden J. Evaluation of body experience questionnaires in eating disorders in female patients (AN/BN) and nonclinical participants. International Journal of Eating Disorders. 2008;**41:**657-665. DOI:10.1002/eat.20531

[37] Fox K. Self-esteem, self-perceptions and exercise. International Journal of Sport Psychology. 2000;**31:**228-240. DOI:10.4324/9781315880198.ch3

[38] Maïano C, Bégarie J, Morin AJS, Ninot G. Assessment of physical self-concept in adolescents with intellectual disability: Content and factor validity of the very short form of the physical self-inventory. Journal of Autism and Developmental Disorders. 2009;**39:**775-787. DOI:10.1007/s10803-008-0686-z

[39] Vancampfort D, Wyckaert S, Sienaert P, De Herdt A, De Hert M, Rosenbaum S, Probst M. Concurrent validity of the international physical activity questionnaire in outpatients with bipolar disorder: Comparison with the Sensewear Armband. Psychiatry Research. 2016;**237:**122-126. DOI:10.1007/s40279-016-0574-1

[40] Rosenbaum S, Ward PB. The simple physical activity questionnaire. The Lancet Psychiatry.2016;3:e1, Jan. DOI:http://dx.doi.org/10.1016/S2215-0366(15)00496-4

[41] Vandensande A, De Herdt A, Probst M. Patiënten-tevredenheid in de psychomotorische therapie: ontwikkeling van een vragenlijst. [Patient Satisfaction in Psychomotor Therapy; The Development of a Questionnaire]. In Simons J, editor. Actuele themata uit de psychomotorische therapie. Leuven: Acco; 2013

[42] American College of Sports Medicine, editor. ACSM's Health-Related Physical Fitness Assessment Manual. Lippincott Williams & Wilkins; 2013.

[43] Vancampfort D, Stubbs B, Ward PB, Teasdale S, Rosenbaum S. Why moving more should be promoted for severe mental illness. The Lancet Psychiatry. 2015;**2:**295. DOI:10.1016/S2215-0366(15)00099-1

[44] Vancampfort D, Sienaert P, Wyckaert S, De Hert M, Stubbs B, Soundy A, De Smet J, Probst M. Health-related physical fitness in patients with bipolar disorder vs. healthy controls: An exploratory study. Journal of Affective Disorder. 2015;**177:**22-27. DOI:10.1016/j.jad.2014.12.058

[45] Vancampfort D, Rosenbaum S, Schuch F, Ward P, Richards J, Mugisha J, Probst M, Stubbs B. Cardiorespiratory fitness in severe mental illness: A systematic review and meta-analysis. Sports Medicine. 2017;**47**:343-352. Doi:10.007/s40279-016-0574-1

[46] Vancampfort D, Stubbs B, Ward PB, Teasdale S, Rosenbaum S. Integrating physical activity as medicine in the care of people with severe mental illness. Australian & New Zealand Journal of Psychiatry. 2015;**49:**681-682. DOI:10.1177/0004867415590831

[47] American SM, Wilkins LW, Kaminsky LA. American College of Sports Medicine. 3rd ed. Philadelphia: Wolters Kluwer Health/Lippincott Williams & Wilkins Health; 2009

[48] Cooney GM, Dwan K, Greig CA, Lawlor DA, Rimer J, Waugh FR, McMurdo M, Mead GE. Exercise for depression. Advances in Psychiatric Treatment. 2014;**20**;2. DOI:10.1192/apt.20.1.2

[49] Ekkekakis P. Honey, I shrunk the pooled SMD! Guide to critical appraisal of systematic reviews and meta-analyses using the Cochrane review on exercise for depression as example. Mental Health and Physical Activity. 2015;**8**:21-36. DOI:10.1016/j.mhpa.2014.12.001

[50] Rimer J, Dwan K, Lawlor DA, Greig CA, McMurdo M, Morley W. Exercise for depression. Cochrane Database of Systematic Reviews. 2012. DOI:10.1002/14651858.CD004366.pub5

[51] Josefsson T, Lindwall M, Archer T. Physical exercise intervention in depressive disorders: Meta-analysis and systematic review. Scandinavian Journal of Medicine & Science in Sports. 2013;**24**:259-272.

[52] Schuch F, Vancampfort D, Richards J, Rosenbaum S, Ward P, Stubbs B. Exercise as a treatment for depression: A meta-analysis adjusting for publication bias. Journal of Psychiatric Research. 2016;**77**:42-51. DOI:10.1016/j.jpsychires.2016.02.023

[53] Richardson CR, Faulkner G, McDevitt J, Skrinar GS, Hutchinson DS, Piette JD. Integrating physical activity into mental health services for persons with serious mental illness. Psychiatric Services. 2005;**56**:3. DOI:10.1176/appi.ps.56.3.324

[54] Craft LL, Landers DM. The effect of exercise on clinical depression and depression resulting from mental illness: A meta-analysis. Journal of Sport and Exercise Psychology. 1998;**20**:339-357. DOI:10.1123/jsep.20.4.339

[55] Van de Vliet P, Auweele YV, Knapen J, Rzewnicki R, Onghena P, Van Coppenolle H. The effect of fitness training on clinically depressed patients: An intra-individual approach. Psychology of Sport and Exercise. 2004;**5**(2):153-167. DOI:10.1016/S1469-0292(02)00044-4

[56] Knapen J, Van de Vliet P, Van Coppenolle H, David A, Peuskens J, Pieters G, Knapen K. Comparison of changes in physical self-concept, global self-esteem, depression and anxiety following two different psychomotor therapy programs in nonpsychotic psychiatric inpatients. Psychotherapy and Psychosomatics. 2005;**74**:353-361. DOI:10.1159/000087782

[57] Knapen J, Vancampfort D, Moriën Y, Marchal Y. Exercise therapy improves both mental and physical health in patients with major depression. Disability and Rehabilitation. 2015;**37**:1490-1495. DOI:10.3109/09638288.2014.972579

[58] Vancampfort D, Probst M, Skjaerven LH, Catalán-Matamoros DC, Lundik-Gyllensten A, Gómez-Conesa AG, Ijntema R, De Hert M. Systematic review of the benefits of physical therapy within a multidisciplinary care approach for people with schizophrenia. Physical Therapy. 2011;**92**:11-23. DOI:10.2522/ptj.20110218

[59] Vancampfort D, De Hert M, Skjerven LH, Gyllensten AL, Parker A, Mulders N, Nyboe L, Spenser F, Probst M. International organization of physical therapy in mental health consensus on physical activity within multidisciplinary rehabilitation programmes

for minimising cardio-metabolic risk in patients with schizophrenia. Disability and Rehabilitation. 2012;**34:**1-12. DOI:10.3109/09638288.2011.587090

[60] Probst M, Diedens J. The body in movement. In: Jáuregui-Lobera I, editor. Eating Disorders. Zagreb: Intech; 2017

[61] Vancampfort D, Probst M, Adriaens A, Pieters G, De Hert M, Stubbs B, Soundy A, Vanderlinden J. Changes in physical activity, physical fitness, self-perception and quality of life following a 6-month physical activity counseling and cognitive behavioral therapy program in outpatients with binge eating disorder. Psychiatry Research.2014;**219:**361-366. DOI:10.1016/j.psychres.2014.05.016

[62] Vancampfort D, Rosenbaum S, Probst M, Connaughton J, Plessis CD, Yamamoto T, Diedens J, Stubbs B. Top 10 research questions to promote physical activity research in people with binge eating disorder. Eating Disorders. 2015;**24:**326-337. DOI:10.1080/10640266.2015.1123988

[63] Poot G. Psychomotorische therapie op een psychoanalytisch georiënteerde afdeling [Psychomotor therapy in an psychoanalytical oriented unit]. In: Probst M, Bosschere RJ, editors. Ontwikkelingen in de Psychomotorische Therapie [Developments in Psychomotor Therapy]. Zeist: Cure & Care Publishers; 2001. pp. 37-50

[64] Bandura A. Self-efficacy: Toward a unifying theory of behavioral change. Psychological Review. 1977;**84:**191-215. DOI:10.1037/0033-295X.84.2.191

[65] Vancampfort D, Vansteelandt K, Scheewe T, Probst M, Knapen J, De Herdt A, De Hert M. Yoga in schizophrenia: A systematic review of randomised controlled trials. Acta Psychiatrica Scandinavica. 2012;**126:**12-20.

[66] Vancampfort D, De Hert M, Knapen J, Maurissen K, Raepsaet J, Deckx S, Remans S, Probst M. Effects of progressive muscle relaxation on state anxiety and subjective well-being in people with schizophrenia: A randomized controlled trial. Clinical Rehabilitation. 2011;**25:**567-575. DOI:10.1177/0269215510395633

[67] Sheldon KM, Williams G, Joiner TE. Self-determination theory in the clinic: Motivating physical and mental health. New Haven, CT: Yale University Press; 2003. DOI:10.12987/yale/9780300095449.001.0001

[68] Firth J, Rosenbaum S, Stubbs B, Vancampfort D, Carney R, Yung AR. Preferences and motivations for exercise in early psychosis. Acta Psychiatrica Scandinavica. 2016;**134:**83-84.

[69] Faulkner G, Biddle S. Exercise and mental health: It's just not psychology! Journal of Sports Sciences. 2001;**19:**433-444. DOI: 10.1080/026404101300149384

[70] Twemlow SW, Fonagy P, Sacco FC. Embodying the mind: Movement as a container for destructive aggression. The American Journal of Psychoanalysis. 2008;**62:**213-235

[71] Fonagy P, Gergely G, Jurist EL, Target M. Affect regulation, mentalization, and the development of the self. New York: Other Press; 2002

[72] Probst M, Majewski ML, Albertsen M, Catalan-Matamoros D, Danielsen M, De Herdt A, Duskova Zakova H, Fabricius S, Joern C, Kjolstad G, Patovirta M, Philip-Raverty S, Tyyska E, Vancampfort D. Physiotherapy for patients with anorexia nervosa. Advances in Eating Disorders; Theory, Research and Practice. 2013;**1**:224-238. DOI: 10.1080/21662630.2013.798562

[73] Probst M. Onderzoek in de psychomotorische therapie: de perceptie van de psychomotorische therapie door patiënten met eetstoornissen [Perception of psychomotor therapy in patients with eating disorders]. In Simons J, editor. Actuele themata uit de psychomotorische therapie. Leuven: Acco; 2007. pp. 133-151

5

Occupational Therapy in Oncology and Palliative Care

Sedef Şahin, Semin Akel and Meral Zarif

Abstract

Cancer is a chronic disease that may occur in both children and adults. Occupational therapy focuses on the activity limitations and participation problems in their life. Oncology rehabilitation involves in helping an individual with cancer to regain maximum physical, psychological, cognitive, social, and vocational functioning with the limits up to disease and its treatments in an interdisciplinary team concept. These treatment options are associated with the risk of some side effects, including fatigue, pain, cognitive problems, decrease in bone density and muscle endurance, weight loss, and stress- or anxiety-related psychosocial problems. Occupational therapy approaches are a holistic view in a client center and use training in activities of daily living, assistive technology, education of energy conservation techniques, and management of treatment-related problems, such as pain, fatigue, and nausea. In palliative and hospice care, occupational therapists support clients with cancer by minimizing the secondary symptoms related to cancer and its treatments. At the end of life, occupational therapy offers to identify the roles and activities that are meaningful and purposeful to the client with cancer and try to determine the barriers that limit their performance. Clients with cancer who have childhood cancer or adult cancer can face problems about body structure and functions, activity, and participation, which may limit their participation to their daily life.

Keywords: oncology, rehabilitation, palliative care, occupational therapy

1. Introduction

Cancer is defined as the growth of abnormal cell structures in the body uncontrollably, without purpose, and with a large number. Cancer develops faster when the body's normal defense and control mechanisms do not work. Old cells do not die; instead, they become uncontrolled and replace new cells that are abnormal. These abnormal cells may be called a tumor, while some cancers do not form tumors such as leukemia [1]. Cancer can be anywhere in the body. Cancer is a chronic disease of various types and characteristics in all ages and genders. According to the literature, the most common cancer is breast cancer in females and prostate cancer in males. Moreover, lung and colorectal cancer affect both men and women at high rates [2]. The most common types of cancer in children between 0 and 14 years of age are acute lymphocytic leukemia (ALL), brain and other central nervous system (CNS) tumors, and neuroblastoma. Although pediatric cancer mortality rates have declined by about 70% in the last four decades, it is still one of the most common causes of death in children [3].

There are five primary categories of cancer: carcinomas, sarcomas, leukemia, lymphomas, and central nervous system cancers. This categorization is made according to the body structure involved. For example, carcinomas begin in the skin or tissues, whereas sarcomas start in the bone, cartilage, fat, muscle, or other connective tissues. Leukemia develops in the blood and bone marrow, lymphomas start in the immune system, and central nervous system cancers start in the brain and spinal cord [4].

The survival rate after cancer treatment is increasing day by day due to advances in children, adolescents, and adults [5, 6]. Cancer survivors also can face the risk of cancer recurrence, metastases, or symptoms such as cancer-related pain, fatigue, stress, or lymphedema, etc. More than 60% of cancer survivors with ages between 5 and 19 years reported at least one serious symptom [7]. Some of the treatment options for cancer clients include surgery, chemotherapy, hormonal therapy, radiotherapy, immunotherapy, and targeted therapy. These treatments contain some risks that are closely related to the individual and the treatment dosage. Some side effects of treatments such as fatigue, pain, cognitive problems, decreased bone density, weight loss, and stressful psychosocial problems as well as hot pressures may occur [8]. It is known that due to these side effects, there is a decrease especially in the physical functions, daily activities of life (ADL), and quality of life in clients with cancer [9].

Occupational therapists (OTs) specialized in oncology does not only need to have high quality of skills but also knowledge about cancer, side effects, and evaluation of the treatments of cancer. This perspective requires a holistic and client-centered approach to provide personal care. OTs working in oncological rehabilitation aim to increase quality of life by facilitating physical, mental, emotional, social, occupational and cognitive needs, goal setting, and participation in meaningful occupations [10]. The main goal of OTs is to provide clients to participate in daily activities of life (ADL). OTs change their occupation or environment to better support occupational engagement in an interdisciplinary team concept. With oncologic rehabilitation, care is given to various age groups in a variety of care settings, including hospital, home, inpatient palliative care, or community-based services [11].

2. Cancer rehabilitation

Cancer rehabilitation is defined by Cromes as "helping a client with cancer to help to reach the maximum physical, social, psychological, and vocational functioning within the limits of disease and treatments" [12]. The functioning is important while engaging in activity and is related with all performance components [13]. In a more contemporary view, the function is a broad vision that encompasses the physical, emotional, cognitive, and psychological states of the individual [14]. The World Health Organization's International Functioning, Disability and Health Classification (ICF) defines a framework in which this multidimensional or biopsychosocial approach focuses on an extensive understanding of the interactions between function, capacity, and performance [13–15]. Cancer treatment itself also can lead to functional problems or impairments in physical, sensorial, or cognitive (body functions and structures), potentially leading to limitations in ADL or instrumental ADL (activity) and participation restriction (participation) [16]. Therefore, as ICF covers all of these domains, it suggests framework and approach regarding diagnosis and evaluation. This framework can also guide treatment programs [17].

Cancer rehabilitation goals are classified as restorative, supportive, palliative, and preventive according to progression of cancer. Generally, restorative care purposes at maximal recovery of residual function of the client. Supportive care aims to increase daily life and mobility by using effective methods such as reducing functional difficulties and compensating for permanent deficits. Palliative care reduces symptoms such as pain and shortness of breath. Preventive care includes in the area of power maintenance and movement after treatment. This process starts right after the diagnosis [18].

Client should be evaluated in terms of goal-oriented activity performance and participation in all contextual areas. Thus, OTs can provide a top-down approach to the clients [19]. **Table 1**

Body functions and body structures
Functions
Sensation of pain
Energy and innerdrive functions
Emotional functions
Voice functions
Respiration functions
Swallowing functions
Structures
Structure of mouth—pharynx-larynx-head and neck region
Activities and participation
Daily routine activity (Self-care-Eating-Drinking)
Social activity (Family and friends relationships)
Productivity activity (Economic self-sufficiency-preparing foods)
Personal factors
Type a or b personality
İnterest
Motivation level
Environmental factors
Products or substances for personal consumption
Immediate family
Health professionals
Work environment

Table 1. Impairment of functional health in neck cancer.

shows an example of functional health impairment areas in neck cancer that should be analyzed by OTs [20]. In occupational therapy (OT), rehabilitation generally focuses on these topics:

- Symptom control
- Activity training
- Client education
- Motor training
- Sensory training
- Cognitive training
- Vocational rehabilitation

3. Occupational therapy role in symptom control

Some clients experience symptoms during the first phase of diagnosis or treatment, while others experience these symptoms due to side effects or long-term outcome of treatment during the treatment phase. The appearance of symptoms can be basically examined in five different phases. The pretreatment phase is first experienced with symptoms of fatigue, pain, and anxiety. In this phase, the client will have difficulty in accepting the idea of the disease, their sleep patterns and routines begin to deteriorate, and problems occur in occupational and social relationships. The second phase is the primary treatment phase; in addition to the symptoms mentioned above, some other symptoms such as inappetency, fever, vomiting, dry mouth, etc. can occur as a result of chemotherapy or other modalities. ADL are interrupted. The post-treatment phase is the third one; the client with cancer experience treatment-related symptoms such as pain, weakness, or constipation after surgery. The influence on the activities and routines are very apparent at this phase. The fourth phase, where the symptoms experienced due to tumor growth occur, is the recurrence phase. Clients with cancer often feel depressive, anxious, fear, and unhappy for repetition. ADL and routines are disrupted with negative emotions and thoughts about their future. In the last phase, the end-of-life phase, the most common symptoms are fear of death and alienation to everything. Client usually cannot even get out of the bed and have lost all interest and the desire to live [13].

Symptoms are multidimensional and changeable in cancer clients. The OT's role in management of symptoms is crucial and important. They must maintain up-to-date professional knowledge of the symptoms and its treatments. They must also investigate the meaning and the impact of the symptom not only to the individual, but also to the caregivers. Besides, in the following sections of this chapter, every title includes client and their family educations for these symptoms, especially. They must search how this situation limits them in carrying out their required objectives in life. Thus, as a priority, realistic and achievable intervention plan can be made for people with cancer to control the symptoms. There are some approaches to control symptoms such as problem-solving strategies, restoration activity, compensation activity, and environmental modification that will be defined in the following sections.

3.1. Problem-solving strategies

Cooper describes problem solving as "analyzing of the client's needs and enabling the client to cope with dysfunction" in approach to symptom control. OT must help to identify physical, emotional, social, and psychological problems and try to resolve them. For solving the problems caused by the symptoms can include: identifying the main problem, discussing another event that may contribute to the induction of the problem, brain storming through occupational therapy models to cope with the problems, setting achievable goals for individual, discussing methods—techniques to cope with the problems, practicing the developed strategies, and checking up the results of problem solving. OT can use problem-solving strategies mostly for clients with HIV/AIDS, cancer, and palliative care [21].

If cancer client have some difficulties on lifestyle, fatigue, and self-esteem, OT could help them to determine their priorities of life, to use energy levels, to recognize that a client's inner feelings and values, to change behavior, and to adapt to their changed lifestyle.

3.2. Restoration activity

Clients have different activities related to their routines in their life. The focus of the restorative approach is to develop client skills and abilities or increase the activity performance and participation of the client with cancer. In this stage, grading of the activity level can be done according to the following parameters [22]:

- Physical assistance: providing physical support with relaxation and breath training to manage symptoms such as fatigue or anxiety. Thus, patients' skill to complete task may be increased. You must remember that the support does not mean that caregiver do all of the tasks instead of the client.
- Supervision and cuing: contain a number and types of cues to support client. It can be supplemented with verbal, tactile, and written material tips to help cognitive impairment of cancer-induced client activities.
- Activity demands: the activity can be changed due to the necessity of performance skills. It will be better to select an activity with appropriate level demands for clients. In activity education, the motor and cognitive demands of the activity can be increased step by step.
- Sequencing of activity: recognize and determine the client's activity priority. Clients' motivation should be supported to participate in activities. The number of steps in tasks and the total number of steps can be increased. Thus, cancer client can complete the activity easily with motivation, without symptoms.
- Type of activity: during activity education, activities can be graded from familiar to unfamiliar or from former to new. This method can help the clients to decrease cancer-related symptoms.
- Environment: the activity environment can affect participation in activities. Usually due to the treatments they receive, they are affected by the environment in which they perform activities in connection with their roles. They are often present in isolated environments

such as hospitals and homes. In order to reduce symptoms and improve the performance of the activity, awareness of the activities that they can perform in the environment they are in is extremely important in terms of occupational therapy intervention.

3.3. Compensation activity

The compensation approach focuses on using the patients' skills to achieve the highest possible stage of functioning in the activities. Despite the symptoms, OTs may teach new methods to increase performances. If the client still needs help, OTs can suggest using assistive equipment. These equipments can decrease symptoms, such as fatigue and pain of cancer, and increase participation in the activities.

3.4. Environmental modification

Environmental modifications consist of compensation, modification, and adaptation strategy. The compensation approach directly influences client functioning. However, environmental modification approach influences patients' functioning indirectly. OT could give advice to the client with cancer to redesign environments, such as home, work, and school, where the client wants to be. Modifications must be low cost and easily accessible.

4. Occupational therapy in childhood cancer

Nearly over 300,000 children develop cancer worldwide each year [23]. As many as two-thirds of children with childhood cancer are likely to experience at least one side effect, one-fourth of survivors experiencing a late effect that is severe or life threatening [24]. There are many studies showing that childhood cancer client experience many specific squeal after cancer diagnosis and treatment such as: hair loss, pain and fatigue, loss of fertility, and other changes in body image [25–27]. In children, it is important to be aware of growth and development stages in evaluation and intervention planning. Different from adults, their development can be affected in all components and more from the therapy. As children are also still dependent on caregivers, they are not fully functioning and still developing physical, social, cognitive skills, etc. Sometimes, to save life, surgeries may be harsh resulting with loss of a limb. Therefore, they may struggle to develop with that loss. The majority of the existing studies have shown that children with childhood cancer have increased anxiety, depression, and distress compared to their healthy peers and the general public [28, 29]. In a recent systematic review by Quinn et al., it is emphasized that psychological symptoms often result in impaired quality of life (QoL) [30].

Long-term treatments affect children's ability in the areas of self-care, productivity, and leisure activity. Treatments of cancer, especially treatments, cause a decrease in motor skills [31]. Gross and fine motor skills play an important role in the development of cognitive, academic, and social skills in children [32, 33]. In childhood cancer, the basic problems can be seen in social relationships, educational attainment, and school functions such as writing skills or reading skills, etc. [33]. Understanding the degree of the motor difficulty that the child faces is important for the efforts to improve their quality of life.

Assessment is needed at the beginning and end of rehabilitation to evaluate body structure and functions, activities, and participation. As all areas are affected, the level of success in terms of rehabilitation goals can be detected by systematic evaluation. **Table 2** shows the rehabilitation goals and assessment tools used by OTs in childhood cancer. It is important to recognize these rehabilitation goals while planning treatment.

Rehabilitation goals	**Evaluation instruments**
Improvement of functional disorders of the musculoskeletal system	Range of motion, muscle test
Determining of function-related treatment goals	Goal assessment scale (GAS)
Reducing post-surgical problems (scars discomfort, seroma)	Clinical observation
Reducing symptoms after radiotherapy (cystitis, proctitis)	Micturition, Chair Diary
Reducing hormone deficiency symptoms (vasomotor reactions, osteoporosis)	Visual analog scale (VAS) *Osteodensitometry must be checked
Reducing symptoms after cytostatic chemotherapy (polyneuropathy)	Common Toxicity Criteria of the National Cancer Institute (NCI-CTC), sensitivity measurement, vibration sense
Reduction of fatigue	The PedsQL™ Multidimensional Fatigue Scale (PedsQL–MFS), Visual Analog Scale-numeric (VAS), Faces Rating Scale
Reducing pain	Faces Rating Scale, Visual Analog Scale- numeric (VAS), Pain Diary South California sensory Integration Tests (AYRES), Semmes Weinstein monofilament test
Assessing sensory process	
Improving balance	The Berg Balance Test (Berg), South California sensory Integration Tests (AYRES)
Maintaining/increasing independence of daily life	Detailed activity analysis, Wee Functional Independence Measure (WeeFIM), Barthel Index (BI), Instrumental Activities of Daily Living Scale (IADL), Role Checklist (RL)
Improvement of cognitive performance	Dynamic Occupational Therapy Cognitive Assessment (DOTCA), Mini mental state examination-child
Activity Performance and Participation	Canadian Occupational Performance Measurement (COPM), Children's Assessment of Participation and Enjoyment (CAPE), Preferences for Activities of Children (PAC), The Children's Leisure Activities Study Survey (CLASS)
Coping with stress and anxiety depressive states and relaxation	Beck Depression Inventory (BDI), Beck Anxiety Inventory (BAI), Spielberger's State Trait Anxiety Inventory (STAI), and Visual Analog Scale (VAS)

Rehabilitation goals	Evaluation instruments
Increasing Gross & Fine Motor Skills	Bruininks Oseretsky Test of Motor Proficiency (BOTMP-2edition), Purdue Pegboard, Jebsen Hand Function Test, Nine Hole Peg Test
Supporting/developing Quality of Life	SF-36, Quality of Life for Cancer Survivors, Childhood Health Assessment Questionnaire (CHAQ)
Family or peer problems	Interview
Reduction of insomnia	Diary
Construction of meaning and objective perspectives	Interview
Improving of school function	The Evaluation Tool of Children's Handwriting (ETCH), Minnesota Handwriting Test, School Function Assessment (SFA)

Table 2. Rehabilitation goals and the evaluation instruments mostly used for childhood cancer.

It is always beneficial to use a framework while planning the treatment. As we prefer person- environment-occupation or Canadian Model of Occupational Therapy in children, we analyze all parameters according to the model. It is useful to train all skills by using play. Play is formed according to the skill loss of the children. OTs should be more creative while working with children. In literature, as we would like to increase motivation, do not bore and tire the child, all components can be trained with play [34]. The most preferred plays are jenga, monopoly, and dart throwing in our clinic. It is because children have joy while playing and these plays can be used to increase proximal stabilization, gross and fine motor skills, sensory skills, cognitive skills, social skills, and bilateral integration.

In motor training it is important to be aware of fine motor skills. Hand strengthening with putty, speed improvement with competitive plays, and endurance training by increasing the time in activities are examples of mostly used trainings. Of course, children should develop in gross motor skills as they participate in school and sports activities. Jumping and climbing are important skills that children should improve. In hospital setting, however, it is harder to train gross motor skills, and via activity, we may train gross and posture muscles.

In sensory training both hyper- or hyposensitivity should be trained. Desensitization or sensory reeducation should be done with materials children are familiar with. If a child has severe problem, caregiver should be well educated to prevent injuries like burn, cut, etc. Motor training can be combined with sensory training. For example, while training grasping, materials can be covered with different materials and the child can be asked to differentiate the feature.

In cognitive training attention is an important component. In development stage, attention is needed for children to be successful in all areas of daily living but especially in school functioning. For example, attention should be handled in terms of selective attention, shifting attention, and divided attention. These attention parameters can be added while skills training via meaningful activity, e.g., singing song while playing jenga. Processing speed, short-long term memory, and sequencing ability should also be trained. Memory cards, history telling, making animation, and memory training by watching cartoon and asking questions can be examples. However, every impairment should be recognized and trained well in a structural planning.

It is important for the children to gain problem-solving skills, confidence, self-esteem, etc. Therefore, children should take responsibility in treatment; parents also should let the child to participate in activities. Some brainstorming home works are useful for both child and family education. ADL training is needed, and we should be aware of the sociocultural form of the family. If the child had never learned the skill, we may teach the parameters of the activity [35]. Children should develop social skills. We may form a social environment for the child and let him/her participate in group activities. Children always develop more by playing with their peers like communication, language, etc. Environment also should be assessed and needed adaptations should be provided.

In addition, OTs should be more creative in therapy applications. They should use creativity-containing methods such as art, music, and dance therapy to increase activity performance and participation in children with cancer [36].

5. Occupational therapy in adult cancer

There are a total of 14.1 million cancer cases that result in 8.2 million deaths according to the global cancer statistics [37]. Survivors of cancers may have physical, social, cognitive, and emotional problems. For example, in breast cancer which is the most common type of woman, they might experience chronic lymphedema, sexual dysfunction, and cognitive impairment [38, 39]. As well as client with prostate cancer may experience urinary incontinence, peripheral neuropathy, weakness of muscle, sexual problems, and fatigue [22]. Among cancer survivors, psychosocial problems are prevalent and may include economic difficulties related to repetition and fear of death, anxiety and depression, feelings of alienation or isolation, job loss, and discrimination in employment [40]. Because of these reasons, researchers focus on quality of life issues after cancer treatment [41]. The common rehabilitation goals and a couple of examples of instrument for assessing the achievement of this goal are shown in **Table 3**.

According to ICF parameters, **Table 3** shows some examples of the rehabilitation goals and the evaluation instruments which are mostly used by OT for cancer client in adults. Clients with cancer need sensory-motor-cognitive training, breathing and relaxation training, fatigue and pain management, and vocational rehabilitation to support independent, healthy life. It is also important to promote occupational balance and appropriate planning of daily routine in adults. Different than children, adults may have more problems in gaining motivation; they are mostly very pessimistic and sometimes it is hard to initiate the rehabilitation program. Therefore, therapist should use therapeutic skills for communicating well.

In sensory training, it is good to support body image, body awareness, and deep sense. Mindfulness, body awareness training, proprioceptive-kinesthetic training can be added to rehabilitation program. Sensory education should be given for both upper and lower extremity. Many clients have problems in perception of foot sole. Sensory input should be given

Rehabilitation goals	Evaluation instruments
Increasing of physical performance	WHO Activity Index, Karnofsky Performance Score, Harvard Step Test, Ergometry, Muscle Strength Measurement (Vigorimeter, Digimax Muscle Testing), Functional Assessment of Cancer Therapy (G: General, F: Fatigue, P: Prostate-FACT)
Reducing post-surgical problems (scars discomfort, seroma)	Clinical observation, Visual Analog Scale (VAS)
Reducing hormone deficiency symptoms (vasomotor reactions, osteoporosis)	Clinical observation, Visual Analog Scale (VAS)
Reducing sensory symptoms after treatments	Sensitivity Measurement, Vibration Sense, Semmes-Weinstein monofilament
Reduction of fatigue	Multidimensional fatigue Inventory (MFI), Cancer Fatigue Scale (CFS), Piper Fatigue Scale (PFS), Functional Assessment of Cancer Therapy, Fatigue (FACT-F), Visual Analog Scale (VAS), EORTC-QLQ-C30, Fatigue Module
Reducing pain	Visual Analog Scale (VAS), Pain Diary
Reduction of lymphedema	Clinical observation, rating scale
Improvement in urinary incontinence	Biofeedback, diary
Dealing with sexual dysfunction, improvement of erectile dysfunction	Diary, International Index of Erectile Function (IIEF)
Improvement of functional disorders of the musculoskeletal system	Range of motion Muscle strength test
Maintaining/increasing independence of daily life	Detailed activity analysis, Functional Independence Measure (FIM), Barthel Index (BI), Instrumental Activities of Daily Living Scale (IADL), Role Checklist (RL)
Increasing motivation and interest in activities	OQ (Occupational Questionnaire), Interest Checklist and Activity Checklist (ICAC)
Improvement of cognitive performance	d2-test (Attention stress test), Benton test (visual memory-BT), Multiple Choice Vocabulary Intelligence Test (MWT-B), Loewenstein Occupational Therapy Cognitive Assessment (LOTCA), Mini mental state examination
Promoting disease management, improving self-awareness and self-acceptance, emotional stabilization	EORTC, SF-36, Functional Assessment of Cancer Therapy (G: General, F: Fatigue FACT)
Coping with stress and anxiety depressive states and relaxation	"Stress thermometer," Hospital Anxiety and Depression Scale (HADS-D), Beck Depression Inventory (BDI), Beck Anxiety Inventory (BAI), Visual Analog Scale (VAS)
Reduction of Progression Improving of Hand Function	Fear of Progression Questionnaire Purdue pegboard, Jebsen Hand Function Test
Improving of Quality of Life	QLQ-C30, cancer-related modules
Breakdown of family and partnership problems	Interview, Couples climate scales
Enabling reintegration, initiating professional promotions	CIO Community Integration Questionnaire, ISSI (Interview Schedule For Social Interaction)

Rehabilitation goals	Evaluation instruments
Obtaining participation in life, increasing activity performance	Reintegration to Normal Living Index, Instrumental Activities of Daily Living Scale (IADL), Canadian Occupational Performance Measurement (COPM)
Reduction of risk behavior (smoking alcohol abuse, overwork)	Life Habits Assessment (LIFE-H), Questionnaires
Providing vocational rehabilitation	Worker Role Interview, Valpar Component Work Samples (VCWS)

Table 3. Rehabilitation goals and the evaluation instruments mostly used for adults cancer.

form planter surface of the foot. Education in upper extremity should be given in a functional manner. Materials and exercises should be selected according to the meaningful activities.

In motor training, according to the areas of weaknesses, muscle strength gain should be aimed. Clients mostly have problems in endurance and control. In hospital setting, activity training should be planned in this manner. For example, for the clients who do not wanted to participate to therapy and can only sit in bed for 5 minutes, we decided to use dart throwing exercise. We asked him to sit in a wheelchair and stand up and throw the dart. First day, he did only one throw; however, second day he stood up three times, and at the end of the week he started walking and participated to the therapy. We should always support antigravity muscles by activities. Endurance and fatigue management should be our priority, afterwards we can aim speed.

Cognitive training will differ according to the effect among cancer clients. However, mostly, programs may include memory, attention, orientation, and executive function. If the client is elderly, cognitive problems may be more visible as with ageing cognitive abilities are decreasing. In working adults, executive functioning gains importance for working skills. It is advisable to start cognitive training as quick as possible because its effect on symptom and fatigue control has been shown.

Breathing and relaxation training consist of learning breathing technique, body/mind relaxation technique, somatic experience technique, and relaxation exercises [21, 22]. The common goal of these techniques is to ensure that people are both physically and cognitively less likely to feel stressed and more comfortable to maintain and participate in their activities.

Fatigue and pain management are most important in rehabilitation. Because nearly every client struggles with fatigue and pain, and these symptoms affect treatment success. Management of these symptoms will closely influence the performance and participation of activities of individuals in their daily lives. OTs should give priority to teach the client to state, sequence, and divide the activity for them to enable to cope with these symptoms. Energy conservation techniques and activity planning should become a part of their lifestyle, so that they can keep their energy for longer or use it more appropriately. In addition, planning sleep routines and daily routines is an intervention that OTs should not forget in adult cancer clients [21].

Leisure activities can also be suggested to these clients. As we aim occupational balance, this area of occupational performance should not be forgotten. Gardening, doing hand crafts, painting, yoga, dance, and pilates are mostly preferred activities. As these activities give joy to clients, some chemicals like serotonin can be released and immune system can be supported. Therefore, we may say that these activities can also have a healing effect.

Adult client may whether continue with their old job or are ready to return to work or whether they will be able to get a new job or not. Thus, vocational rehabilitation may be needed in treatment plan. OTs can make suggestions on improving the physical, psychological, and cognitive skills of the worker about the work, and give suggestions about designing the working activity or modify the work environment. In conclusion, occupational therapy should carry out a holistic approach including improv-ing endurance and muscle strength, preserving energy for daily living activities, decreasing stress, improving activity performances, and participation in adults' cancer [22, 42].

6. Rehabilitation in palliative care and hospice care

The role of occupational therapist in palliative care and hospice care is quite similar and important. In these care services, occupational therapists support mostly the secondary symptoms related to cancer client, cancer types, and treatments. End-of-life care of children and adults can include the management of physical, emotional, social or cognitive symptoms, limitations of performance, meaningful roles and activities, family, and social support. They analyze the current activity preferences and the personal and environmental resources to increase client participation. Hospice care generally has been little experienced with children, while it is mostly used as an approach to care during the last stages of life in adults [24]. The main aim of OTs is to improve the quality of life according to the values of the client and to maximize lasting functional skills [43].

7. Conclusion

OT clinical trial evaluation and interventions focus on functioning and participation by improving the abilities of cancer clients. The care of cancer client prolongs from the start of treatment to the end of the client life. They provide evidence-based interventions in inpatient care, outpatient care, education, and home care and in hospital care settings. Cancer clients may usually need support for ADL, using breathing and relaxation training, lifestyle redesigning and fatigue management, self-esteem, motor skills, cognitive therapy, vocational rehabilitation, and client and caregiver education. The OTs mainly focuses on these subjects and activity and participation restrictions in the rehabilitation community.

Author details

Sedef Şahin*, Semin Akel and Meral Zarif

*Address all correspondence to: sedefkarayazgan88@hotmail.com

Faculty of Health Sciences, Occupational Therapy Department, Hacettepe University, Ankara, Turkey

References

[1] Makar AP, Tropé CG, Tummers P, Denys H, Vandecasteele K. Advanced ovarian cancer: Primary or interval debulking? Five categories of client in view of the results of randomized trials and tumor biology: Primary debulking surgery and interval debulking surgery for advanced ovarian cancer. The Oncologist. 2016;**21**(6):745-754

[2] Jemal A, Bray F, Center MM, Ferlay J, Ward E, Forman D. Global cancer statistics. CA Cancer Journal for Clinicians. 2011;**61**:69-90. DOI: 10.3322/caac.20107

[3] Siegel RL, Miller KD, Jemal A. Cancer statistics, 2016. CA: A Cancer Journal for Clinicians. 2016;**66**(1):7-30

[4] Ward E, DeSantis C, Robbins A, Kohler B, Jemal A. Childhood and adolescent cancer statistics, 2014. CA Cancer Journal for Clinicians. 2014;**64**(2):83-103

[5] Keegan TH, Ries LA, Barr RD, et al. Comparison of cancer survival trends in the United States of adolescents and young adults with those in children and older adults. Cancer. 2016;**122**(7):1009-1016

[6] Phillips SM, Padgett LS, Leisenring WM, et al. Survivors of childhood cancer in the United States: Prevalence and burden of morbidity. Cancer Epidemiology, Biomarkers & Prevention. 2015;**24**(4):653-663

[7] Heidenreich A, Bastian PJ, Bellmunt J, Bolla M, Joniau S, Kwast TV. EAU guidelines on prostate cancer. Part 1: Screening, diagnosis, and treatment of clinically localised disease. European Urology. 2011;**59**:61-71. DOI: 10.1016/j.eururo.2013.09.046

[8] Rietman JS, Dijkstra PU, Hoekstra HJ, Eisma WH, Szabo BG, Groothoff JW, Geertzen JHB. Late morbidity after treatment of breast cancer in relation to daily activities and quality of life: A systematic review. European Journal of Surgical Oncology (EJSO). 2003;**29**(3):229-238

[9] Chasen MR. Cancer nutrition and rehabilitation–its time has come! Current Oncology. 2008;**15**(3):2-7

[10] Taylor K, Currow D. A prospective study of client identified unmet activity of daily living needs among cancer client at a comprehensive cancer care centre. Australian Occupational Therapy Journal. 2003;**50**:79-85

[11] Occupational Therapy Australia. Position Paper: Occupational Therapy in Palliative Care. 2015. Available from: http://www.otaus.com.au/sitebuilder/advocacy/knowledge/asset/files/21/positionpaper-occupationaltherapyinpalliativecare%5Baugust2015%5D-occupationaltherapyaustralia.pdf [Accessed: February].

[12] Fialka-Moser V, Crevenna R, Korpan M, Quittan M. Cancer rehabilitation. Particularly with aspects on physical impairments. Journal of Rehabilitation Medicine. 2003;**35**:153-162

[13] Chasen MR, Jacobsen PB. Chapter 37. Rehabilitation in cancer. In: Olver Ian N., editor. TheMASCC Textbook of Cancer Supportive Care and Survivorship. USA: Springer; 2011;pp. 389-396

[14] Dalton SO, Johansen C. New paradigms in planning cancer rehabilitation and survivorship. Acta Oncologica. 2013;**52**(2):191-194. DOI: 10.3109/0284186X.2012.748216

[15] Egan MY, McEwen S, Sikora L, Chasen M, Fitch M, Eldred S. Rehabilitation following cancer treatment. Disability and Rehabilitation. 2013;**35**(26):2245-2258. DOI: 10.3109/09638288.2013.774441

[16] Weis J, Giesler JM. Rehabilitation for cancer client. In: Goerling U, editor. Psycho-Oncology. Berlin, Heidelberg: Springer; 2014. pp. 87-101

[17] Holm LV, Hansen DG, Kragstrup J, Johansen C, dePont Christensen R, Vedsted P. Influence of comorbidity on cancer patients' rehabilitation needs, participation in rehabilitation activities and unmet needs: A population-based cohort study. Supportive Care in Cancer. 2014;**22**(8):2095-2105

[18] Dietz JJ. Adaptive rehabilitation in cancer. Postgraduate Medical Journal. 1980;**68**:145-153

[19] Lehmann C, Beierlein V, Hagen-Aukamp C, Kerschgens C, Rhee M, Frühauf S. Psychosocial predictors of utilization of medical rehabilitation services among prostate cancer client. Die Rehabilitation Journal. 2012;**51**(3):160-170. DOI: 10.4414/smw.2015.14214

[20] ICF Research Braunch. Available from: https://www.icf-research-branch.org/images/ICF%20Core%20Sets%20.Download/Brief_ICF_Core_Set_for_Head_and_Neck_Cancer.pdf] (Accessed: February)

[21] Cooper J. Occupational therapy in oncology and palliative care. In: Cooper J, editor. Occupational Therapy Approach in Symptom Control. USA: John Wiley Sons; 2006. pp. 27-40.

[22] Huri M, Akel BS, Şahin S. Rehabilitation of client with prostate cancer. Prostate. 2016;**6**:8

[23] Burstein HJ, Krilov L, Aragon-Ching JB, Baxter NN, Chiorean EG, Chow WA, Epstein AS. Clinical cancer advances 2017: Annual report on progress against cancer from the American Society of Clinical Oncology. Journal of Clinical Oncology. 2017; 35 (12):1341-1367.

[24] Ward E, DeSantis C, Robbins A, Kohler B, Jemal A. Childhood and adolescent cancer statistics, 2014. CA: a cancer journal for clinicians. 2014; 64(2), 83-103.

[25] Leuteritz K, Friedrich M, Nowe E, Sender A, Stöbel-Richter Y, Geue K. Life situation and psychosocial care of adolescent and young adult (AYA) cancer client–study protocol of a 12-month prospective longitudinal study. BMC Cancer. 2017;**17**(1):82

[26] Zebrack BJ, Casillas J, Nohr L, Adams H, Zeltzer LK. Fertility issues for young adult survivors of childhood cancer. Psycho-Oncology. 2004;**13**(10):689-699

[27] Geue K, Sender A, Schmidt R, Richter D, Hinz A, Schulte T, Stöbel-Richter Y. Gender-specific quality of life after cancer in young adulthood: A comparison with the general population. Quality of Life Research. 2014;**23**(4):1377-1386

[28] Dyson GJ, Thompson K, Palmer S, Thomas DM, Schofield P. The relationship between unmet needs and distress amongst young people with cancer. Supportive Care in Cancer. 2012;**20**(1):75-85

[29] Larsson G, Mattsson E, Von Essen L. Aspects of quality of life, anxiety, and depression among persons diagnosed with cancer during adolescence: A long-term follow-up study. European Journal of Cancer. 2010;**46**(6):1062-1068

[30] Quinn GP, Gonçalves V, Sehovic I, Bowman ML, Reed DR. Quality of life in adolescent and young adult cancer client: a systematic review of the literature. Client Related Outcome Measures. 2015;**6**:19

[31] Wright MJ, Halton JM, Martin RF, Barr RD. Long-term gross motor performance following treatment for acute lymphoblastic leukemia. Pediatric Blood & Cancer. 1998;**31** (2):86-90

[32] Davis EE, Pitchford NJ, Limback E. The interrelation between cognitive and motor development in typically developing children aged 4-11 years is underpinned by visual processing and fine manual control. British Journal of Psychology. 2011;**102**(3):569-584

[33] De Luca CR, McCarthy M, Galvin J, Green JL, Murphy A, Knight S, Williams J. Gross and fine motor skills in children treated for acute lymphoblastic leukaemia. Developmental Neurorehabilitation. 2013;**16**(3):180-187

[34] Schover LR. Article motivation for parenthood after cancer: A review. Journal of the National Cancer Institute Monographs. 2005; 34: 1-5.

[35] Compas BE, Connor-Smith JK, Saltzman H, Thomsen AH, Wadsworth ME. Coping with stress during childhood and adolescence: Problems, progress, and potential in theory and research. Psychological Bulletin. 2001;**127**(1):87

[36] Favara-Scacco C, Smirne G, Schilirò G, Di Cataldo A. Art therapy as support for children with leukemia during painful procedures. Pediatric Blood & Cancer. 2001;**36**(4):474-480

[37] Patel V, Wang Z, Chen Q, Rusling JF, Molinolo AA, Gutkind JS. Emerging cancer bio-markers for HNSCC detection and therapeutic intervention. In: Kuriakose, Moni Abraham, editor. Contemporary Oral Oncology. USA: Springer International Publishing. 2017;pp. 281-308

[38] Ahles TA, Saykin AJ, Furstenberg CT, et al. Neuropsychologic impact of standard-dose systemic chemotherapy in long-term survivors of breast cancer and lymphoma. Journal of Clinical Oncology. 2002;**20**:485-493

[39] Boquiren VM, Esplen MJ, Wong J, Toner B, Warner E, Malik N. Sexual functioning in breast cancer survivors experiencing body image disturbance. Psycho-Oncology. 2016;**25** (1):66-76

[40] Hewitt M, Rowland JH, Yancik R. Cancer survivors in the United States: Age, health, and disability. The Journals of Gerontology Series A: Biological Sciences and Medical Sciences. 2003;**58**(1):M82-M91

[41] Huri M, Huri E, Kayihan H, Altuntas O. Effects of occupational therapy on quality of life of client with metastatic prostate cancer: A randomized controlled study. Saudi Medical Journal. 2015;**36**(38):954-961. DOI: 10.15537/smj.2015.8.11461

[42] Pekçetin S, Bumin G, Güngör T, Tunç S. Kemoterapi Alan Jinekolojik Kanserli Hastalarda Algılanan Aktivite Performansının Toplumsal Katılım ve Yaşam Kalitesi Üzerine Etkisi. Ergoterapi ve Rehabilitasyon Dergisi. 2013;**1**(2):31-41

[43] Prochnau C, Liu L, Boman J. Personal–professional connections in palliative care occupational therapy. American Journal of Occupational Therapy. 2003;**57**(2):196-204

6

Community Participation in People with Disabilities

Gokcen Akyurek and Gonca Bumin

Abstract

Despite the fact that participation is an important building and a valuable target, the conceptualization, identification and measurement methods vary widely. This chapter tried to gain an insider's perspective from the obstacles that summarize what meaning participation means, how to characterize it, and what prevents and supports participation. Participation is seen as a right and a responsibility attributed to and attributed to both the person and the community. Participation does not take place in a vacuum; the environment dynamically influences participation. The effects of this conceptual framework are discussed for change at the level of evaluation, research and systems to support the participation of the people with disability.

Keywords: participation, disability, occupation, function and quality of life

1. Introduction

Being disabled is defined as being out of "normal" as a biological sense, while in social sense, it is defined as the social and cultural obstruction of the individual's ability to live independently and easily in society [1]. Therefore, appropriate sociocultural environment is essential to enable disabled people to develop their skills and gain a place in social life. For example, the parent of person of a disability does not have an interest in him because he does not trust him or herself and shows an extreme protectionist attitude [2].

In order to enable individuals with disabilities to find jobs, marry, spend their leisure time, and continue their education and vocational training in the society they live in, relations with various social institutions, social status gains and integration with society are important factors [3]. Community participation activities are those that relate to organizing behaviors that arise during interaction with others in a particular social system: family, peers, or friends [4, 5].

The quality of life, which is defined as the way people perceive health as a result of the constraints of social and professional life, is also negatively affected [6–8]. In addition, the limitation of daily life activities due to functional disabilities also affects the community participation negatively [9]. It should not be forgotten that the physical, psychosocial and economic level of the people with disabilities affects the quality of life and there is a relationship in which the degree of dependence of the person is inversely related to the quality of life [10] (**Picture 1**).

Adolph Mayer, the author of occupational therapy "People organize themselves to participate in activities throughout their lifetime and use their time" [11]. Participation from the perspective of occupational therapy is to be a part of everyday life. Participation is the main goal of occupational therapy. The World Health Organization (WHO) also focuses on participation as an important goal for all the people. The World Health Organization has defined areas of participation as knowledge learning and practice, general tasks and desires, communication, movement, self-care, interpersonal interaction, home and work habits, community life, social life and citizenship [12].

The nature, quality and/or duration of participation are personality and, even if it has the same health status, two different people cannot be compared at all. Participation examines the situation in the social environment rather than activity. The main problem of participation is the limitations bring to life of certain health problems and environment [13]. Community participation is sufficient for the individual to participate in the activities in his/her field. There are those who say that social skills are participation of everyday life, but according to the experts, social participation is more complicated than communication [14].

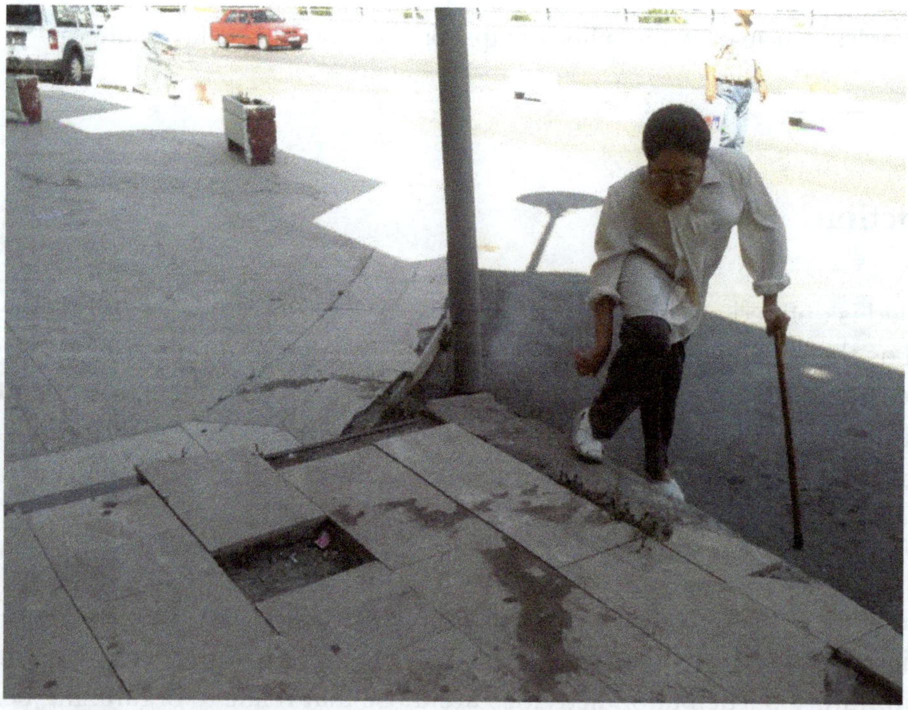

Picture 1. Health and well-being negatively affected of the inappropriate environment.

2. Philosophy of occupational therapy and community participation

The philosophy of a profession is based on three components; first, the metaphysical component "What is human nature?" deals with the question. Second, etymology component "nature of human science, the starting point and the boundaries of" dealing with "How do we know everything?, How do we know what we know?" search for answers to their questions. Third, value teaching component, two types of questions One is "what is beautiful or valuable" which is related to esthetics, and the other is "what are the standards or rules of correct behavior" related to ethics? [15].

Occupational therapy is a scientific discipline that uses purposeful and meaningful activities therapeutically. Activity is the essence of being good. Meaningful activity is used to develop the capacity for internal motivation. Human life is in a continuous adaptation process. Adaptation is the change in the functions and directs the person to survive and develop. Biological, psychological, and environmental factors can disrupt adaptation in the life cycle. Decrease in function occurs when adaptation is impaired. Meaningful activity helps the adaptive process to regenerate [16].

The main goal of occupational therapy is to ensure that people participate in daily life activities and improves their performance. Occupational therapy provides a client-centered approach to health and well-being. At the same time, occupational therapy focuses on increasing the competence of people by organizing people, activities, the environment or some or all of them in order to increase social participation [16].

The handling of occupational therapy in all directions of humankind is called *holistic approach*. Holistic approach emphasizes the organic and functional relationship between whole and parts. This approach assumes the person as a whole as biological, psychological, sociocultural and spiritual [17].

Occupational therapy sees man as an active being. Man can determine and control his own behavior and even change it at will. Moreover, there is constant interaction between the human and environment. To survive, everyone has to do certain activities for himself or someone else, such as feeding himself or someone else [18].

According to occupational therapy, every person has the ability to be adaptive. Adaptation is the change in function for survival and self-renewal [11]. Occupational therapy also increases activity adaptation [19]. When Gail Fidler and Jay Fidler describe adequacy, they say that "adapting, the ability to cope with problems in daily life and fulfill roles depends on the richness of one's relationships with both people and the environment" [20]. Adaptation depends on the person. The role of the occupational therapist in this process is to regulate the environment in order to facilitate the emergence of a specific adaptive response [21].

Occupational therapy aims to increase the quality of life of people whose functional ability is limited or impaired. To this end, it helps to improve performance independence in any area of the person: Strengthening the person's body for the necessary roles, improving the coordination for activities, improving the hobbies to make the person happy, or improving the social skills of the person to increase their participation in these aims. Thus, the meaning and value of the activity and the quality of life will increase [17].

Occupational therapy is based on the philosophy of humanism, which sees the applicants as human rather than as an object. The humanistic point of view is the basic approach of this profession. Today, this approach is called person-centered approach. The therapist understands the importance of the person, family, and other individuals in his/her life in the treatment approach. The person has an active role both in the treatment modalities and in defining the goals and preferences for the treatment [17].

3. International classification of functioning, disability and health-ICF and community participation

International classification of functioning, disability and health (ICF) is a system that forms a standard language for defining health and health-related situations for the measurement, classification and conceptualization of disability and functioning [13].

In the past, the disability began at the place where the health had ended and anyone with any kind of heart was seen as second class. This way of thinking has evolved to support and improve the collective participation of the person with a disability who changes over time. ICF is a measure of the functioning of the individual in society, regardless of the cause of the disorder [22].

In the ICF classification, factors affecting the health status of a person are stated to be body functions and structures, activity, participation and environment. The consequences of these factors are functional and structural disorders, activity and participation limitations [23].

ICF reveals body function and structure, activity, participation, and personal and environmental factors. The content of occupational therapy is performance components, activity performance, participation and environmental factors [24].

ICF can be used for evaluation, intervention, and in service. The occupational therapist examines body functions and structures so performance components, to evaluate the primary target according to the individual. It interferes with functional impairment by focusing on the occupational performance. If malfunctions are encountered, it affects the person's participation and quality of life. Therapists should be familiar with these principles and should use them when planning services [24].

The language and content of ICF and Occupational therapy Frame of Reference are very similar. The frame is based on the ICF. This is particularly evident when the classification system in the ICF and the classification of the body functions in the frame are compared. The relationship between the activity areas of the frame and the activity participation areas of the ICF is indirect but overlaps with each other. Moreover, the ICF includes activities and areas of participation that can be compared to the performance capabilities listed in the frame. Most of the performance abilities in the frame have parallel codes in ICF [25].

The mobility field in the ICF is parallel to the motor skills. The communication/interaction skills and social interaction skills in the frame and the communication, interpersonal interaction and relationships in the ICF are parallel. Finally, the activity and performance areas of the framework and the ICF's activities and areas of participation are similar [25].

4. Occupational therapy models for evaluation of participation

Models provide people with a sense of how they choose their activities and their experiences with them. It also specifies the problems of the people's activities and the rational solutions that can be brought to them [26].

- Occupational therapy' applications lead the occupational therapists to ask the following questions:

1. How can the physical and cognitive disorders of people's daily activities be minimized?
2. How can people's despair and sensitivity be understood when they are accustomed to their lives and lose the capacities they need? And how to get more control over their lives? [12].

- Purpose and structure of models;

A model involves a dynamic knowledge development process. A model is a way of thinking about applications, always reviewing and developing them [26].

4.1. Model of human occupation (MOHO)

This model was developed from Reilly's activity behavior model. This model focuses on function and activity. It guides in restructuring the activity, because this model focuses on person's roles and habits and determines the person's perspective and will. Person is seen as a dynamic system influenced by the physical and social environment. This model provides information on the occupational therapist's performance capacity [12].

Main elements of this model;

- The roles and habits of the person (habituation)
- Volition for activities and tasks (volition)
- Performance and environmental (performance capacity) (**Figure 1**)

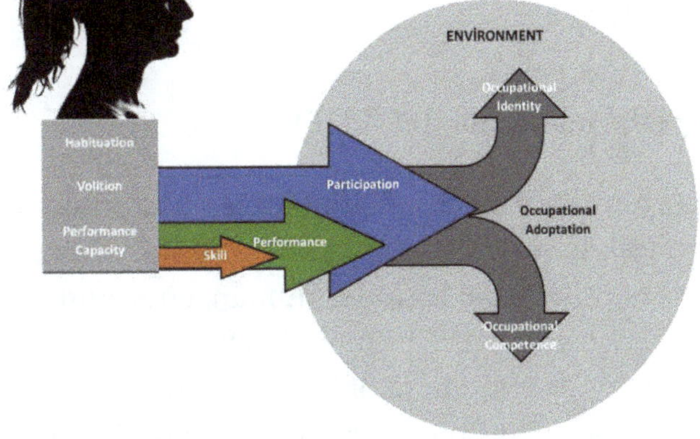

Figure 1. Model of human occupation scheme.

Habituation: Habits arise when organizing behavior in repetitive patterns keeps pace with the social world. Repeated movements in special cases constitute a habit pattern. The habit pattern grows with time and strengthens the organization and communication habits of the person with daily, weekly and seasonal routines [27]. Every person has one or more roles, and they have to do with those roles. Sometimes a person is a worker, sometimes a parent. This role guides other people's anticipations and how the natural person of the social system should behave. The roles are shaped by behavior. The person can reflect on their role activities, movements or clothing style [30–32].

Volition: The volition of the person for activities and duties depends the activity of the person, the importance of the activity for the person, and the satisfaction from this activity. Motivation is shaped by one's previous experiences and is closely linked to the future. It also influences motivation, causes, values and interest [27].

1. Personal reasons reflect the importance of the activity to the person and the capacity of the person. The person uses capacity in relation to cultural observations and demands of the environment. Because people think about doing the activity when they are confident in their physical, social and mental abilities. Some people are talented in sports, music, while others are successful in human relationships. After all, people shape their activities using their environment and capacities [27].

2. The choice of activity is also influenced by the values. Values consist of beliefs and concepts of well right importance as defined by society [29] and are felt by the individual as necessity. This obligation turns into a sense of belonging and social righteousness for the person when he or she acts according to the value of the person [27].

3. Activity brings together the fulfillment and satisfaction of interest [30]. Each individual has different interests, depending on the opportunities for dealing with the activity and the mood [27].

Performance capacity: It is influenced by body systems (such as musculoskeletal system, cardio-pulmonary system, neurological system), mental and cognitive abilities (such as memory and planning abilities) [27].

MOHO also emphasizes how to use the body to maintain daily performance and how to benefit from body experiences [27].

4.2. Ecology of human performance model (EHP)

The ecology of human performance model assumes that environmental factors and/or natural phenomena such as physical, temporal, social and cultural influence the performance of the person [33]. The structure of this model includes human, environment and performance variables and the interaction between them. This model defines the person as a three-dimensional model we have observed in his environment of him. The client-cantered approach defines the activities and tasks of the person. This model helps the therapist to develop special strategies for overcome the barriers that limit the performance of the person.

The main elements of this model are as follows:

- Activities and tasks of the person in the living environment
- Understanding the social, cultural and physical environment and its impact on the performance of the patient [28].

This model has expanded the range of interventions by addressing the environment. This model offers five intervention approaches: restoration, adaptation, replacement, prevention, and creation. Restoration intervention indicates changing the skills and abilities of the person. Adaptation and change are for the conditions and tasks. Prevention and creation strategies can focus on person, circumstances or relative but must be used before the problem arises. These forms of intervention remove the therapist from focusing solely on the individual and reveal a wide range of situations in which the environment can affect participation [4] (**Picture 2**).

The difference between other models and EHP is the use of terminology. In this model, authors preferred to use the term "task" rather than activity. The first reason is to work and collaborate with other disciplines. Second, the task word is more common on the day-to-day basis. In this model, there are three main structures: person, task and environment [28].

The *person* is in a dynamic and specific environment. So it is not possible to understand a person without knowing the environment of the person. The person affects the environment, and the environment also affects the person. The activity performance of the person determines the interaction between the person and the environment, environmental stimuli and the obstacles in the environment [28].

In the EHP model, the *task* is a series of behaviors. When tasks are combined, the person participates in the activity they want to achieve. The task is to determine the specific behavior required for successful participation. The person's skill, ability and interest will be combined with the characteristics of the participation and conditions to determine which task to use [34].

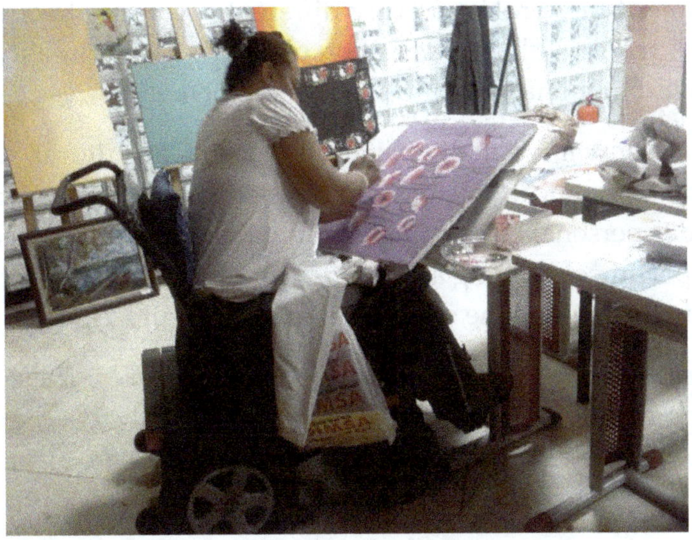

Picture 2. A leisure activity of a woman in adaptive environment.

There are two aspects of the environment in terms of time and environment. The temporal orientation is due to social and cultural connections. It is chronological. And it is maintained at every stage of development, affected by the phases of life and disability. The environmental aspect influences the performance of the physical environment (accessibility to unmanned environmental conditions), the social environment (the individual's accessibility to meaningful expectations), and the cultural environment (dressing, life patterns, beliefs, behavioral standards). As a result, the ecology model provides a way for the individual to understand their natural affairs, activity performance and environment. Finally, according to this model, the performance of a person depends on the person (ability, skill and motivation) and the environment (support and obstacle) [34].

4.3. Person-environment-occupation (PEO)

This model assesses the person, environment, activity, and interaction with each other. This is one's own daily life. Developers of this model have indicated that activity performance cannot be separated from environmental influences, temporal factors, physical and psychological characteristics of a person. They also define that in this model, environments, tasks, activities, and roles change constantly. They clearly stated the importance of focusing on the client's goals and creating a partnership that would help him/her to give his rehabilitation responsibility to the patient [12].

The main elements of this model are;

- Choosing the person's choices and goals for the activity
- Physical and psychological characteristics of the person
- Social, cultural, physical and institutional environmental factors affecting performance
- Time orientation and stages of life [12].

In this model, *human* beings are considered as part of every role and change. The importance, duration and meaning of these roles are very different according to environment and time. The human mind is a whole with a composition of body and spirituality. Human's qualities are physical, cognitive, emotional, and life experiences [29].

In this model, the *environment* is equally balanced in terms of cultural, social, physical, institutional, political and economical. It is the environment where environmental behaviors are practiced and provides personal information about what to do with expectations. These components may be supporting or limiting activity performance. With this model, it is also important how the individual perceives the environment [29] (**Figure 2**).

Activity encompasses all self-care, producers and leisure activities. These represent the activities that one is engaged in for life [29]. When the activity is analyzed, the characteristics of the tasks, the duration of the activity, the complexity, and the need are examined [34].

Activity performance occurs at the intersection of these three conglomerates and is dynamic, and the performance experience varies according to the variation of these three components.

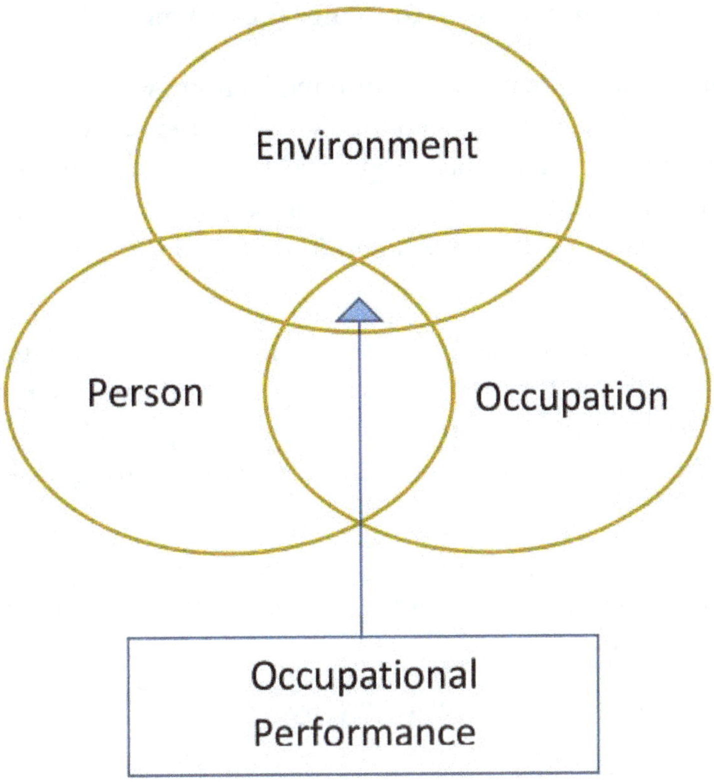

Figure 2. Person-environment-occupation scheme.

The change of these three components in the PEO model over time determines the area of activity performance. If the closeness of these components is appropriate, the performance of the activity is optimal. Therefore, the basis of occupational therapy intervention is the adjustment of the activity performance of the changes in these components [29] (**Figure 3**).

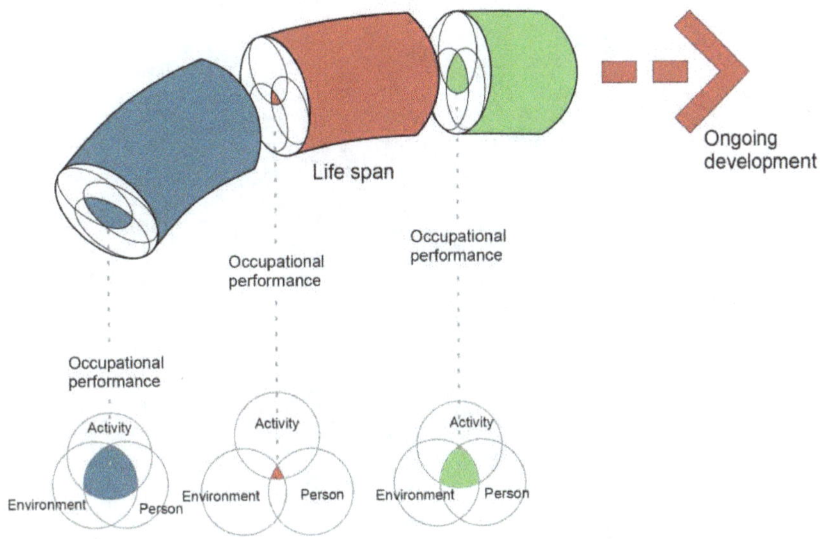

Figure 3. Development of person-environment-occupation in life span.

4.4. Person-environment-occupation-performance (PEOP) model

The person-environment-occupation-performance model acknowledges that the activity performance of a person cannot be separated from the client-centered and environmental effects. This model uses internal factors (psychological, cognitive, physiological, and neurobehavioral) and environmental factors (physical, cultural, social, social policies, and attitudes) to perform important activities, roles and tasks for the person and to understand the capacity of the person [12] (**Figure 4**, **Picture 3**).

In addition, one's own image, abilities, self-understanding and motivation are assessed in a dynamic partnership with the therapist [perhaps family and cat, others involved in his/her life]. This approach requires the therapist to determine the person's roles, duties and activities. This model predicts intervention by meaningful activities during health or recovery [12].

The main elements of this model are as follows:

- Activities, tasks and roles are important for people, organization and society. His image is his activity.
- Inner factors supporting performance are psychological, cognitive, physiological and neurobehavioral factors.
- External factors that support or hinder the occupational performance are the physical, cultural, social environment, social policies and attitudes [12].

4.5. Canadian model of occupational performance (CMOP)

It is known as the model that sets the basis of client-centered treatment. This model defines the relationship between person, person's environment and occupation, and intervention. Spiritually, the innate essence of man is the center of this model [12].

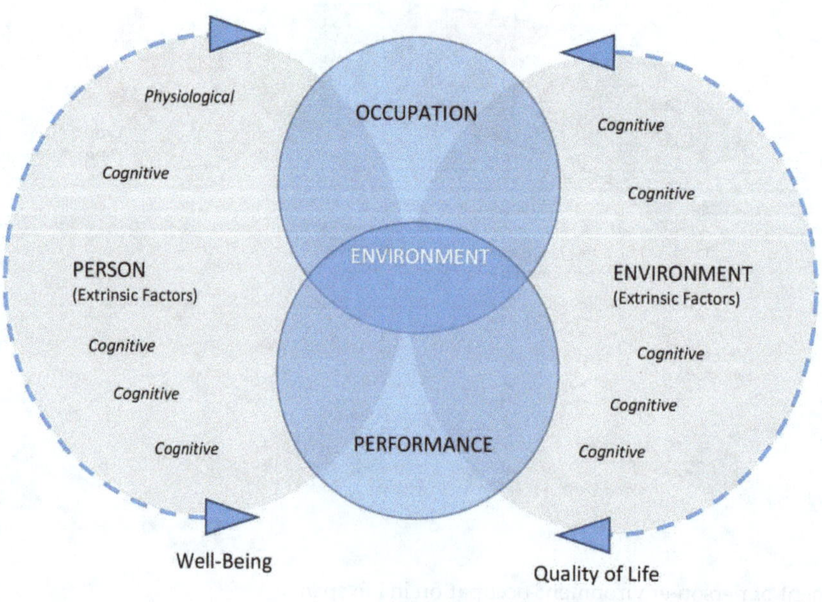

Figure 4. Person-environment-occupation-performance (PEOP) model scheme.

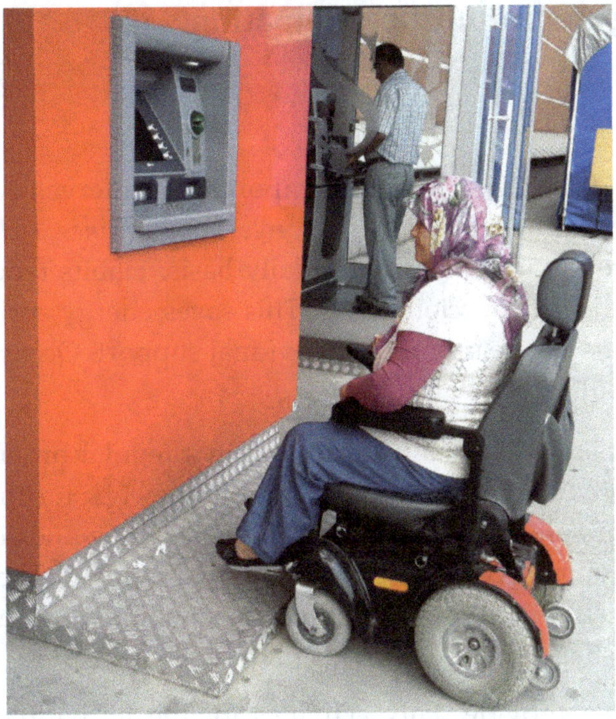

Picture 3. Environment: the determinates of participation for people with disabilities.

The main elements of this model are as follows:

- Occupation that is important to the person (self-care, production, leisure)
- Internal resources of the person (physical, cognitive, emotional)
- The environment of the person (physical, institutional, social, cultural)
- Spiritual factors (internal structure) [12]

This model has two focal points: The first is the treatment process and the client-centered practice that expresses the relationship between the treatment and the person. The second is the occupational performance which is done for self-care, enjoyment of life, participation in social and economic life, organize and satisfy them with respect to age, culturally appropriate and meaningful work [35].

This model includes factors that affect occupational performance and beliefs that affect the conceptualization of occupational therapy. Values and beliefs influence person's environment, health and client-centered practices [35].

Examples of values related to the activity are as follows:

- Activity is meaningful to life.
- It is necessary for health and well-being.
- Organize behaviors.
- Change over time and evolve.
- It shapes the environment and is shaped by the environment.
- Has a therapeutic effect [35].

5. Factors affecting community participation

5.1. Personal factors

When these structures deteriorate, it is very important to intervene and evaluate the intervention. Performance constructs include *habits, roles, and routines. Habits* are the models and talents that will engage the individual on a daily basis. Habits tend to automate and are usually automated at the subconscious level. This saves energy and allows us to focus on higher-level tasks. Habits can be useful for individual support. Occupational therapists con-Figure it to intervene [36].

Routines are things that an individual usually does in a regular order. Routines bring order sensibility and an individual or a group forms the framework for their daily lives. Studies have shown that routines are made at certain times of the day and somehow provide daily rhythm or biological rhythm according to the individual's biological clock. Routines are also shaped by society and culture at the same time. When children return from school, doing homework is a routine shaped by society and culture [36].

Both habits and routines provide daily activities for the individual. Habits and routines help an individual to have a certain lifestyle. Lifestyles are a sign of health and well-being. Individuals with routine preventive measures, habits, and daily walking or non-smoking routines will have a healthier lifestyle. The occupational therapists should be aware of the work of their patients and the meaning of these things in relation to the patient [14].

5.2. Performance skills

It defines certain abilities and features that the person typically combines to complete a functional ability. These include sensory, motor, emotional, cognitive, and communication/interaction skills [14].

The main examples are as follows:

- **Motor and praxis skills***:* The ability of an individual to interact with his environment and occupation, or with the objects in the environment [14].
- *Posture:* The ability to achieve a steep position even if the balance and balance of the individual is disturbed. This ability includes body trunk stabilization, alignment of the individual's body in a vertical position, and bringing the body to a safe and controlled position after completing the activity [36].
- *Mobility*: Ability of the individual to act to complete an occupation or activity. This ability includes walking on rough surfaces without stumbling, using foot tools or ancillary tools such as walking sticks, walkers or wheelchairs. If the individual is able to walk, the ability can also include situations such as being able to successfully reach the object with arms or with an apparatus and to tilt the body according to the task [36].
- *Coordination:* The capacity to use more than one extremity in relation to the task or activity. This ability includes the use of two or more limbs to stabilize or manipulate the object. The

individual must use small muscle groups for controlled movements such as object manipulation, speed or hand skill [36].

- *Strength and effort:* Move the objects against gravity as if it were the sum of muscle power used to counteract the movement or in the case of lifting an object standing on the ground. The individual must use the grip strength necessary to hold objects tight and adjust their speed, magnitude [36].
- *Energy* is to sustain and maintain certain durability and speed throughout the entire task without showing any signs of fatigue [36].
- **Process skills:** Individuals use skills to make the necessary movements to complete their daily life skills [14].
- *Energy:* The ability to focus on the workflow that continues over a period of time. This skill includes that the person adjusts his/her own speed and maintains attention throughout the mission [36].
- *Knowledge:* It is enough to research, acquire, and use knowledge for the task. This is the skill of the individual to select, use and protect the tools and materials related to the task. The individual has to learn more by asking questions or reading the guidelines to effectively complete the task [36].
- *Temporal organization*: The ability to plan, organize, and applicant stages of a task in turn. This capability includes initiating and continuing the task in succession and stopping or pause the activity when required [36].
- *Organizing space and objects:* It is the ability to organize the duration of the occupation or the task. This skill encompasses the ability of the individual to research tools for successful occupational performance, the ability to gather the tools needed for the task, and the ability to place tools in a logical and orderly manner. When the task is over, the individual must clean the work area and put the tools he uses in appropriate storage locations. This skill is also an ability to overcome an obstacle and also means that the individual moves his body or wheelchair around any object [36].
- *Adaptation*: The skill of the individual to learn something from his mistakes during his performance. This is the skill of recognizing the problem and the ability to adapt or change the movements of the individual to the situation of the task-related objects during or before the problem. This skill also requires that the individual comply with the work environment before or during the problem [36].
- **Sensory perceptual skills:** The ability to describe, interpret and respond to sensory information. These skills also require the individual to remember perceptual events. Sensory information can be interpreted in many ways, including auditory, visual, tactile, smelling, tasting, proprioceptive, and vestibular [36]:
- *Body position:* This is capable of bringing the individual's body to a proper position for a movement.
- *Hearing*: The ability to receive and recognize the auditory information.

- *Visualizing:* The ability to use visuals to interpret information.
- *Locating:* This ability comes into play when the individual begins to use sensory information to relocate objects. This ability is about stereognosis.
- *Timing*: The individual is able to self-adjust for a motor task or activity.
- *Discerning*: Using sensory ability to describe the differences between objects. An example is that an individual can tell the difference in temperature between foods.
- **Emotional regulation skills:** The ability to use movements or behaviors to express feelings when interacting with individuals or groups, or to deal with them [36]:
- *Responding*: It is the ability to understand and react to others' feelings.
- *Persisting*: Despite the difficulties, it is the capacity to continue the tasks.
- *Controlling*: Controlling feelings or anger about other individuals.
- *Recovering*: The individual is used when he is disappointed or when his feelings are hurt.
- *Displaying*: To have the ability to express appropriate feelings about a situation or experience.
- *Utilizing:* The ability to use some skills and techniques to resist emotional situations.

Cognitive skills: To use ideas or behaviors to design an activity or task [36]:

- *Judging*: the task is the ability to decide what is important or necessary for completion. An example is when an individual decides not to prioritize jobs that run the length of time.
- *Selecting*: Ability to select appropriate tools for a specific task.
- *Organizing*: Having the ability to complete the activity in the given order and time.
- *Prioritizing*: The ability to define the steps and solutions needed to complete a task.
- *Creating*: Can participate in fun activities.
- *Multitasking:* At the same time, the ability to do multiple jobs.

Communication/social skills: It is enough to explain the needs and ideas of the individual to others in a social environment and in an acceptable way [14].

- *Physicality*: The ability to use the individual's body or body language for communication. This skill involves physically touching others, bringing your body into a position or turning it into a direction in relation to eye contact and others.
- *Information exchange*: Ability to inform others and get information from them. This skill includes explicit self-expression, asking for information, and being able to include a meaningful word. Thus, the individual can communicate his/her feelings in the direction of information they share.
- *Relations*: Ability to continue relationships. This skill requires that the individual has the ability to interact with other people, to connect with people who have ordinary interests, or to have the ability to catch relationships at a certain level with everyday interactions [36].

5.3. Performance areas

Different living spaces were defined in the social participation of the individual. These include activities of daily living (ADL), instrumental activities of daily activities (IADL), work, education, play and leisure. The occupational therapist should take into account the person's role, social support, and occupational performance in different time and space [37].

The activities of the individual affect the activity of the roles in determining the role of his life. Christiansen and Baum have defined roles as "expected responsibilities and privileges in society" [34]. For example, in a reading activity, a mother reads a book for a 5-year-old child and has different activities to read a report. while she is in a job. That is, both the content and the printing scales of the material to be read will be different. While reading a book requires reading, a voice reading a report does not require it [38].

Activities can be divided into smaller tasks. For example, the account payment activity includes a series of tasks such as calling a waiter, requesting an account, reading the amount, putting the required amount in the account box. One uses the abilities and skills when doing these tasks. The skills required for these tasks include good motor skills, visual perception, selection, and oral motor function [38].

Activities of daily living (ADL): ADL skills include self-care, functional mobility, communication, and management of pharmaceutical and health routines. While defining activities of daily living, different terms can be used, such as simple daily life activities and personal daily life activities. Despite the different definitions of the ADL definition, it is people take care of yourself. ADL is an example of bathing, bowel control, dressing, eating, functional mobility, personal care, sexual activity, and toilet cleaning. Bathing activity, for example, is the acquisition and use of bathroom accessories such as soap, towels. The essence of this activity is to transfer into and out of the bath or bath with the ability to get the proper bath position and adjust the safe water temperature. Dressing activity includes the ability to dress up and choose clothes according to time, season and activity in our mind. Eating activity is the ability to graze, chew, and swallow food. Functional mobility is the ability to move from one position to another or from one place to another. Personal care activity is the provision and use of tools for the care of skin, ear, eye and nails. It is also necessary for this activity to scan the person's hair, use a toothbrush and toothpaste for mouth cleaning, toilet hygiene activities, in-and-out transfer, preparation of toilets, and post-toilet cleaning activities [37, 38]

Instrumental activities of daily living (IADL): Lawton and Brody have described "secondary tasks necessary for independent living in the community" as instrumental activities of daily living. IADL, consist of money management, telephone use, medication use, travel, shopping, food preparation, laundry and housework. It is recognized that IADL is important for the quality of life and well-being of the disabled individual. But there is no consensus about what activities are needed for independent community life. Barer and Nouri classify leisure activities (gardening and other hobbies) as transportation (use of transportation vehicles, walking on the street, getting in and out of the car and driving), home activities (laundry jobs, food preparation and housework) [37].

The application of IADL is complex multi-step activities. It requires the use of special tools such as telephones. Practices can occur inside and outside the house. Independent practice requires mental, physical and social skills such as decision-making, problem solving, initiation and sequencing. The evaluation of IADL is especially important for those who are prepared to return to community life. In addition, this assessment provides meaningful information about a person's cognitive status. In persons with cognitive impairment, disturbances are observed in IADLs, especially in telephone use, transportation, drug use, and money management [37].

Work/school activities: Job-based activities are the focus of one's life. Work-related activities are an important way to demonstrate the "adequacy" of an individual. The occupation as an employee depends on a successful interaction with the interpersonal, environment and business. The job evaluation of the person leads the therapist to specific tasks in the business area. The assessments in this area are used as an important source of information for the state. The best person to do the same job analysis as the job analysis can be identified [37].

Assessing the child, adolescent or young adult's ability to provide education is important [22]. It provides information about the child's participation in school activities, occupational performance and supports the child uses [37].

Leisure activities/play: Leisure activities are non-essential activities that are freely chosen, mostly occurring in nature, and providing individual satisfaction, relaxation, recreation and self-expression. Individuals are delightful and rewarded with inner rewards. Individuals with experience in leisure activities believe that events are on their control and will result in free choices of the outcome of the activity. These events and characteristics affect the person's ability to make choices. It has also been shown that participation in leisure has a positive impact on health [37].

The play is the first activity in childhood and youth. The play is a versatile phenomenon. The play improves internal motivation while providing relaxation and entertainment. Factors such as what players do, how players like the selected game activity, how the players' approach to the activities are, how the players play the games, and how the game supports the play are important [37].

5.4. Environmental conditions

In previous years, it was thought that the person with a disability had a disability in daily activities, participation in education, play and work, and these problems were related to the person. Later, awareness of environmental factors has also led to difficulties experienced by people with disabilities [39, 40].

First, the focus was on the physical and structural environment, and a lot of effort was spent on ramps, elevators, etc. on the pavements. The people with disabilities began to participate more in collecting [37].

Environmental conditions include three major factors:

1. Physical conditions (structural, natural and technological environment),
2. Social support,
3. Social conditions (socio-economic, cultural and political environment) [37].

Physical conditions: Physical conditions are classified in the building (man-made environment), technology (auxiliary devices, fixtures and software) and natural environment categories used by ICF [13].

1. There are two simple approaches to modifying the *building environment*. The first is the regulation or addition; the second is the addition of environmental products such as displacement or fixing devices. Reorganization of the building, the addition of a building to the home or community area, or the reshaping of the natural area may be expensive but necessary. On the other hand, the arrangement of the furniture in the rooms can be achieved with less cost. The second approach focuses on regulating whether the toilet or bath can be raised or lowered. Thus, one can make the right decision about his abilities and practice the task successfully. Connell and Sanford found that persons with disabilities who modified their homes had moderate difficulty or independence in activities of daily living. Gitlin and colleagues found a decrease in the rates of functional dependence and attachment to careers with house modification. Mann and colleagues reported that in the old age, the use of assistive technology and increased environmental regulation has reduced spending on personal care and health care [37].
2. Another important method of regulating the environment is the provision of *assistive technology and products*. Products consist of modifications for adaptive software or environmental control. Assistive technology is defined as systems and products that improve the functional capacity of people with disabilities. This technology is designed for environmental barriers that prevent someone from achieving maximum occupational performance. Sitting and moving devices provide connectivity to the community. A wide variety of assistive devices and systems are available, such as computer interface systems, communication enhancing devices, adaptive driving devices and environmental control units. Vehicles with high technology may cost more. These are not covered by health insurance nowadays, and the person may stop using the assistive device due to reasons such as the person does not want using or being embarrassed. These factors may have an impact on the individual's independence [37].
3. Usually, the properties of the *natural environment* cannot be changed. For example, the Taurus Mountains in the Mediterranean, snow and ice in Agrı city, temperature and humidity in Antalya. The characteristics of the natural environment such as climate, atmospheric pressure, and population density can affect the performance of the disabled individual. Although these features cannot be modified, modifications can be made. There are also legal regulations for improving the performance of the activity. For example, providing air conditioning for risky individuals in extreme temperatures or providing access to parking spaces and lifts makes a difference between activity and disability. Where the natural environment for the handicapped cannot be changed, information becomes the most important thing. A map can provide information about the area, rest areas, or alternative methods [37].

Support, relevance and effectiveness of occupation: The use of social support as both formal (programs and services) and informal (family and friends) is a strategy used to compensate for environmental barriers. In a therapeutic perspective, social support for people with disabilities is often defined by their care, their love, and their ability to trust others. Social support is a concept that includes practical support, informative support and emotional support. *Practical support* is a physical support. Supporting transfers, preparing meals, or taking them to a doctor are examples of practical support. This type of support may be informal (if given by a family member or loved one) or formal (if given by a paid caregiver or someone interested in personal care). *Informative support* is generally considered to be advice or guidance. For example, an individual can be referred to as advice or information to teach ways of saving energy or to take supplies for the bathroom. Family or friends, as well as professionals or peers, provide this kind of information. Emotional support generally includes feelings of belonging or respect. Despite the fact that the professionals provide this kind of support, *emotional support* is a role that falls on the family and peers to become a group member or morale in difficult times [37].

Social support can improve physical fitness, harmony between person and environment. For example, the activity of eating in the life of an individual who temporarily uses a wheelchair for mobility may be disrupted. The person may not be able to move enough in the kitchen due to the narrow space in the kitchen, the lack of space for return, unreachable cabinets, and environmental obstacles such as not being able to see what is being cooked in the kitchen. By increasing the surface area, it can be a strategy to change the area of motion by removing furniture, cabinets, and an angled mirror over the oven to create more space. Teaching to use a microwave oven set at a level that can reach the person is also an alternative. A third solution would be to use a home-cooked meal service (official practical support). The fourth alternative might be to inform the family or friends of the individual and provide assistance (unofficial practical support) to the disabled individual during the preparation and preparation of food [37].

The effect of socio-economic and political direction on environment and occupation: *Culture* is values, norms, beliefs, traditions, behaviors and perceptions shared by a group or society. Culture can be related to people, organization, community, and community level. Individually, the culture can determine the level of independence of the individual's wishes. For example, the exchange of an elder's clothes can be accepted for the culture. The culture is also influential in home modifications. In Turkey, for example, when entering the house, the shoes are removed and the house is one step higher than the area from which the shoe is removed. This tradition creates difficulties for the wheelchair user to enter the home [37].

Policies that provide funding for programs that help people with disabilities, services, may play a role in whether there is funding. In the United States and some European countries, individuals with disabilities regulate home modifications. Insurance schemes in these countries cover home caregivers, home health benefits, and regulations that will increase the freedoms of people with disabilities. Many practical programs and attitude changes affecting the environment have been carried out to a large extent as a result of legislation. These laws shape the programs and policies affecting participation, as well as profoundly affecting the professional productivity of people with disabilities [37].

The Turkish Institute of Statistics has established the "Turkey Disability Survey" in order to solve the problems of people with disabilities in Turkey and disability issues. According to the results of the research, it is seen that the proportion of the disabled population is 12.29% of the total population. Accordingly, there are approximately 8.5 million people with disabilities in our country. The most disadvantaged part of the society, the disabled, health, education, employment, care, rehabilitation, accessibility and so on. It is important that many socio-cultural and economic problems are resolved. With this in mind, Law No. 5378 on the Amendment of Decrees on Disability and Some Laws and Decrees on the Law has entered into force on 07.07.2005. On December 3, 2008, the Assembly approved the United Nations Convention on the Rights of Persons with Disabilities, which is World Disability Day. Thus, the right of all disabled citizens to live equal, free and dignified is guaranteed [41].

Persons with disabilities are less likely to receive education and work than healthy people. The cost of non-income disability is twice as expensive as the disability. In this case, even laws cannot save from the obstacle of social exclusion. In a survey conducted, it was reported that the employer did not have the courage to give obstructive employment and some of them refused to do business [37] (**Picture 4**).

Beliefs about disabled people also affect the occupational performance. Laws, policies and beliefs, shape society and beliefs are the most influential external factor in the lives of the disabilities. In the past, there were practices that discriminated in the workforce, in public participation, and in education. Negative beliefs against disability affected participation in all phases of life. Protecting and increasing the reputation of the disabled will be provided by changing social attitudes, lifting social barriers and legal approaches [37].

5.5. Quality of life and community participation

Aristotle, who defines happiness as a virtuous activity of the soul, states the concept of quality of life. Happiness is said to be for a short time, a feeling of goodness temporarily felt by daily affairs. There may be many areas to describe the quality of life. These are cultural, psychological, social, religious, economic, political, temporal and philosophical fields. The quality of life is a dynamic perception because it changes with people and the environment [42].

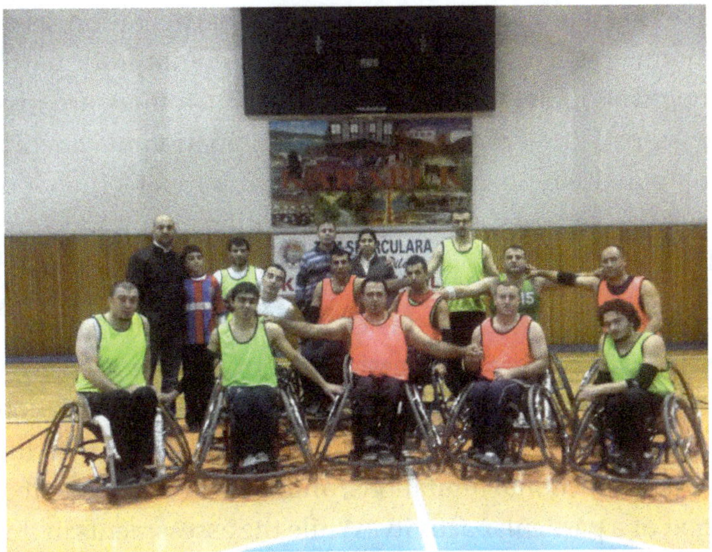

Picture 4. Sports affects participation as a work and leisure activities.

World Health Organization (WHO) has defined the quality of life as "Positive perception of person's aims, expectations, standards and values related to it and its life in culture." This definition clearly shows that occupational therapists believe that the quality of life will increase in meaningful connection with the person, family and society and occupation. That is, meaningful community participation is associated with good quality of life [42].

Occupation and quality of life: A meaningful activity is directly associated with a good quality of life. Because the activity encourages the person, at the same time, it changes and strengthens the character of the person. Constrained activity also limits the potential for activity remaining for the individual. People are prevented from participating in necessary activities and contributing to the meaning of life with the reasons of disability and occupational deprivation. The effect of occupational deprivation includes feelings of loneliness, emotional distance from one's self and others, and despairs that will distract the person from the quality of life. As a result, meaningful occupation significantly affects person's quality of life [42].

Not long ago, many people with disabilities encountered great obstacles to meaningful occupation and there were limited occupational available to them. These constraints in activism stemmed from the prejudices of the society about superstitions, disaggregation in institutions and the capacity and potential of people with disabilities. Such barriers have significantly reduced the chances of eliminating the abilities, and self-potential of disabilities. In today's society, many people with disabilities are still faced with such occupational obstacles that lower quality of life. For this reason, the search for quality of life may present additional difficulties, especially in the area of occupational. Therefore, occupational therapists pay particular attention to the quality of life for the handicapped [42, 43].

6. Evaluating of community participation

We understand the forms of community involvement by gathering experiences of our clients' occupations that make up their daily lives. Community participation, as defined, is a versatile and contextual phenomenon. These basic attributes of community participation imply that there is more than one way to determine whether our customers are involved (i.e., whether they are multi-dimensional) and that our clients' participation may actually vary depending on what they are doing and where they are doing it. It happens (i.e., it depends on the content). For this reason, it is best to gather useful information about how our different clients are involved among all relevant occupations and settings.

The assessment approaches addressed in this chapter support the use of a top-down and customer-focused approach to our clients' professional performance needs. When using a bottom-up approach, it first focuses on getting the client's community participation profile by defining what the customer wants to do, what to do, or what to expect. And then they organize services that deal with distortions, functional limitations, and contextual factors that limit levels of participation in the context of a particular activity. While the assessments in this section will enable us to systematically acquire the community participation profiles of our customers, we do not concentrate on the subset of activities that have the most restrictions on their participation.

Many of these measures have been developed over the past decade and have provided ideas for thinking and measuring lifelong involvement of people with disabilities. These measures differ in terms of their completeness, how they are implemented, how long they are completed, the intended population of the target population, and their intended purposes. In this section, we will consider the participation assessments developed for young children, children and adolescents, adults and older adults. The table below gives an overview of what each assessor can do to help you collect information as you start the assessment process with your clients [42, 43] **[Tables 1, 2]**.

The Preschooler Activity Card Sort	(Berg & LaVesser, 2006) [44]
The Asset-Based Context Matrix (ABCM)	(Wilson, Mott, & Batman, 2004) [45]
The Assessment of Preschool Children's Participation (APCP) scale	(Law, King, Petrenchik, Kertoy, & Anaby, 2012) [46]
The Routines-Based Interview (RBI)	(McWilliam, Casey, & Sims, 2009) [47]
The Children's Participation Questionnaire (CPQ)	(Rosenberg, Jarus, & Bart, 2010) [48]
Children's Assessment of Participation and Enjoyment (CAPE)	(King et al., 2006) [49, 50]
The School Function Assessment (SFA)	(Coster, Deeney, Haltiwanger, & Haley, 1998) [51]
The Pediatric Activity Card Sort (PACS)	(Mandich, Polatajko, Miller, & Baum, 2004) [52]
The Child and Adolescent Scale of Participation (CASP)	(Bedell, 2009) [53]

Table 1. Selected Participation Measures for Young Children.

The Meaningful Activity Participation Assessment (MAPA) [54]	
The Participation and Environment Measure for Children and Youth (PEM-CY)	(Coster, Law, & Bedell, 2010) [55]
The Engagement in Meaningful Activity Scale (EMAS)	(Goldberg, Brintnell, and Goldberg, 2002) [56]
The Activity Card Sort (ACS)	(Baum & Edwards, 2008) [57]
The Community Integration Questionnaire (CIQ)	(Corrigan & Deming, 1995; Sander et al., 2007; Willer, Rosenthal, Kreutzer, Gordon, & Rempel, 1993) [58, 59]
The Craig Handicap Assessment and Reporting Technique (CHART)	(Whiteneck, Charlifue, Gerhart, Overholser, & Richardson, 1992) [60]

Table 2. Selected Participation Measures for Adults and Older Adults.

Author details

Gokcen Akyurek* and Gonca Bumin

*Address all correspondence to: gkcnakyrk@gmail.com

Department of Occupational Therapy, Faculty of Health Sciences, Hacettepe University, Ankara, Turkey

References

[1] Burcu E. Türkiye'de Özürlü Birey Olma Temel Sosyolojik Özellikleri ve Sorunları Üzerine Bir Araştırma. Ankara: Hacettepe Üniversitesi Yayınları; 2007

[2] Polat ÇS. Engelliliğin Atasözü ve Deyimlere Yansımasının Sosyolojik Analizi Ulıslararası Türkiye-Mısır ilişkileri Sempozyumu ve Güzel Sanatlar Sergisi, 2-7 Kasım, Kahire/Mısır. 2009

[3] Burcu E. Özürlülük Kimliği ve Etiketlemenin Kişisel ve Sosyal Söylemleri, Hacettepe Üniversitesi Edebiyat Fakültesi Dergisi. 2006;**23**(2):61-83

[4] American Occupational Therapy Association. Occupational therapy practice framework: Domain and process. American Journal of Occupational Therapy. 2002;**56**(6):609-639

[5] Mosey AC. Applied Scientific Inquiry in the Health Professions: A Epistemological Orientation. 2nd ed. Bethesda, MD: AOTA; 1996

[6] Bullinger M, Schmidt S, Petersen C. The Disabkids Group. Assessing quality of life of children with chronic health conditions and disabilities: A Europen approach. International Journal of Rehabilitation Research. 2002;**25**:197-206

[7] Küçükdeveci AA. Rehabilitasyonda Yaşam Kalitesi. Türkiye Fiziksel Tıp ve Rehabilitasyon Derneği. 2005;**51**(B):23-29

[8] Uyanik M, Kayıhan H, Düger T, Bumin G, Ergun A. Hemiplejik hastaların günlük yaşam aktivitelerini değerlendirmede standardize dört testin karşılaştırması. Fizyoterapi ve Rehabilitasyon. 2001;**12**(2):67-74

[9] Kimler DD, Abresch TD, Fowler WM. Serial manuel muscle testing in duchenne muscular dystrophy. Archives of Physical Medicine and Rehabilitation. 1993;**74**(11):1168-1171

[10] Spilker B. Quality of Life. Assessments in Clinical Trials. New York: Raven Press; 1996

[11] Meyer A. The philosophy of occupation therapy. Archives of Occupation Therapy. 1922;**1**(1): (Reprinted in American Journal of Occupation Therapy. 1977;**31**(10))

[12] Law M, Baum C Measurement in Occupational Therapy. In: Law M, Baum C, Dunn W. Measuring Occupational Performance: Supporting Best Practice in Occupational Therapy. 2nd ed. Thorofare, NJ: Slack Inc. 2005.

[13] World Health Organization (WHO). International Classification of Functioning, Disability and Health. Geneva, Switzerland: 2001; p. 18

[14] O'Sullivan B. Practice framework and activity analysis. 2nd ed. In: Sladyk K, editor. OT Study Cards in a Box. Thorofare, NJ: SLACK Incorporated; 2003;**2**:1-32

[15] Shannon PD. Philosophy and core values in occupational therapy. 4th ed. In: Sladyk K, Ryan SE, editors. Ryan's Occupational Therapy Assistant: Principles, Practice Issues, and Techniques, Thorefare: Slack; 2005

[16] American Occupational Therapy Association. The philosophical base of occupational therapy. American Journal of Occupation Therapy. 1979;**33**:785. (Reviewed by COE and COP in 2004)

[17] Hussey SM, Sabonis-Chafee B, O'Brien JC. Introduction to Occupational Therapy; 3rd ed. St Louis, MO: Mosby Elsevier; 2008

[18] Reed KL, Sanderson SN. Concepts of Occupational Therapy. 4th ed, Philadelphia: Lippincott William and Wilkins; 1999

[19] Fidler GS. From crafts to competence. American Journal of Occupation Therapy. 1981;**35**:567

[20] Fidler GS, Fidler JW. Doing and becoming: Purposeful action and self actualization. American Journal of Occupation Therapy. 1978;**32**:305

[21] King KJ. Toward a science of adaptive responses. American Journal of Occupation Therapy. 1978;**32**:14

[22] Towards a Common Language for Functioning, Disability and Health. 2002. Available from: http://www.who.inc.int/classifications/icf/site/beginners/bg.pdf

[23] www.ozida.gov.tr/siniflandirma/icf.htm

[24] Karaduman AA, Özberk ZN. Uluslar arası Fonksiyonellik, özür ve sağlığın sınıflandırması-ICF. Fizyoterapistler için ICF temel eğitim çalıştayı.

[25] Fisher A. Overview of Performance Skills and Client Factors. In: Pendleton HM, Schultz-Krohn W. Pedretti's Occupational Therapy: Practice Skills for Physical Dysfunction. 6th ed. St Louis: Mosby/Elsevier. 2006.

[26] Kielhofner G. Conceptual Foundations of Occupational Therapy. 3rd ed.; 2004. ch5. pp. 73-74

[27] Kielhofner G, Forsyth K, Barrett L. The model of Human Occupation. In: Crepeau EB, Cohn ES, Schell BAB, editors. Willard and Spackman's Occupational Therapy. 10th ed. Philadelphia: Lippincott Williams and Wilkins; 2003.

[28] Dunn W, McClain LH, Brown C, Youngstrom MJ. The Ecology of Human Performance. In: Crepeau EB, Cohn ES, Schell BAB, editors. Willard and Spackman's Occupational Therapy. 10th ed. Philadelphia: Lippincott Williams and Wilkins, 2003.

[29] Stewart D, Letts L, Law M, Cooper BA, Strong S, Rigby PJ. The Person Environment Occupational Model. In: Crepeau EB, Cohn ES, Schell BAB, editors. Willard and Spackman's Occupational Therapy. 10th ed. Philadelphia: Lippincott Williams and Wilkins, 2003.

[30] Sarbin TR, Scheibe KE. A model of social identity. In: Sarbin TR & Scheibe KE, editors. Studies in Social Identity. New York: Praeger Publiching, 1983.

[31] Grossack M, Gardner H. Man and men: Social psychology as social science. Scranton: International Textbook. 1970

[32] Matsutsuyu JS. The interest chech list. American Journal of Occupation Therapy. 1970;**24**:93-101

[33] Dunn W, Brown C, McGuigan A. Ecology of human performance: A framework. American Journal of Occupation Therapy. 1994;**48**(7):595-607

[34] Dunn W. Ecology of human performance model. In: Dunbar SB, editor. Occupational Therapy Models for Intervention with Children and Families. Thorofare, NJ: Slack Incorporated; 2007. pp. 127-157

[35] Law M, Polatajko H, Baptiste S, Townsend E. Core Concepts of Occupational Therapy; In: Townsend E, editor. Enabling occupation: An occupational therapy perspective. Ottawa, ON: CAOT Publications ACE; 1997

[36] Sladyk K, Jacobs K, MacRae N. Occupational therapy essentials for clinical competence. Occupation, Activity, Skills, Patterns, Demands, Context and Balance. Thorofare, NJ: SLACK, Incorporated; 2010.

[37] Christiansen C, Baum C, Bass-Haugen J. Occupational therapy: Performance, participation and well being. Thorofare, NJ: Slack Incorporated; 2004

[38] Oksuz C, Akel S, Bumin G. Effect of occupational therapy on activity level and occupational performance in patients with neuromuscular disease. Fizyotrapi Rehabilitasyon. 2011;**22**(3):231-239

[39] Cook AM, Polgar JM. A framework for assistive Technologies. In: Cook AM, Polgar JM, editors. Cook and Hussey's Assistive Technologies: Principles and Practice. 3nd ed. St. Louis, MO: Mosby Elsevier; 2008.

[40] Bumin G, Akyürek G. Environmental perception and social participation of amateur and professional athletes with disabilities. 16th congress of the World Federation of Occupational Therapists in Collaboration with the 48th Japanese Occupational Therapy Congress and Expo, 18-21 June 2014; Japan

[41] http://www.ozida.gov.tr/yenimezuat/mevzuat.pdf Erişim tarihi: 11.02.2017

[42] Pizzi MA, Renwick R. Quality of life and health promotion. In: Scaffa ME, Reitz SM, Pizzi MA. Occupational therapy in the promotiong of health and wellness. Philadelphia, FA Davis Plus, 2010

[43] Akyürek G, Bumin G. Investigation of factors that affect community participation of people with disabilities. The 13th International Conference on Mobility and Transport for Elderly and Disabled Persons (TRANSED 2012); September 17-20, 2012; New Delhi; India

[44] Berg C, LaVesser P. The preschool activity card sort. Fall. 2006; 26 (4): 143-51.

[45] Wilson LL, Mott DW, & Batman D. The Asset-Based Context Matrix (ABCM). TECSE 2004; 24(2): 110-20.

[46] Law M, King G, Petrenchik T, Kertoy M, & Anaby D. The Assessment of Preschool Children's Participation (APCP) scale: Internal consistency and construct validity. Physical and Occupational Therapy in Pediatrics 2012; 32 (3): 272-87.

[47] McWilliam RA, Casey AM, & Sims J. The Routines-Based Interview (RBI) A method for gathering information and assessing need. Infants & Young Children 2009: 22 (3): 224-33.

[48] Rosenberg L, Jarus T, & Bart O. Development and initial validation of the Children's Participation Questionnaire (CPQ). Disability and Rehabilitation 2010; 32 (20): 1633-44.

[49] King GA, Law M, King S, Hurley P, Hanna S, Kertoy MK, et al. Measuring children's participation in recreation and leisure activites: Construct validation of the CAPE and PAC. Child: Care, Health & Development 2006; 33 (1): 28-39.

[50] Bumin G and Akyalcin S. The effect of activity participation in quality of life in children with cerebral palsy. Arch Phy Med Rehab. 2016; 97 (10): e29.

[51] Coster W, Deeney T, Haltiwanger J, & Haley S. School Function Assessment user's manual. San Antonio, TX: The Psychological Corporation, 1998.

[52] Mandich AD, Polatajko HJ, Miller LT, Baum C. Paediatric Activity Card Sort (PACS). CAOT Publications ACE, Ottawa; 2004.

[53] Bedell G. The Child and Adolescent Scale of Participation (CASP). Dev Neurorehabil. 2009; 12(5): 342-51.

[54] Eakman AM, Carlson ME, Clark FA. The Meaningful Activity Participation Assessment (MAPA): A measure of engagement in personally valued activities. Int J Aging Dev 2010; 70 (4): 299-317.

[55] Coster W, Bedell G, Law M, Khetani MA, Teplicky R, Liljenquıst K, Gleason K, Kao Y. Psychometric evaluation of the Participation and Environment Measure for Children and Youth (PEM-CY). Developmental Medicine & Child Neurology, 2011; 976-977.

[56] Goldberg, Brintnell, and Goldberg. The Relationship between engagement in meaningful activities and quality of life in persons disabiled by mental illness. Occupational Therapy in Mental Health. 2002; 8 (2): 17-44.

[57] Baum CM, & Edwards DF. Activity Card Sort (ACS): Test manual (2nd Ed). Bethesda, MD: AOTA Press. 2008.

[58] Willer B, Rosenthal M, Kreutzer JS, Gordon WA, Rempel R. Assessment of community integration following rehabilitation for traumatic brain injury. J Head Trauma Rehabil. 1993;8:75-87.

[59] Akyürek G, Salar S, Bumin G, Kayıhan H. Turkish Adaptation of The Community Integration Questionnaire (CIQ) and Its Validity And Reliability in people with SCI. Arch Phy Med Rehab. 2016; 97 (10): E41.

[60] Whiteneck GG, Charlifue SW, Gerhart KA, Overholser JD, & Richardson GN. Quantifying handicap: a new measure of long-term rehabilitation outcomes. Arch. Phys. Med. Rehabil. 1992; 73; 519-526.

7

Early Intervention in Pediatric Occupational Therapy

Serkan Pekçetin and Ayla Günal

Abstract

Early intervention is services for infants and toddlers who have developmental deficiency or considered high risk due to the environmental or biologic factors. The aim of the early intervention is increasing the physical, cognitive and emotional capacities of infants/toddlers with protecting them from the environmental or biological risk factors. Early intervention should start as soon as possible for obtaining the best results for the child and family. First 3 years of life are critical period of the child development because neurologic development still continues. Infants and toddlers are providing physical, cognitive, sensory and social development with different experiences and various sensory stimuli from the environment in this period. Occupational therapists evaluate and implement interventions to activity, environment, infant/toddlers and their families for minimizing the developmental risks. For these reasons, occupational therapists are considered important members of early intervention team.

Keywords: early intervention, occupational therapy, sensory motor performance, play therapy, cognitive, feeding disorders, social development

1. Introduction

1.1. High risk infant

This term is using for the infant who has increasing risk for disability, but the exact disability is not actualized yet. The risk factors of infants can be divided into two main subheadings. The first subheading is biological risk factors. These are: intracranial hemorrhage, diabetic retinopathy, sepsis, necrotizing enterocolitis, apnea, asphyxia, intraventricular hemorrhage and the brachial plexus injury. The second subheading is environmental risk factors. These are: adolescence pregnancy, low socioeconomic status, mental health problems of parents, substance abuse of parents and the lack of family caregiving skills [1].

1.2. Occupational therapy intervention in neonatal intensive care unit

Many high risk infants begin to the first days of their lives in Neonatal Intensive Care Unit (NICU) for provision of medical treatment. The occupational therapist should consider biological risk of infants, NICU's environmental risk factors and early separation problems of infant caregivers when planning their assessments and interventions. Due to this reason, occupational therapy interventions in the NICU should involve infants, families, NICU staffs and environmental factors.

The early mother and infant separation are risking the mother-infant bonding, which is critical role in infant development. Thus, occupational therapy intervention for high risk infants should start as soon as possible after the infant born. Occupational therapy intervention in NICU should include infant, family and environmental factors. Occupational therapist should motivate the parents to take care of their infants in NICU. This intervention provides positive social interaction between mother and infant at an early period. Occupational therapy program in NICU should include increasing the confidence of caregiving skills of mothers and establish strong relationship between infant and mother with increasing mother's observation skills to infant behaviors. These interventions' aim is providing the mother's positive feeling to infants. Then occupational therapists should give opportunity to observe the infant. Family should sensitive to infant's reaction to environmental stimuli and tries to provide a positive response from them. Thus, mother's self-confidence increase with ability to understand the response of the infant and mother can provide appropriate sensory stimuli to her infant [2].

Kangaroo care is another important intervention of occupational therapists working in the NICU. Kangaroo care is a technique that nude infant is positioned between the breast and under the clothes of his/her mother or primary caregiver in a vertical position to provide skin-to-skin contact. Mother sits on a rocking chair and swing rhythmically to provide vestibular stimulus to infant. Kangaroo care's aims are providing mother-infant bonding and preventing sensory processing disorders of infants. Due to that reason, kangaroo care should be initiated as early as possible even in the delivery room and infant-mother separation should be finished [3].

NICU environmental risk factors and immaturity of infants' biologic and neurologic systems are lead to sensory processing disorders in infants or even if loss of sense. All sensory interventions for infants who are taking medical treatment in the NICU, priority should be given to reduce sensory stimuli rather than provide sensory stimuli. Due to the reason, environmental adjustments in the NICU gain an important role for occupational therapists. Occupational therapist should adjust the environmental factors of NICU's light and sound. NICU lighting design should include: (1) infants should be kept out of the direct light, (2) incubator must have covered with a thick blanket for reduction of light, (3) the provision of day-night cycle by changing the light levels at specific times of day; this will be supporting the infant rapid eye movement (REM) sleep, and (4) levels of lighting instruments should measure and reduction of light exposure should be provided. Sound level design in NICU should include: (1) noise reduction should be provided in NICU, (2) NICU's sound level should not exceed 50 decibels, (3) temporary sound level in NICU should not exceed 70 decibels, (4) equipment noise level in NICU should not exceed 40 decibels, and (5) NICU staff training should be done for decreasing noise level [4].

Another important intervention of occupational therapist in the NICU is providing minimal touch to infant. Occupational therapists should coordinate taking blood samples, imaging techniques, aspiration, and chest physiotherapy for providing minimal touch and give a formal warning to other health care providers regarding the provision of enough and quiet rest time to infant.

Occupational therapy interventions in the NICU provide infant's medical status get better, and infants can early discharge from the NICU. After discharge from NICU, parents should be educated for taking care at home for high risk infant and developmental follow-up must be done. At this period, occupational therapists should evaluate and implement interventions for infant's sensory processing disorders, social-emotional development, feeding problems, motor development, cognitive development and playing skills.

1.3. Sensory processing disorder

Dr. J. Ayres developed sensory integration theory in the 1970s. She defined sensory integration as a neurological organization process enabling the effective use of one's body through stimulus from his body and the environment [5].

Ayres' the most important contribution to the understanding for the child's development is highlighting the importance of senses, but especially proximal senses (vestibular, tactile and proprioceptive). From the point of sensory integration view, it was emphasized that proximal senses are very important. Child uses these senses for interacting with environment at early stages of life, because these senses are primitive and basic senses. The distal senses such as vision and hearing gain more importance as the child grows and gets more critical. Ayres hypothesis was that proximal senses are providing basic to child complex activities [5].

When infant behavior is examined from the sensory integration theory, both environmental and biological factors are effective on the of infants' behavior. Infant's related factors, "Four As" (arousal, attention, affect and action), the sensory threshold and self-regulation skills. Each of these factors is interrelated and affects each other. "Four As" was defined by the Anzalone. These factors are:

1. *Arousal:* Arousal is the ability to maintain infant's vigilance and manage to pass between situations.
2. *Attention:* Attention is the ability to give selective attention to stimulus or task by infant.
3. *Affect:* Affect is the emotional components of behavior.
4. *Action:* Infants' ability to perform purposeful behaviors [6].

Sensory threshold, ideally, this threshold is high enough that we can tolerate the complexity and stimulation inherent in the environment, yet low enough that we can perceive subtle changes and novelty in the environment. This threshold varies both between and within individuals. Infant's threshold range will determine infant's behavior organization level.

Self-regulation is a process that involves the infant's capacity to modulate mood, self-calm, delay gratification and tolerate transitions in activity.

Environmental factors are sensory stimuli from infant's physical and social environment [7].

1.3.1. Evaluation tools of infant/toddler sensory processing disorders

There are three specific tests for determining sensory processing problems in the range of 0–3 years. These tests are: Test of Sensory Functions in Infants (TSFI), Sensory Rating Scale (SRS) and the Infant/Toddler Sensory Profile (ITSP) tests. The SRS and ITSP are both parent-reported questionnaires, whereas the TSFI is a performance-based assessment [8].

1.3.2. Sensory integration interventions for infant/toddler

Sensory integration interventions can be applied in three different ways for infants/toddlers. The first type of these interventions is individualized sensory integration therapy. The second type of sensory intervention is the sensory diet. The third type of this intervention is family education [9].

1.3.2.1. Individualized sensory integration interventions

Sensory integration interventions should include these parameters; desensitization of hyper-reactive response, increasing the hyporeactive response, ensures attention continuity, providing purposeful activity and ensures appropriate behavior to sensory stimuli. The most important principle of sensory integration therapy is gaining ability to organize and process senses to provide purposeful activity. The occupational therapist uses individualized sensory integration interventions for treating atypical responses to sensory stimuli. For example, brushing techniques can be used for desensitization of hypersensitivity to touch or for gaining appropriate response to vestibular stimulus; hammock can be use in therapy. Such sensory integration techniques will help to normalize the child's response to sensory stimuli [9].

1.3.2.2. Sensory diet

A sensory diet is individualized home program that is carefully planned and has a positive effect on functional skills to regulate sensory stimulus. It is important to specify the intensity, duration and timing of sensory-based activity to obtain optimal performance from the sensory diet.

One of the most important principles in the treatment of sensory processing disorder for infant/toddler is including sensory integration intervention into the activities of daily living and play activities. It can provide with modifying child's daily routine, functional activities and play materials to meet the child's sensory needs. House environment also should be configured in sensory diet [10].

Sensory integration theory provides the basic principles for the treatment of sensory modulation disorder. Sensory diet of children will provide optimum sensory modulation and optimum sensory modulation facilitates the appropriate adaptive response. This is an indirect treatment method for sensory modulation disorder. Sensory diet for infants should be included in activities of daily living such as bathing and feeding. Normal sensory response will gain with changing daily routines and the sensory parameters of home environment that ensuring optimum sensory stimulation [11].

1.3.2.3. Family education

Family education is often used for regulation disorders caused by sensory processing disorder, and constitutes an important part of the treatment process. There are two important benefits of family education. First, family will understand that sensory processing disorders are underlying factor of infant/toddlers' behavioral problems. By this way, it helps the mother and infant bonding. Second, family education teaches coping strategies to families for infant/toddler's behavioral problems [12].

1.4. Social-emotional development

Social-emotional development process begins with infant-primary caregiver bonding in infancy period. Infants' first interaction is with their primary caregiver. Infants express needs with crying or gaze at something. Primary caregiver meet the infant's needs and infant calm down; thus infant carry out first social communication. Children increase the social development interacting with other family members, peers and teachers. Social skills may be negatively influenced from the factors related to primary caregiver such as mother's mental health problems or factors related to infants such as insufficient cognitive skills. Negative experiences in infancy may cause insufficient social skills in childhood [13].

1.4.1. Evaluation tools of social-emotional development for infants/toddlers

Social-emotional development in infancy can be evaluated with The Social-Emotional Assessment/Evaluation Measure, Ages & Stages Questionnaire: Social-Emotional (ASQ: SE), Brief Infant-Toddler Social-Emotional Assessment (BITS), the Temperament and Atypical Behavior Scale (TABS), Infant-Toddler Social-Emotional Assessment (ITSEA), the Functional Emotional Assessment Scale (FEAS), Bayley Scales of Infant Development, Infant Behavior Record, Parent-Child Early Relational Assessment (PCER), the Devereux Early Childhood Assessment Clinical Form (DEC-C), Social Skills Rating System (SSRS), Preschool Learning Behaviors Scale (PLBS) and Infant/Toddler Symptom Checklist [14, 15].

1.4.2. Occupational therapy intervention for social-emotional development of infants/toddlers

Occupational therapy interventions in this area can be classified in three subheadings. First is touch-based interventions for providing self-regulation of infant and infant-caregiver bonding. Second is relation-based interventions for providing positive mother-children interaction. Third is increasing attention skills.

Touch-based interventions include kangaroo care, deep pressure and massage interventions. These interventions' aims are ensuring calming the infant and promotion of mother-infant bonding.

The occupational therapists frequently use DIR-Floortime method for relationship-based intervention. DIR is the developmental, individual-differences and relationship-based model that was developed by Dr. Stanley Greenspan and Dr. Serena Wieder. Dr. Greenspan stated the goal of DIR model, as increasing social, emotional and intellectual capacities of children. *Developmental* in this model represents that the intervention should be appropriate to developmental milestones. There are six milestones defined in this model. These are (1) *Self-Regulation and Interest in the World* (0–3 months): Being calm and feeling well enough to attend to a caregiver and surroundings. (2) *Forming Relationship, Attachment and Engagement* (2–7 months): Interest in another person and in the world, developing a special bond with primary caregivers. (3) *Two-Way Purposeful Communication* (3–10 months): Simple back and forth interactions between child and caregiver. (4) *Complex Sense of Self* (9–18 months): Engaging complex organized problem solving interactions. (5) *Representational Capacities* (18–30 months): Meaningful and creative use of ideas and words. (6). *Representational Differentiation* (30–48 months): to establish relationships between ideas. *Individual differences* in this model represent all individuals' perception of environment are different from each other. In particular, attention is drawn on differences between sensory processing capacities of each child.*Relationship-based* part of the model emphasizes the developments of the human being bring results with interaction with other people. With young children, these playful interactions may occur on the "floor," and these interactions should be purposeful. In this model, the parents who play with child should know six major milestones of the early development stages. In this therapy method, parents should play 20 or more minutes with their children on the floor. However, there are two important points that therapists should pay attention. First, the parents should follow the leadership of the child and the second, all the interactions between the child and parent should support developmental process. DIR model is holistic approach that addresses the both family and child strength and needs. This model is not focus only on the child's development; it also aims to improve the overall functioning of the family. DIR-floortime effectiveness can be provided with cooperation between therapists and families, and parents must be committed to the program [16, 17].

Joint attention is the process in which an infant learns to recognize the direction of an adult's gaze, orient their own gaze to follow it, and then look in the same direction. Attention skills are critical for social development, and it seems related to language development [18].

Socio-emotional behavior is a key factor of understanding the child because it will affect the other performance areas. Occupational therapist should help to determine the parents which behavior of the child most problematic in home environment for improving the fit between the child and the environment. The determined behaviors constitute the objective of intervention, and later therapist can make suggestions for compensation to cope with this behavior [19].

1.5. Feeding disorders in infants/toddlers

Swallowing is one of the two vital functions of humans along with respiration. Feeding disorders are occurring approximately 50% of high risk infants and toddlers. Feeding disorders may continue to older ages for most of the infants who experienced these disorders during infancy period [20].

Sucking: Swallowing function begins with sucking at 36 weeks' gestation. Tongue, upper lip, mandible and the hyoid first move to up and down and later forward and backward as a unique unit to provide the positive and negative pressure, thus milk bolus ingestion provided. This nutritive sucking occurs in term infants per second [21, 22].

Sucking swallowing breathing: Sucking-swallowing-breathing reflex is essential for successful sucking because infant has to coordinate especially swallowing and breathing. Prematurity, neurologic disorders in infancy or respiratory disorders have higher risk for the developmental process of this reflex [23].

Chewing: At almost 6 months of age, infants begin a munching type of oral-motor activity, using back-forth tongue movement and up-down movements of the jaw. An infant can eat pured or soft foods after achieving munching. The next developmental stage of chewing is lateral motion of the jaw and seen at 9 months of age. At this stage, lateral movement of tongue start and infant can transfer the food to masticatory surface. The final developmental stage is rotatory movement of the jaw. This stage can be seen between 18 and 30 months of age. At this stage, infant can eat most of the hard foods [24, 25].

1.5.1. Evaluation methods of infant/toddlers feeding disorders

Evaluation methods are: Neonatal Oral-Motor Assessment Scale (NOMAS), Pediatrics Feeding Behavioral Assessment Scale (BPFAS), Pediatric Eating Assessment Tool (Pedi-EAT), Fiberoptic Endoscopic Evaluation of Swallowing (FEES) and Videofluoroscopic Swallow Study (VFSS) for infants and toddlers [23, 26].

The VFSS test is the gold standard for the diagnosis of oropharyngeal dysphagia. VFSS is a radiographic procedure that provides a direct, dynamic view of the oral, pharyngeal and upper esophageal function. Barium bolus is given to the clients during VFSS, and the movement of bolus is observed. Each episode of deglutition starting from the oral phase to until the end of the swallowing function is recorded, all phases of swallowing can be assessed at this time. VFSS provides the most detailed evidence to swallowing problems and provides specific recommendations about the content of food, feeding position (for reducing the aspiration and to provide oral motor skills) [27].

1.5.2. Occupational therapy interventions for feeding disorders

Intervention should plan according to the strength and weakness of infants/toddlers that informations gained from the evaluation process. Therapists' first goal should be providing safety during the intervention session.

1.5.2.1. Enabling swallowing

Occupational therapist can activate swallowing muscles of infants with cold application on the tongue and palate with frozen pacifier. This application helps swallowing muscles to get ready and swallowing duration time get shortened. Occupational therapist can use frozen popsicle or an ice for providing cold application to toddlers. Another method for enabling swallowing is cold or sour bolus (e.g., lemon juice). Therapist should carefully evaluate, and if needed, the cold applications should be carried out for providing swallowing [28, 29].

1.5.2.2. Oxygen support and positioning adaptations

Respiratory disorders may cause problems in coordination sucking-swallowing and breathing (SSwB) of infants, because increased respiratory rate leads to pausing sucking for breathing and cause problems in SSwB coordination. Oxygen support should be provided for infants with low oxygen level during feeding. Thus, respiratory rate gets normal range, and infant can swallow easier [30].

Infants with respiratory disorders usually struggling during the feeding. Because they cannot coordinate SSwB. As a result, breathing becomes an urgent requirement, infants cough or vomit. Glass and Wolf suggest "external pacing" technique for providing external support to SSwB coordination disorders. Occupational therapist should know the suck-swallow-breathe requirements for feeding by bottle and can determine the problems in SSwB coordination. After third to fifth suck without spontaneous suck, break the suction by inserting finger into corner of mouth while leaving the nipple in place, tilt the bottle downward to stop flow of liquid and remove the bottle. Therapist gives an opportunity for breathing and relaxation to infants with the interruption of the sucking [21].

Occupational therapists should consider age, motor developmental level, feeding skills of children to decide best feeding position. Because appropriate positioning provides necessary support during feeding. For newborns and infants, side-lying position in caregiver's arm is appropriate during breast feeding or bottle feeding. Supine position on caregiver's thigh is another appropriate feeding position for infants. This position provides neutral alignment and midline orientation to infants. The caregiver's both hands are free during this position. An another advantage of this position is providing caregivers and infants' eye contact that can promote social interaction during feeding. For toddlers with good sitting posture, high chair or booster seat can be appropriate. The toddler can sit the table, and thus, social and communication skills may increase [19].

1.5.2.3. Sensory integration interventions for feeding disorders

Infants/toddlers with feeding disorders are generally hyper responsive to touch near or within the mouth. Oral hypersensitivity is usually correlated with experiences during neonatal period. Newborns who experienced medical interventions in NICU such as intubation, orogastric or nasogastric tube feeding and the toddlers who cannot experience oral feeding for a prolonged period may exhibit oral hypersensivity. Preterm infants usually have increasing risks for sensory modulation disorders and may experience hyper responsive to tactile stimuli. Cerabral palsy, autism, developmental disorders, genetic disorders and neurologic disorders may lead to exhibition of oral hypersensitivity too [31, 32].

Occupational therapist generally uses desensizitation techniques for intervention to hypersensitivity to touch. Oral desensizitation activities for infants should begin with discovering the mouth with his/her fingers. Therapist may help to infant to take his/her hand to infant's mouth and let the infant to suck the hand. NUK brushes, toothbrushes can use for providing tactile stimulation. Therapist can apply firm pressure to infant's palate for decreasing oral hypersensitivity. Towel's texture touch is easy to manage for infants/toddlers with oral hypersensitivity. Thus, therapist should use towel for brushing or applying pressure and let the infant/toddler suck or chew the towel [31].

Sensory integration activities should contain new flavors and textures for increasing acceptance of foods. Therapist may dip the rubber toy or toothbrush to pured foods or juice for providing oral activities to infants/toddlers. These activities should provide challenge but not disencourage feeding attempts [31].

Positioning adaptations should be done considering the sensory processing disorders in addition to these sensory-based activities. Therapist should provide head and neck support when positioning infants/toddlers to make feel stable and safe, but not constraint whole body movements. Infants/toddlers with general sensory processing disorders may be more undisturbed when sitting on a chair rather than being held by mother's hands, because human touch provides intense sensory stimuli [31].

1.5.2.4. Transition from non-oral feeding to oral feeding

Non-oral feeding methods are using when the infant/toddlers cannot meet his/her nutrition or hydration orally. These methods are nasogastric and orogastric feeding, pharyngostomy, esophagostomy and gastrostomy. They may be used because of dysphagia, infant/toddler's medical problems or infants/toddlers cannot feeding orally to provide adequate growth [33].

Infant/toddlers' medical status and readiness to transition of oral feeding should be evaluated carefully by multidisciplinary team. The team should discuss with the family all the stages of transition process and show respect to family's decisions about transition process (such as beginning time to transition). Occupational therapists should provide assistance to family during all the stages of transition [34].

Oral motor intervention is the first stage of the transition process. Infant/toddler should try to succeed the oral feeding. Occupational therapist should desensitize the near or within the mouth. Therapist tries to increase oral-motor skills during the sensory-based play activities. Desenzitation activities may involve sucking and chewing the rubber toys, NUK brushes and textured fabrics [35]. Babbling activities and blows toys may be other activities to provide oral motor activity. Therapist must emphasize all of the success of infants/toddlers and provide working toward the goals of interventions together with infants/toddlers and their families [36].

The families sometimes have an anxiety about feeding separate from infant/toddlers' medical status or weight loss problems and show increased attention on feeding. This process sometimes cause to infants/toddlers' avoidance or behavioral problems during feeding. Behavioral techniques should be implemented when the feeding problem originated from the behavioral problems of infants/toddlers [37].

The achievement of transition process is dependent on the providing support both infant/ toddlers and their families. The prolonged non-oral feeding duration causes difficulties in transition to oral feeding. The family support groups may be efficient for providing shortened transition to oral feeding [37].

1.6. Motor development

High risk infants usually have problems in motor, cognitive and behavioral responses areas when compared with term infants. These problems may cause negative effects on both child's school success and adolescent period even in adulthood [38, 39].

Motor system includes posture, muscle tonus, reflexes, movements and activities [40, 41]. Characteristically, hypotonia is observed in premature infants. Hypotonia's severity is related to gestational age of infants [42, 43]. For example, an infant who was born at 28 weeks of gestation has wider range of motion than a full-term infant and has more flexibility in shoulders, elbows, hips and knees. Typical positions of premature infant's extremities are extension and abduction. There is an impairment in the midline orientation and flexor patterns. Random movements are generally decreased. Primitive reflexes are decreasing and disappearing or emerging in a contrary manner [44]. Functional motor skills and both gross and fine motor skills delay in premature infants when compared with term infants [45, 46].

Newborn motor skills are influenced by many factors such as autonomic instability, stress, environmental heat, infection, electrolyte irregularity, jaundice, respiratory distress and drugs [40]. One of the most important roles of neonatal occupational therapists is to determine the developmental level of the infant and plan the occupational therapy intervention. In particular, in the first 2 years of life, it is very important to determine the developmental impairment and problems in early motor development for providing early intervention [47].

Motor control or effective use of the body for infants means mobility, discovering the environment and increasing communication skills before talking. Motor control is often on the basis of most intervention programs because of the influence on the social, cognitive and emotional system [48].

1.6.1. Evaluation tools of motor development for infants/toddlers

Motor development in infants and toddlers can be evaluated with Pretechl's Qualitative Assessment of General Movements, Naturalistic Observations of Newborn Behavior, Brazelton Neonatal Behavioral Assessment Scale [40], The Bayley Scales of Infant Development, Psychomotor Developmental Index I-II, Griffiths Locomotor Subscale, Test of Infant Motor Performance, Alberta Infant Motor Scale, The Peabody Developmental Motor Scales, The Vineland Adaptive Behavior Scale, Denver II Gross Motor Sector, Wee Functional Independence Measure, Infant Motor Aktivite Log [49]. Canadian occupational performance measure is used to determine the motor developmental level of infants from the primary caregiver's point of view [50, 51].

1.6.2. Occupational therapy intervention for motor development for infants/toddlers

1.6.2.1. Neurodevelopmental treatment

This intervention was developed by Bobath to provide motor control for children with cerebral palsy. It is a treatment approach widely used by the members of interdisciplinary team [52]. This intervention method is convenience during infancy period [53]. The aim of intervention is to improve function of infant and provide quality of movement with special handling techniques. The therapist and family members provide the physical movement of infant with handling techniques. In addition to therapeutic handling, the therapist can modify the infant's environmental factors to improve function. Environmental adaptations can be simple (using a roll blanket in the cradle to facilitate side-lying positioning) or complex (such as using an infant seat). Adaptations should design according to targets of both family and infant and also matched with treatment principles. For example, if the infant cannot achieve sitting position properly, the sitting adaptations should be done. Adaptations are particularly effective when only meet the goals of the family. The role of the occupational therapist in this intervention is shaping the philosophy in accordance with the function of the other team members [48].

1.6.2.2. Neonatal positioning

Preterm infants often have positional problems that lead to different posture and movement problems. For example, the shoulder protraction and the posterior pelvic tilt occur because the preterm infant cannot perform the neonatal flexion position precisely. If these positions are not corrected, it may not be possible to bring the infant's hands to the midline. These problems lead to delays in the area of fine motor skills and insufficiency in midline hand play. Positioning is not merely to provide of infant comfort, but also focuses on flexion and midline orientation. Positioning can reduce stress and provide psychological stability. This will provide the arrangement of sleep, which is vital for development and weight gain. Each infant's specific positioning needs should be decided on the basis of individuality. The main criterion for selecting the position is infant's presenting problems such as low muscle tone, prolonged extension position, and impaired movements caused by the infant [40].

Positioning techniques: Positioning is carried out in consideration of the individual needs of the infant along with the medical and developmental advantages and disadvantages of each positioning techniques [40].

Prone position: This position facilitates flexion, head control and hand-to-mouth activity. In this position, the bed should be inclined by 15° in order to raise the infant's head. The hip and knees are in the flexion, the arms are near the head in the flexion, the head is on one side, and the hand is on the face near the mouth [40].

Supine position: In this position, this is easy to meet the infant's medical needs and facilitates visual discovery of infant. The infant's knees and hips should be in the right flexion to the abdomen and the feet in this border, the elbows should be on the flexed side of the body, the head should be on midline or on the side where the infant feels comfortable [40].

Side-lying position: It facilitates the midline position of the head and extremities. It also facilitates hand and hand-to-mouth activities, the flexion and adduction of the legs, and prevents the external rotation of the legs. The infant's hips and knees should be in flexion. The arms should be forward and comfortably flexed. The head should be on the midline and a slight flexion if possible. The back should be supported well to maintain the position [40].

Seated position: It is an alternative position for older babies when they are awake. The hip and knees should be positioned symmetrically on the flexion, shoulders on the front and head in the same line as the body or slightly flexed [40].

Positioning is to prevent head flattening: In preterm infants, head tilt is occurring due to the head not being able to hold on the midline, which causes pressure on the sitting side of the head weight, causing a typical head flatness in the soft cartilaginous skull. To prevent this condition in preterm infants, lateral supports can be used in the supine position. It is also suggested to replace water beds, gel pillows and change of head position [40]. All these positioning are very important both in improving neurodevelopmental outcomes and in decreasing infant stress and facilitating sleep. The role of occupational therapist is to give suggestions and train the early intervention team about positioning [40].

1.6.2.3. Modified restricted movement therapy

This intervention suggests the restriction of the unaffected arm's movements and providing the intense use of the affected arm. There are four main steps in the treatment of infants: (a) 24/7 casting of the less affected upper extremity for 23 days, followed by 4 days without casting; (b) intensive occupational therapy sessions for 4 weeks, 5 days a week; (c) family education to improve the use of the affected upper limb and (d) providing treatment services for infant's home. The therapy sessions include functional, play-based, sensory, and force-enhancing activities to enhance the movement of the affected upper limb. The therapist ensures consistent and positive reinforcement for consistency of motor ability. Specific sensory-motor targets can be created for each infant. Play activities are selected by considering the level of infant ability, motivation, environment and goals of the family. Therapists can often use the play in a supine, crawling and supported sitting position with the aim of weighting the affected limb. The tasks selected here are carried out according to the motor learning and are selected for the purpose of releasing the repetitive motions and motor patterns targeted in the therapy. The family is trained to perform targeted activities. These are the activities of the therapist and can be adapted to put in the routine of the family (such as facilitating eating or bathing with the affected hand) [54].

1.6.2.4. Newborn individualized developmental care and assessment program

The basic movements revealed by infant should not be regarded as neurological function only. It should be kept in mind that these movements may be signs of pain and stress. These stress responses may appear as signs of incompatibility between the developmental capacity of the preterm infant and the environment. Occupational therapists can handle this situation with the Newborn Individualized Developmental Care and Assessment Program (NIDCAP) [55].

The NIDCAP can be integrated easily with the Person-Environment-Occupation Model, because NIDCAP assesses infant's psychological and behavioral responses to different handling types together with the environment [56]. Movements observed in NIDCAP are categorized as stress signals or stability signals. These are general extremity movements, specific extremity movements and specific hand movements. In this approach, occupational therapists help preterm infants to self-organizing and to provide engagement in their own environment [56, 57].

In children receiving developmental intervention, it has been shown that there is an increase in the organization of autonomic, motor and state systems and self-regulation. In addition, infants receiving developmental intervention are in a decreased state of alert, and this leads to an increase in the quality of social and environmental interactions. Flexion posture is gained instead of extension posture with the intervention program [40, 58]. In this approach, which is a special developmental intervention, the environment is defined as an important area. The nature of the environment, especially the quality of the home environment, also affects gross motor function [46].

1.6.2.5. Goal activity motor enrichment intervention

The intervention is based on active motor learning, family-based care, family coaching and environmental enrichment. Family goals and environmental enrichment for motor learning are customized according to the child's motor skills. This approach involves the activities according to the targets defined to increase of motor practices and the family with home programs [50]. Together with the family, the basic goals related to motor development are defined. The therapist helps the family to set realistic goals in terms of both developmental and temporal aspects. In this intervention, the family should learn how to help the child, the deviations from the target and the needs of the child. The family also should learn how much help they should offer to the child according to needs. The environment for the child is enriched with the right toy selection to find out the motor movement desired in the treatment. If the therapist sees appropriate, siblings take part in treatment. Therefore, the environment is enriched with mother, siblings, therapist and toys [51].

1.7. Cognitive development

According to Jean Piaget's cognitive development theory, there are four stages of logical thinking: (1) sensory-motor stage (0–2 years), (2) preoperational stage (2–7 years), (3) concrete operational stage (7–11/12 years), and (4) formal operational stage (11/12 years and over) [59].

Sensory motor phase (0–2 years): The infant tries to understand the environment with his/her senses and motor skills. They start to use simple symbols. The information about the world in that the infant is in is very limited, but he learns about the surroundings with motor movements. When they are about 7 months old, they lose the object permanence. This acquisition is especially important because it shows memory development. When children reach their second birthday, they start to use symbols to think and communicate. Language skills develop during this period. They can evaluate the events from a self-centered point of view. They can classify objects. Symbolic plays take an important place in the daily life of the child [60].

This defined cognitive development may be delayed in premature infants. Immaturity in neurologic systems and mother infant separation causes impairments in executive functions in premature infants [61]. However, it has been reported that there is a deficiency in verbal and nonverbal abilities in cognitive development in these infants [62].

1.7.1. Evaluation tools of cognitive development for infants/toddlers

Occupational therapists try to determine the factors that disrupt successful activity performance in the framework of activity performance. Occupational therapist can obtain information about cognition by observing performance, asking questions to family members and using standardized cognitive tests. The standardized cognitive measures used by occupational therapists are usually related to functional tasks and/or daily objects. These are Wee Functional Independence Measure. Peabody Picture Vocabulary Test-Revised, Bayley Scale of Infant Development-2nd edition [63].

1.7.2. Occupational therapy intervention for cognitive development for infants/toddlers

Early intervention methods to increase cognitive skills of infants, which are applied by occupational therapists are family-based approaches, developmental interventions and kangaroo care [64–68].

1.7.2.1. Developmental interventions

These interventions can be applied at neonatal intensive care unit, at home, child care services and kindergarten. Developmental interventions result in gains in early cognitive development (e.g., infant and preschool age) with inconclusive evidence for gains through school age [64].

1.7.2.2. Kangaroo care

Kangaroo care contributes to the neural maturation of prematurity in the neonatal period. There is a increase in autonomic function, maternal attachment and decrease maternal anxiety after care. This leads to the development of cognitive development and executive functions of the child [65].

1.7.2.3. Creating opportunities for parent empowerment

The education of families of preterm infants is very sensitive to the needs of infants and is very responsive to increased cognitive and attention interaction. The theoretical framework of the intervention is based on the theory of self-regulation and control. Being able to cope means cognition and behavioral change in order to meet specific internal and external demands. This concept of coping involves arranging emotional responses and problem solving. It is also very important to assess the ability of the mother to cope and its consequences. In such a program, mothers will be informed about their infants' behavior and will be able to better understand their infants and what they can do. This will increase the infant and mother interaction in an appropriate manner. In the early period, high-quality family-infant interaction influences cognitive and social-emotional development positively. Negative mode of mother, family stress and low level family confidence are problems in child development and behavior in the later period [66].

At the beginning of the practice, infant's characteristics, stage of development, behaviors, and the intensive care unit where the infant is located are evaluated and recorded by mother. Then therapists should do recommendations to provide caregivers participation in the care and development of the infant, the identification of the infant's signs of stress and communication readiness, the identification of strategies for calming, and the implementation of the strategies learned in the hospital in the post-discharge period at home [66–68].

In home-based therapy, occupational therapist learns how to interact with the infant's environment and infant's development of adaptations. More realistic and helpful approaches are offered. Targets are defined according to the needs of the infant, in accordance with the socio-economic situation of the family. These goals are facilitating the play development, normal sensory-motor development, and socio-economic development of infant with the family-infant interaction. At the same time, it is discussed with the family in relation to premature infants, general development, risk factors of premature infants and play development in children in this treatment [62].

1.8. Play development

In the context of occupational behavior, play is considered as the primary activity of the child and precondition for the fight/competition of occupational roles in the next life. Observation of the play is easy, but it is difficult to define it theoretically. The play is multidirectional behavior. Internal motivation and enjoyment are often considered in the construction of the play. Play has competing and exploration component. Work and play are developmental continuity; play continuity provides adaptive function in adulthood. During the play, children have the opportunity to explore the surrounding objects and people, how they affect it, develop and test their social and occupational roles. When children move around, they discover the world, receive information from the senses, learn about the properties and nature of the objects, understand their space and time localization. These abilities evolve during the play as children respond to the demands of the environment and interact with them. This provides perceptual, conceptual, intellectual and linguistic development, resulting in the final combination of the cognitive abilities [69]. Child establishes an interactive relationship with peers and learn different roles such as imagining scenarios and preparing food, being a cop or being a firefighter. The success of the role of the player gives meaningful occupational connection and increases the quality of life for child [70].

Children learn by playing games. One of the first steps in the learning process is that the child is self-aware. After that, he is ready to practice and learn other things related to him. Then, the child moves one step and learns the names of the parts he touches. Then he may explain, "My mouth is under my nose, my ears on the sides of my head." Then the child uses what they learn and relate to his toys. The baby moves and crawls to recognize both the space and the body. As a result, the child uses this information when feeding, washing and starting to self-dress.

At the same time, the child must learn and understand the world around him. Children learn differences between shapes and structures by playing plays. He does this when he starts taking objects into his mouth. While child learn what to do with the objects in the environment; also he learns to make sound from their toys, shoot and build them. Although the child learns all these and more while playing, as he grows asking questions, practices, learns the wrongs, and improves his skills [71].

1.8.1. *Evaluation tools of play development for infants/toddlers*

Evaluation should be made in the natural environment of infant. The evaluation should be done in consideration of the infant's position and the time spent in that position, play development, repertoire, play phase, play interests [41, 72]. However, play frequency, current toy variety, physical environment, social interaction with peers and caregivers should be considered in these processes. The cultural structure also affects the value of the play. The occupational therapist should use structured measures as well as the child observes in the unstructured environment. However, the occupational therapist should evaluate the play over as many as five factors: (1) What the infant/toddlers do. (2) Why the infant/toddlers enjoy chosen play activities. (3) How the infant/toddlers approach to the play? (4) Infant's capacity to play. (5) The relative supportiveness of environment. Standard scales that can be used for play assessments are: Play history, test of playfulness version 4, Revised Knox Preschool Play Scale, Child-Initiated Play Assessment, Transdisciplinary Play-Based Assessment, Test of Environmental Supportiveness, Home Observation for Measurement of the environment [63].

1.8.2. *Occupational therapy intervention for play development for infants/toddlers*

Occupational therapist working in sensory integration, neurodevelopmental, occupational behavior and developmental contexts describe the social, constructive and sensorimotor benefits of play and widely use as a treatment modality [69]. Occupational therapists may encounter difficulties in combining plays with different treatments. For example, a spastic diplegic infant's muscle tone may be exacerbated by effort spent. The therapist can benefit from the play of regulating the tone without disturbing the motivation, curiosity and discovery necessary for the play. Alternatively, it may facilitate cognitive and social development without producing abnormal motion patterns. The clinical decision requires that actual treatment targets be met within infinite total needs [48] or an infant who is hypersensitive to touch may not want to play textured toys. In this example, the occupational therapist can provide the toy that can be adapted to the sensory preference of the child, and giving information to the family about the toy preference of child during the play participation [73].

Occupational therapists define play as a therapeutic intervention, a way of strengthening intervention, a way of developing role. They also use the play as an evaluation tool [74]. Infants and toddlers spend most of their time with playing during the time they are awake. Therefore, play is a very important issue for occupational therapists. Research reveals clearly the relationship between play and learning as well as play and development [75].

According to infant space theory, infant's play development happens in four stages up to 18 months. The first stage of development is visual play. During the first 2 months, infants are scanned with mothers, then, object tracking outside the visual field, choosing objects, playing with hiding, using eyes and hands together. The second stage of development is mapping and changing the infant's house view. The third stage of development is play with a fixed object, and the fourth stage of development is play with a mobile object [76].

In play development, the first stage of playing with an object is called an exploratory play. Exploratory play (2–10th months) is the way to evaluate the environment to gain information from objects or toys for infants. The second phase is the relational use of objects (10–18th months). At this stage, objects are combined and defined by hand. Then, the use of functional objects (12–18th month) is learned. Finally, symbolic play is learned (18–30th month) [77]. As a result, therapists should consider treatment plans in view of all these developments.

Occupational therapists use play-related approaches with interdisciplinary approaches. Piaget's cognitive and play development theories and Gesell's motor development theory are among them. It is stated that children show the best performance for play in their natural habitats. In the structured circles, it is stated that the play has less effect on the development than the play in the home environment. It is not easy to create natural environmental opportunities to develop infant skills, but it is very important for development. Occupational therapists use natural play opportunities to create enriched playing environment for infant. Occupational therapists find out what is limiting and makes the necessary adaptations for infant. However, how the spatial structure of the clinical and educational environment affects, development is also assessed. All approaches should be done with the family involvement [76].

The occupational therapist should fully understand the individual and environmental factors, the role of the player, and the time required for the play, in order to facilitate the infant's play experience and specialize in the player role. The role of the occupational therapist is to improve the child's potential and abilities for play, to ensure participation in play, to organize the cultural, social, temporal and physical environment that supports the play. The child's abilities and interests are influenced by the barrier and support of the playing neighborhood, the difficulties and convenience of the play [69].

Playing without constraints allows the infant to discover his own capacity, experiment with objects, make decisions, understand cause-effect relationships, learn, insist and understand the results. This kind of play strengthens the child's creativity and improves social development, especially when played with a peer. It also provides the child to learn how to cope with anxiety, frustration and fatigue. Unfortunately, a disabled infant is deprived of the benefits of playing regularly. As a result of this situation, being dependent on another individuals, low motivation, loss of confidence, reduced social skills in unstructured situations can occur for infants. These results will adversely affect the development of the child both early and later in life. Preventing secondary problems is a very important role for the occupational therapist [72, 75].

Many obstacles are defined in front of non-constraint play. The obstacle created by the caregiver (not knowing exactly what the child will do, risk of injury, etc.), physical and individual limitations of the child (such as inadequate mobility and communication, difficulty in reaching and understanding, impaired sensory responses, reduced internal motivation and concentration), environmental (limitations on home and playground) and social barriers (peer and family interaction problems), cause to the children be deprived from the play.

The occupational therapist has the opportunity to work with these children at home, in the field of treatment, or in a wide range of social settings. Occupational therapist can facilitate this consulting process by being aware of the obstacles frequently encountered by the child and by defining the child's abilities at the same time [69, 75].

In this context, opportunities for free play should be created. Play should be actualized at home, in the community, or during therapy. Opportunities must be created for the child to choose, explore, create, and respond to change in order to be free. At all possible times, the family should be encouraged to explore the child and to establish an independent relationship. The family must understand the value of the play as well as the importance of the play in terms of health and development [69].

The relationship between the family and child should be mutual. Family's anticipations and beliefs will affect the quality of the play. Sometimes parents see negatively motivation, self-concept development, and very active participation. In that case, it may be useful to increase the participation of siblings or peers at home or on the playground. The occupational therapist clearly displays the practices that the family will do at home and matches the objects and spaces in the house appropriately. The goals of typical play development take place in daily life experiences. With the treatment being understandable, the therapist and the family will put it in the target they want to see in the child. Thus, therapist uses the natural objects in the house more effectively, and the family contributes to this improvement by using many small play opportunities in everyday life. In this approach, the occupational therapist can place the objects near the child to develop the child's visual play, follows child to create home memory, and plays along the edges of the room to create spatial development patterns. For playing with stationary objects occupational therapist can use single or combined object plays that can be found in house-rich playgrounds. Any area of the house (curtains, bookshelf, corridors) and objects can be used for therapeutic toys, far from commercial toys. The therapist can actively take part in the typical development of mobile object play interventions such as dancing, climbing, driving and transporting. At the same time, the therapist can train the family on daily activities and routines for the child to explore the home environment and to promote movement [69, 77].

As a result, the play is child-centered, organized in the form of flexible and needs-based interventions with a holistic perspective with participation in the family in occupational therapy approaches.

Author details

Serkan Pekçetin[1*] and Ayla Günal[2]

*Address all correspondence to: serkanpekcetin@gmail.com

1 Department of Occupational Therapy, Faculty of Health Sciences, Trakya University, Edirne, Turkey

2 Department of Physiotherapy and Rehabilitation, Faculty of Health Sciences Gaziosmanpasa University, Tokat, Turkey

References

[1] Reed KL. Quick Reference to Occupational Therapy. 2nd ed. Austin, Tex: An Aspen Publication; 2003. pp. 79-85.

[2] Muller-Nix C, Forcada-Guex M, Pierrehumbert B, Jaunin L, Borghim A, Ansermet F. Prematurity, maternal stres and motherchild interactions. Early Human Development. 2004;**79:**145-158.

[3] Nieder-Heitmann E. The impact of a sensory developmental care programme for very low birth weight preterm infants in the neonatal intensive care unit [master thesis]. Stellenbosch: University of Stellenbosch; 2010.

[4] Vanderburg KA. Individualized developmental care for high risk newborns in the NICU: A practice guideline. Early Human Development. 2007;**83:**433-42.

[5] Bundy AC, Lane SJ, Murray EA. Sensory Integration Theory and Practice. Philadelphia: F. A. Davis Company; 2002. pp. 3-35.

[6] Williamson GG, Anzalone MA. Sensory Integration and Self Regulation in Infants and Toddlers: Helping Very Young Child Interact with Their Environment. Washington, DC: Zero to Three; 2001.

[7] Roley SS, Blanche EI, Schaaf RC. Understanding the Nature of Sensory Integration with Diverse Populations. Therapy Skill Builders; 2001.

[8] Eeles AL, Spittle AJ, Anderson PJ, Brown N, Lee KJ, Boyd RN, Doyle LW. Assessments of sensory processing in infants: A systematic review. Developmental Medicine & Child Neurology. 2013;**55(4):**314-326.

[9] DeGangi GA. An integrated intervention approach to treating infants and young children with regulatory, sensory processing, and interactional problems1. USA: ICDL ClinicalPractice Guidelines; 2000. pp. 215-242.

[10] Dunn W. Supporting children to participate successfully in everyday life by using sensory processing knowledge. Infant & Young Children. 2007;**20(2):**84-101

[11] Yack E, Aquilla P, Sutton S. Building Bridges Through Sensory Integration. 2nd ed. USA: Sensory Resources; 2002. pp. 21-38.

[12] Gomez CR, Baird S. Regulatory disorder identification, diagnosis and intervention planning. Infants and Young Children. 2004;**17(4):**327-339.

[13] Case-Smith J. Systematic review of interventions to promote social–emotional development in young children with or at risk for disability. American Journal of Occupational Therapy. 2013;**67(4):**395-404.

[14] Greenspan SI, DeGangi G, Wieder S. The Functional Emotional Assessment Scale (FEAS) for Infancy and Early Childhood: Clinical and Research Applications. USA: Interdisciplinary Council on Developmental and Learning Disorders; 2001. pp. 131-167.

[15] Halle TG, Darling-Churchill KE. Review of measures of social and emotional development. Journal of Applied Developmental Psychology. 2016;**45:**8-18.

[16] Tibby G. The Developmental, Individual Difference, Relationship-based (DIR) Model. Skyhorse Publishing, New York; 2010

[17] Greenspan SI, Wieder S. The Child with Special Needs. Persues Book, Massachusetts; 1998.

[18] Kasari C, Paparella T, Freeman S, Jahromi LB. Language outcome in autism: Randomized comparison of joint attention and play interventions. Journal of Consulting and Clinical Psychology. 2008;**76(1):**125-137.

[19] Case-Smith J. Pediatric Occupational Therapy and Early Intervention. U.S.A.: Butterworth-Heinemann; 1998. pp. 49-83.

[20] Rommel N, De Meyer AM, Feenstra L, Veereman-Wauters G. The complexity of feeding problems in 700 infants and young children presenting to a tertiary care institution. Journal of Pediatric Gastroenterology and Nutrition. 2003;**37(1):**75-84.

[21] Wolf LS, Glass RP. Feeding and Swallowing Disorders in Infancy: Assesment and Management. Tucson, AZ: Therapy Skills Builder; 1992.

[22] Lau C. Development of suck and swallow mechanisms in infants. Annals of Nutrition and Metabolism. 2015;**66(5):**7-14

[23] Arvedson JC. Swallowing and feeding in infants and young children. GI Motility online. 2006.

[24] Toomey K. Feeding strategies for older infants and toddlers. Pediatric Basics. 2002;**100:** 2-11.

[25] Wilson EM, Green JR. The development of jaw motion for mastication. Early Human Development. 2009;**85(5):**303-311.

[26] Thoyre SM, Pados BF, Park J, Estrem H, Hodges EA, McComish C, Murdoch K. Development and content validation of the pediatric eating assessment tool (pedi-EAT). American Journal of Speech-Language Pathology. 2014;**23(1):**46-59.

[27] Martin-Harris B, Jones B. The videofluorographic swallowing study. Physical Medicine and Rehabilitation Clinics of North America. 2008;**19(4):**769-785.

[28] Alper BS, Manno CJ. Dysphagia in infants and children with oral-motor deficits: Assessment and management. Seminars in Speech and Language. 1996;**17(4):**283-310.

[29] Logemann JA, Pauloski BR, Colangelo L, Lazarus C, Fujiu M, Kahrilas PJ. Effects of a sour bolus on oropharyngeal swallowing measures in patients with neurogenic dysphagia. Journal of Speech, Language, and Hearing Research. 1995;**38(3):**556-563.

[30] Case-Smith J. Pediatric Occupational Therapy and Early Intervention. U.S.A.: Butterworth-Heinemann; 1998. pp. 127-167.

[31] Case-Smith J, O'Brien JC. Occupational Therapy for Children. USA: Mosby; 2010. pp. 446-474.

[32] Cermak SA, Curtin C, Bandini LG. Food selectivity and sensory sensitivity in children with autism spectrum disorders. Journal of the American Dietetic Association. 2010;**110(2):**238-246.

[33] Birnbaum R, Limperopoulos C. Nonoral feeding practices for infants in the neonatal intensive care unit. Advances in Neonatal Care. 2009;**9(4):**180-184.

[34] Bazyk S. Factors associated with the transition to oral feeding in infants fed by nasogastric tubes. American Journal of Occupational Therapy. 1990;**44(12):**1070-1078.

[35] Fucile S, Gisel E, Lau C. Oral stimulation accelerates the transition from tube to oral feeding in preterm infants. The Journal of Pediatrics. 2002;**141(2):**230-236.

[36] Dunbar SB, Jarvis AH, Breyer M. The transition from nonoral to oral feeding in children. American Journal of Occupational Therapy. 1991;**45(5):**402-408.

[37] Manikam R, Perman JA. Pediatric feeding disorders. Journal of Clinical Gastroenterology. 2000;**30(1):**34-46.

[38] Johnson S, Ring W, Anderson P, Marlow N. Randomized trial of parental support for families with very preterm children: outcome at 5 years. Archives of Diseases in Childhood. 2005;**90(9):**909-915.

[39] Marlow N. Neurocognitive outcome after very preterm birth. Archives of Diseases in Childhood Fetal Neonatal Edition. 2004;**89(3):**224-228.

[40] Hutchon B. Occupational therapy in the neonatal intensive care unit. In: Hong CS, Howard L, editors. Occupational Therapy in Childhood. Philadelphia: Whurr Publishers Ltd; 2002. pp. 153-191.

[41] Bumin G. The principles of occupational therapy in pediatric rehabilitation. In: Elbasan B, editor. Pediatric Physiotherapy Rehabilitation. 1st ed. İstanbul: Medical Publishing Scientific Works Series; 2017. pp. 309-320.

[42] Lenke MC. Motor outcomes in premature infants. Newborn and infant. Nursing Reviews. 2003;**3(3):**104-109.

[43] Krusteva MB, Krustev BP, Mileva SA. Neonatal muscle hypotonia-an early manifestation of cerebral palsy. Folia Medica (Plovdiv). 2000;**42(3):**37-40.

[44] GGücüyener K. Neurological examination of high risk infants. In: Elbasan B, editor. Pediatric Physiotherapy Rehabilitation. 1st ed. İstanbul: Medical Publishing Scientific Works Series; 2017. pp. 13-28.

[45] Snider L, Majnemer A, Mazer B, Campbell S, Bos AF. Prediction of motor and functional outcomes in infants born preterm assessed at term. Pediatric Physical Therapy. 2009;**21(1)**:2-11.

[46] Goyen TA, Lui K. Longitudinal motor development of "apparently normal" high-risk infants at 18 months, 3 and 5 years. Early Human Development. 2002;**70(1-2)**:103-115.

[47] Developmental delay: An information guide for parents, The Royal Children's Hospital. Available from; http://recil.grupolusoforapt [Accessed: 20.01.2017]

[48] Gorga D. Occupational therapy treatment practices with infants in early intervention. The American Journal of Occupational Therapy. 1989;**43(11)**:731-736.

[49] Mutlu A. Early neuromotor assessment methods in pediatrics. In: Elbasan B, editor. Pediatric Physiotherapy Rehabilitation. İstanbul: Medical Publishing Scientific Works Series; 2017. pp. 55-62.

[50] Morgan C, Novak I, Dale RC, Guzzetta A, Badawi N. Single blind randomised controlled trial of GAME (Goals-Activity-Motor Enrichment) in infants at high risk ofcerebral palsy. Research Developmental Disabilities. 2016;**55**:256-267.

[51] Morgan C, Novak I, Dale RC, Guzzetta A, Badawi N. GAME (Goals-Activity-Motor Enrichment): protocol of a single blind randomised controlled trial of motor training, parent education and environmental enrichment for infants at high risk of cerebral palsy. BMC Neurology. 2014;**14(203)**:1-9.

[52] Bobath B. The very early treatment of cerebral palsy. Developmental Medicine and Child Neurology. 1967; **9(4)**:373-390.

[53] Kong E. Very early treatment of cerebral palsy. Developmental Medicine and Child Neurology. 1966;**8(2)**:198-222.

[54] Lowes LP, Mayhan M, Orr T, Batterson N, Tonneman JA, Meyer A, Alfano L, Wang W, Whalen CN, Nelin MA, Lo WD, Case-Smith J. Pilot study of the efficacy of constraint-ınduced movement therapy for ınfants and toddlers with cerebral palsy. Physical Occupational Therapy Pediatrics. 2014;**34(1)**:4-21.

[55] Westrup B. Newborn individualized developmental care and assessment program (NIDCAP)-Family-centered developmentally supportive care. Early Human Development. 2007;**83(7)**:443-449.

[56] Holsti L, Grunau RE. Extremity movements help occupational therapists identify stress responses in preterm infants in the neonatal intensive care unit: A systematic review. Canadian Journal of Occupational Therapy. 2007;**74(3)**:183-194.

[57] Als H, McAnulty GB. The newborn individualized developmental care and assessment program (NIDCAP) with kangaroo mother care (KMC): Comprehensive care for preterm infants. Current Women's Health Reviews. 2011;**7(3)**:288-301.

[58] Mouradian LE, Als H. The influence of neonatal intensive caregiving practices on motor functioning of preterm infants. The American Journal of Occupational Therapy. 1994;**48(6)**:527-533.

[59] Piaget J. The theory of stages in cognitive development. In: Green DR, Ford MP, Flamer GB, editors. Measurement and Piaget. New York McGraw-Hill; 1971. pp. 1-11.

[60] Simatwa EMW. Piaget's theory of intellectual development and its implication for instructional management at presecondary school level. Educational Research and Reviews. 2010;**5(7)**:366-371.

[61] Aarnoudse-Moens CSH, Duivenvoorden HJ, Weisglas-Kuperus N, Van Goudoever JB, Oosterlaan J. The profile of executive function in very preterm children at 4 to 12 years. Developmental Medicine and Child Neurology. 2012;**54(3)**:247-253.

[62] Ment LR, Vohr B, Allan W, Katz KH, Schneider KC, Westerveld M, Duncan CC, Makuch RW. Change in cognitive function over time in very low-birth-weight infants. JAMA. 2003;**289(6)**:705-711.

[63] Law M, Baum C, Dunn W. Measuring Occupational Performance: Supporting Best Practice in Occupational Therapy 2nd ed. United States of America: SLACK Incorporated; 2005. pp. 129-149.

[64] Frolek Clark GJ, Schlabach TL. Systematic review of occupational therapy interventions to improve cognitive development in children ages birth-5 years. The American Journal of Occupational Therapy. 2013;**67(4)**:425-430.

[65] Feldman R, Rosenthal Z, Eidelman AI. Maternal-preterm skin-to-skin contact enhances child physiologic organization and cognitive control across the first 10 years of life. Biological Psychiatry. 2014;**75(1)**:56-64.

[66] Melnyk BM, Alpert-Gillis L, Feinstein NF, Fairbanks E, Schultz-Czarniak J, Hust D, Sherman L, LeMolne C, Moldenhauer Z, Small L, Bender N, Sinkin RA. Improving cognitive development of low-birth-weight premature ınfants with the COPE program: A pilot study of the bene®t of early NICU intervention with mothers. Research in Nursing Health. 2001;**24(5)**:373-389.

[67] Benzies KM, Magill-Evans JE, Hayden KA, Ballantyne M. Key components of early intervention programs for preterm infants and their parents: A systematic review and meta-analysis. BMC Pregnancy Childbirth. 2013;**13(Suppl 1)**:1-15.

[68] Colyvas JL, Sawyer LB, Campbell PH. Identifying strategies early intervention occupational therapists use to teach caregivers. The American Journal of Occupational Therapy. 2010;**64(5)**:776-785.

[69] Missiuna C, Pollock N. Play deprivation in children with physical disabilities: The role of the occupational therapist in preventing secondary disability. The American Journal of Occupational Therapy. 1991;**45(10)**:882-888.

[70] Rigby P, Rodger S. Developing as a player. In: Rodger S, Zivani j, editors. Occupational Therapy with Children. USA: Blackwell Publishing Ltd; 2006. pp. 177-199.

[71] Kayıhan H. Play. In: Kayıhan H, editor. Cerebral Palsy Child and Independent Living. Ankara: Hacettepe University Physical Therapy Rehabilitation High School Publications; 1995. pp. 183-221.

[72] Salls JS, Silverman LN, Gatty CM. The relationship of infant sleep and play positioning to motor milestone achievement. The American Journal of Occupational Therapy. 2002;**56(5)**:577-580.

[73] Corbetta D, Williams JL, Haynes JM. Bare fingers, but no obvious influence of "prickly" Velcro! In the absence of parents' encouragement, it is not clear that "sticky mittens" provide an advantage to the process of learning to reach. Infant Behavior Development. 2016;**42**:168-178.

[74] Couch KJ, Deitz JC, Kanny EM. The role of play in pediatric occupational therapy. The American Journal of Occupational Therapy. 1998;**52(2)**:111-117.

[75] Learning Through Play. Available from; http://www.aota.org/about-occupational-therapy/patients-clients/childrenandyouth/play.aspx. [Accessed: 29.01.2017]

[76] Pierce D, Munier V, Myers CT. Informing early intervention through an occupational science description of infant-todler interactions with home space. The American Journal of Occupational Therapy. 2009;**63(3)**:273-287.

[77] Baranek GT, Barnett CR, Adams EM, Wolcott NA, Watson LR, Crais ER. Object play in ınfants with autism: Methodological ıssues in retrospective video analysis. The American Journal of Occupational Therapy. 2005;**59(1)**:20-30.

8

Assistive Technology in Occupational Therapy

Gokcen Akyurek, Sinem Kars, Zeynep Celik,
Ceren Koc and Özge Buket Cesim

Abstract

In this chapter, occupational therapists from leading specialists exploring ways they can collaborate with assistive technology (AT) users to help them get the most out of these devices. By gratefully acknowledging the advances in technology of the last century, people with disabilities can live independent lives, contribute to their communities, attend regular schools, and work in a career. This technological development means medically switching to a social model of technology presentation, where users are as much focused on social reintegration as their physical abilities. This change means that field workers will not be able to focus on delivering technology on their own but will have to go one step further and partner with consumers and communities to ensure that the aids are used in the best possible way.

Keywords: assistive technology, disabilities, performance areas, funding, disability

1. Introduction: assistive technology definition

Dictionaries provide the following definition of technology: (1) the science or study of the practical or industrial arts and (2) applied science and (3) a method, process, etc., for handling a specific technical problem. However, none of these definitions says anything about a *device*. We call an *assistive technology* for this important concept. It refers to a broad range of devices, services, strategies, and practices that are designed and applied to improve the problems of people with disabilities. One definition of an assistive technology device is used in public law of the United States as follows:

> *"Any items, piece of equipment or product system whether acquired commercially off the shelf, modified, or customized that is used to increase, maintain or improve functional capabilities of individuals with disabilities"* [1].

This definition comprises several important details like such as commercial, modified, and customized devices. But the most important that emphasizes *functional* capabilities of *individuals* with disabilities are the main topics of occupational therapy.

Technology has an important place in our daily life. Occupational therapy uses technology to increase the occupational performance and participation of their clients. Therefore, technology is an important application of occupational therapy services.

Assistive technology services include evaluating the needs, selecting the appropriate device, purchasing the device, providing support to the user and other interested persons in the process of adapting to the device, and training staff.

Occupational therapists use some evaluation methods like activity analysis in the therapy process in order to meet the activity demands of each client in context. They consider the tools used to meet their occupational demands and consider about the skills and abilities of the clients with which tools they use. These tools can be an assistive technology as a definition, if they increase, maintain, or improve someone's functional capabilities. If these tools typically used to improve the performance of the activity do not match the skills and abilities of the client, the therapist adapts or changes them, as he or she will use them. Therefore, providing assistive technology devices and services is an important element of occupational therapy intervention to support individuals, improve their performance, and increase their participation for their activities [2].

2. A historical perspective on assistive technology devices and services

Although industry of assistive technology is very demanding, important developments in this topic began to appear about 30 years ago. If you want to look at its root, it is needed to go old times. Let us imagine we are at the Stone Age; a friend broke his foot in the hunt. However, there was no plaster at that time; therefore, his foot is left to self-healing process. When he began to heal, he started to limp. However, he had to provide food to his clan. So that, he used a stick that would help him walk. In this way, the first assistive technology tool has come up. At that time, a special tool is named as high technology. As time passes, it is decided that assistive technologies respond to other needs also.

After the stick, it is discovered that empty animal horn can be used for loading to voice. Thus, it can be supported to fade hearing. As another example, the wheel that provides the transportation is an invention that is reinvented many times over the years. This device is the most important component of the current wheelchair. The most important thing in these devices at the past is that they were functioning extensively in terms of form or style. The stick that is used as a walking tool is similar with the todays' crutches and canes. The animal horn is only functionally related with the current hearing aids as well. The major point that will carry us to the next step in assistive technology is the similarity between the examples from the past and todays' assistive technology.

2.1. Evolution of the latest assistive technology

Assistive technology always is shaped according to the materials of the time. All the time, the functionality is more important than other features. Therefore, for many years, some applications have been modified little. The stick is an example; although its structure remains same, the material is modified. For sure, the other developments are only feasible as long as technologies are evolved. Over the years, some events that have happened have ensured these developments. For example, the Civil War in the United States especially provided the improvements in lower limb prostheses. In order to create a better fit and to be more functional outcome, sockets were enhanced. A socket developed by Parmelee in 1863 featured the first suction attachment of lower limb prosthesis [3]. Still, this kind of socket is used to prevent alignment problems and the risk of breakage at the joint. Though, there is a little similarity between the materials used in the past and today. As the current prosthesis consists of metal and plastic, Parmelee's component consists of wood and leather.

The miniature electronic circuits that were replaced with animal horn have been reached approximately in the last 35 years. Although this hearing aid was patented in the 1890s, throughout the years its actual function has not been changed. The only thing changed is its structure (fit in to the ear, amplify a wider range of sounds, and more effective). In the last 100 years, much progress has been made in comparison with the improvements made after 1890 with the horn hearing aid produced.

The development in electronics is the reason of gain today. In some conditions, the current assistive technology applications were not possible up to 15 years ago, and especially developments of the computers provide this situation. The biggest development is the existence of the microprocessor electronic circuit named as chip that reduces complicacy in computer design and structure. It is provided that room-sized devices are reduced by microprocessor up to affordable sizes that everyone can get. Moreover, microprocessors have become useful in our life such as microwave ovens and household appliances, not only in computer technology. These chips make possible developments in assistive technology such as synthesized speech, robotic aids, and computer graphics.

The recent improvements in assistive technology devices and the industrial developments in assistive technology have been affected by federal legislation in the United States, and the summary of this legislation is shown below.

2.1.1. Recent major US federal legislation affecting assistive technologies

- Rehabilitation Act of 1973, as amended
- Individuals with Disabilities Education Act amendments of 1997
- Assistive Technology Act of 1998 (replaced Technology-Related Assistance for Individuals with Disabilities Act of 1998)
- The Developmental Disabilities Assistance of Bill Rights Act

- American with Disabilities Act (ADA) of 1990
- Medicaid
- Early and Periodic Screening, Diagnosis, and Treatment Program
- Medicare

This legislation basically mandates the facilitate access to or the use of assistive technologies by providing structure to society by prohibiting discrimination and provides services that may include assistive technologies, in relation to assistive technology.

2.2. Developments in Turkey

In our country, the statistical institution of Turkey in 2002 carried out the first comprehensive research on the people with disabilities. The second research was done in 2010 and the results were analyzed. It has been found that the analysis results in basically five categories (physical, visual, hearing, speech, and mental) of disabilities and about 9 million of the total population.

Disability is not only the person who is experiencing this problem; it is a question that affects his/her family and the surrounding environment economically, socially, and psychologically; and each group with disabilities has different needs.

While it is a disadvantage for some to be advanced and expensive, for some, simple and inexpensive technological tools can reshape their way of life. On this account, their lives can be made more livable and sustainable. Thanks to today's advanced information and communication technologies, approximately one in every eight people in the community is able to survive on better terms, becoming both necessary and feasible for them and for the general health of the community.

In addition, many legal regulations introduce responsibilities for people with disabilities. The Constitution obliges the right to work, education and social security and similar rights of all members of the society directly and indirectly in the 17-I, 42-I, 49-I, 50-I and 50-II, and 61-I materials. The regulation of 61-I, "The state takes measures to protect the people with disabilities and their adaptation to the society's life" is the responsibility of the state to take measures to protect the people with disabilities and to ensure their adaptation to society. On the other hand, Article 5 of the Electronic Communication Law No. 5809 states that "The special needs of people with disabilities, elderly and other people in need of social protection, including the use of technological innovations, are taken into account." In addition, Article 5 of the Consumer Rights Regulation in the Electronic Communications Sector stipulates, "Visually impaired persons have the right to demand subscription contracts and invoices so that they can benefit from them." Again, in our Institutional 2010–2012 Strategic Plan, it was aimed to raise awareness among entrepreneurs in related fields, including how to make access to electronic communication services easier for people with disabilities, such as accessing products and services accessible to other consumers.

3. Ethics and standards of practice

"The study of standards of conduct and moral judgment… and the system or code of morals of a particular… profession" is ethics definition [4]. When applied to a field of professional endeavor such as assistive technology delivery or a profession such as occupational therapy or rehabilitation engineering, the ethical conduct of practitioners is embodied both in code (or canons) of ethics and in standards of practice. Each assistive technology practitioner (ATP) must comply with the code of ethics for his or her discipline (e.g., rehabilitation engineering, occupational or physical therapy, speech-language pathology, or vocational rehabilitation counseling). The professional association serving a discipline generally develops the code of ethics for it. As discussed, ATPs have responsibilities in assistive technology service delivery that are not specified by their individual discipline's code of ethics. For this reason, it is important to have a code of ethics that addresses the specific issues related to the application of assistive technologies. Standards of practice differ from codes of ethics in that they describe more specifically what is and is not considered to be good practice in a given discipline [5].

A standard is a document. Professional practitioner can find everything in this document about providing requirements, specifications, guidelines, or characteristics that can be used consistently to ensure that materials, products, processes, and services are fit for their purpose. ISO standards are an important tool, because they give information about the specifications and guidelines on how to design products and services that are accessible to everybody, to manufacturers, service providers, designers, and policy makers. There are quite a few alternative methods for grouping assistive technology. The most well-known and official classification of assistive technology is the International Classification of ISO 9999 or its European Standard CEN 29999. ISO 9999:2011 establishes a classification of assistive products, especially produced or generally available, for persons with disability. Assistive products used by a person with disability, but which require the assistance of another person for their operation, are included in the classification. The following items are specifically excluded from ISO 9999:2011: items used for the installation of assistive products; solutions obtained by combinations of assistive products that are individually classified in ISO 9999:2011; medicines; assistive products and instruments used exclusively by healthcare professionals; nontechnical solutions, such as personal assistance, guide dogs, or lipreading; implanted devices; and financial support.

There are a number of different usability standards (Bevan 2001ab; Earthy, 2001); some of them are ISO 9241 series, ISO/IEC 9126 ISO 20282 Ease of Operation of Everyday Products, ISO 9241, ISO 14915, IEC TR 61997, ISO CD 9241-151, ISO 13406, ISO 13407, ISO 16982, and ISO WD 20282. These usability standards are about different issues such as a definition of usability; product quality, which defines usability in terms of understandability, learnability, operability, and attractiveness; the usability of the user interface of everyday products; ergonomic requirements for office work with visual display terminals; software ergonomics for multimedia user interfaces; and guidelines for the user interfaces in multimedia equipment for general purpose use [6–9].

3.1. Code of ethics for assistive technologies: the RESNA Code of Ethics

RESNA is an interdisciplinary professional association whose activities focus on assistive technologies. Its members come from many disciplines and a variety of settings, and their activities involve the full scope of assistive technology applications. In 1991 the RESNA Board of Directors adopted the code of ethics shown in **Figure 1**. This code is similar to those of other

RESNA Code of Ethics

RESNA is an interdisciplinary association for the advancement of rehabilitation and assistive technology. It adheres to and promotes the highest standards of ethical conduct. Its members and credentialed service providers:

- Hold paramount the welfare of persons served professionally.
- Practice only in their area(s) of competence and maintain high standards.
- Maintain the confidentiality of privileged information.
- Engage in no conduct that constitutes a conflict of interest or that adversely reflects on the association and, more broadly, on professional practice.
- Seek deserved and reasonable remuneration for services.
- Inform and educate the public on rehabilitation/assistive technology and its applications.
- Issue public statements in an objective and truthful manner.
- Comply with the laws and policies that guide professional practice.

Figure 1. RESNA code of ethics [9].

disciplines involved in rehabilitation and is based on several of them. However, it includes issues related to the provision of technology. It is presented as a reminder of the obligations that a practitioner in the assistive technology industry has to his or her consumers, others who work with and care for them, the general public, and the profession as a whole [10, 11].

Ethical levels	Techno-ethical considerations
Level 1: clinical/AT services*Operational context*Client-practitioner	• Educating consumers of AT services available • Clinical assessment matching consumer to device • Beneficence, non-maleficence, autonomy, fidelity
Level 2: clinical/interdisciplinary*Operational context*Practitioner-practitioner	• Information dissemination • Resource allocation, preservice and in-service training • Justice, fidelity
Level 3: institutional/agency*Operational context*Institution-member	• Adequate AT service provision • Efficient and effective service provision • Justice, fidelity
Level 4: social resourcesPublic policy*Operational context*Legislative-constituent	• Adequacy of resources • Periodic review and assessment • Legal issues • Reciprocal advocacy, justice

Table 1. Techno-ethical considerations within the four-level model prepared by Peterson and Murray.

3.2. Standards of practice

Because each assistive technology practitioner belongs to his or her own discipline, it is important that the standards are often the basis for professional certification programs. RESNA has developed the standards of practice accessed from http://www.resna.org/sites/default/files/legacy/certification/Standards_of_Practice_final_10_10_08.pdf for assistive technology practitioners and suppliers.

A hierarchical model of ethical practice that could be applied in education, supervision, and research is proposed by Tarvydas and Cottone [11]. Peterson and Murray defined that given the ubiquity of AT and its seemingly unlimited applications, a similar approach can be used to discuss ethical considerations with AT and its related applications; critical techno-ethical considerations related to each level are discussed and summarized in **Table 1** [12].

4. Assistive technology's effects on occupational performance areas: self-care, productivity, play, and leisure

The role of assistive technology with disabilities is not to compensate or to adapt for missing or delaying functions; it is also used to support for everyday living in targeted performance areas [13]. The role of assistive technology in performance areas defines the occupational therapy practice framework appropriately. It includes the analysis of the performance skills and patterns of the person and the activity demands of the occupation the person is attempting to perform [14].

Occupational performance areas occurred from routines, tasks, and subtasks performed by people fulfill the requirements of occupational performance roles. These include self-care (activities of daily living, ADLs), school/productivity, and leisure/play activities. Assistive technology assists a person that has functional limitations secondary to some pathology; they may not have the cognitive, motor, or psychological skills necessary to engage in meaningful activity. To assist means to help, aid, or support, not restoration of these activities. This supports an impaired function of the user without being expected to change the native functioning of the person. For example, a wheelchair replaces the function of walking or canes support independent walking but do not improve strength or not change the ability to walk without them [13].

4.1. Technology for daily living or self-care

The ADLs comprise typical tasks required for self-care and self-maintenance, such as hygiene, bathing, feeding, dressing, medication routine, socialization, and communication. Impaired occupational performance may trigger a process that frequently influences people's biopsychosocial context, impaired self-esteem, and the sense of independence. Technological support for everyday living is all pervasive. It is also about adaptive strategies and personal assistance services. Without some combination of this supportive service, a person with a disability may not be able to get out of the house and into bed, eat dinner, take a bath, or put on clothes. The supporting services used may vary according to the needs, time, and circumstances of the person. In that way, this technology is the most challenging of all technological interventions [15, 16].

An individual's need of experience and practice with the devices that may become a part of his or her ongoing support system is frequently ignored. Professional rehabilitation intervention is often not continuing after rehabilitation process in the hospital is finished, usually because of the lack of funding. The distance of rural areas to an occupational service may be another complication. Individuals and families should be informed about the benefits and availability of professional services. Ideally, the process of technology teaching to client should be a part of the first rehabilitation in the hospital. The independent living skills training programs designed for people with disabilities and geriatrics for their social integration are important exceptions. These programs that focus on human-environment interactions should be widespread [16].

The everyday technology usefulness is not limited to any particular group of people. Everyone can use it and easy to understand design is important (**Picture 1**). Because everyone who is in contact with a person with a disability sooner or later touches his or her tool that he or she is using to live, caregivers, assistants, classmates and coworkers, and the everyday contacts should think before choosing the equipment. Another important thing about selection of equipment is that the device is perfectly fit for the person, but it causes stigmatization which creates an obstacle for interpersonal interaction for the people who use it. So everyday technology that works for everyone should be evaluated by occupational therapist in every aspect [17].

A careful match between the abilities and activities of people with disabilities for sensory perception, cognitive processing, and motor capabilities of assistive technologies ensures effective interventions [13].

A person can have different roles simultaneously, and the roles we hold during our lifetime can change such as being a student, parents, a son, a sibling, an employee, a friend, and a

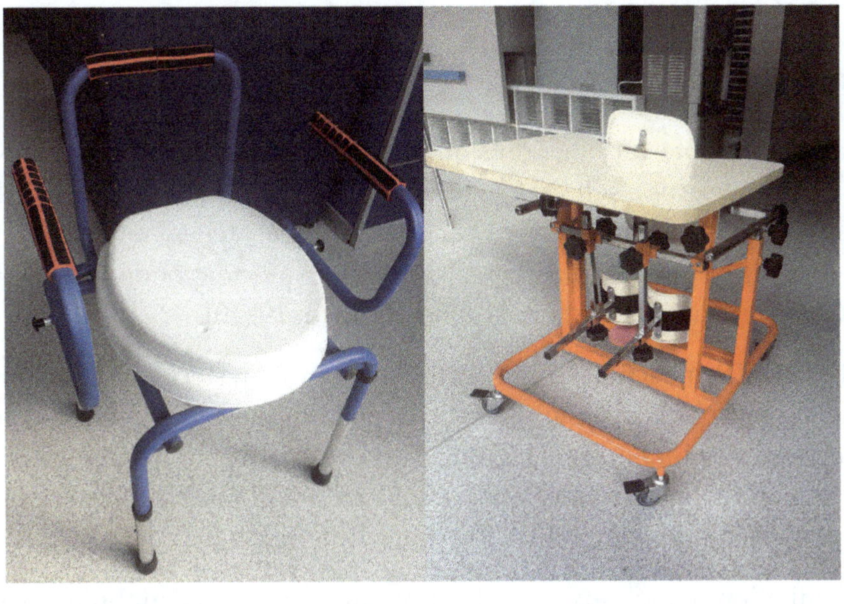

Picture 1. Assistive technology for daily living activities.

homemaker. The life role of the individual influences the activities performed by the individual. As a part of our everyday lives, activities can be learned and are governed by the society and culture in which we live. The activities performed by an individual are determined by the roles of the individual. At the most basic level of daily living activity is the use of the upper extremities, especially fingers and hands for manipulation [18].

Daily living technology includes technological support systems in the following areas: shelter such as access and environmental control; interpersonal relationships such as communicating; personal care such as eating, hygiene, dressing, and health management; home management such as food preparation and cleaning; and functional tasks such as lifting, reaching, holding, and transferring [18].

Low technology for daily living:

General-purpose aids: mouth sticks, head pointers, and reaches

Special purpose aids:

Self-care: a variety of utensils with modified handles, modified plates, and removable rims that are attached to any plate. Zipper pulls, single-handed buttoning, quad grip handles, long handled shoe horn, manual razors, long handled sponges, curved handled brushes, and key holders

Work and school: book holders and mouth stick

Play and leisure: modified shutter release, modified grip scissors, or garden tools

Special purpose electromechanical aids: electrically powered feeders, page-turners, environmental control units, and trainable or programmable devices

Robotic aids: robotic arms, desktop vocational assistant robot, mobile assistive robots, and mobile vocational assistant robot

4.2. Technology for mobility

Mobility is fundamental of every person's quality of life and is necessary for participation in each of the performance areas: self-care, work or school, and play or leisure. The ambulation can be replaced by low-tech aids such as canes, walker, crutches, wheelchair, or systems of various types. Increased mobility can achieve goals such as independence, functionality, positive self-imagination, social interaction, and health care [19, 20].

Disorders that affect the musculoskeletal and neurological systems such as ankylosing spondylitis, osteogenesis imperfecta, osteoporosis, Paget's disease and cerebral palsy, traumatic brain injury, cerebral vascular accident, Guillain-Barre syndrome, Huntington's chorea, muscular dystrophy, Parkinson's disease, polio myelitis, spinal cord injury, stroke, spina bifida, and multiple sclerosis result in mobility disorders [19] (**Table 2**).

The degree of limitation in mobility are full ambulatory, marginal ambulatory can walk short distances; may need wheelchair at times; marginal manual wheelchair users (part of time

Medical condition	Characteristics of conditions	Seating needs
Cerebral palsy (spastic type)	Fixed deformity, decreased movements, abnormal patterns	Correct deformities, improve alignment, decrease tone
Cerebral palsy hypotonus	Subluxations, decreased active movement, hypermobility	Provide support for upright positioning, promote development of muscle control
Athetoid tone	Excessive active movement, decreased stability	Provide stability but allow controlled mobility for function
Muscular dystrophies (Duchenne)	Loss of muscular control proximal to distal	Provide stable seating base, allow person to find balance point
Multiple sclerosis	Series of exacerbations and remissions	Prepare for flexibility of system to follow needs
Spina bifida	Decreased or absent sensation	Reduce high risk for pressure concerns, allow for typically good upper extremity and head control
Spinal cord injuries	Partial or complete loss of function below level of injury, decreased or absent sensation	Reduce high risk for pressure concerns, allow for trunk movements used for function
Osteogenesis imperfecta	Limited functional range, multiple fractures	Provide protection
Poliomyelitis syndrome	Fixed or flexible	If fixed, support; if flexible, correct
Traumatic brain injury	Severity dependent on the extent of central nervous system damage, may have cognitive component	Allow for functional improvement, flexible to changing needs
Geriatrics	Decreased bone mass, decreased strength, incontinence	Provide comfort and visual orientation

Table 2. Conditions that require consideration of seating and positioning.

manual, part of time powered wheelchair users); totally mobility impaired users (dependent mobility base) [19] (**Pictures 2** and **3**).

Factors to consider when selecting a wheelchair:

1. Client's profile: disability, date of onset, size, and weight (**Table 2**)
2. Client's needs: activities, contexts of use, preferences, transportation, reliability, and durability
3. Physical and sensory skills: range of motion, motor control, strength, vision, and perception
4. Functional skills: transfers and ability to propel [19]

These factors need to be evaluated for wheeled mobility. The selection of a wheelchair is a process of matching characteristics to the person's needs and skills [19].

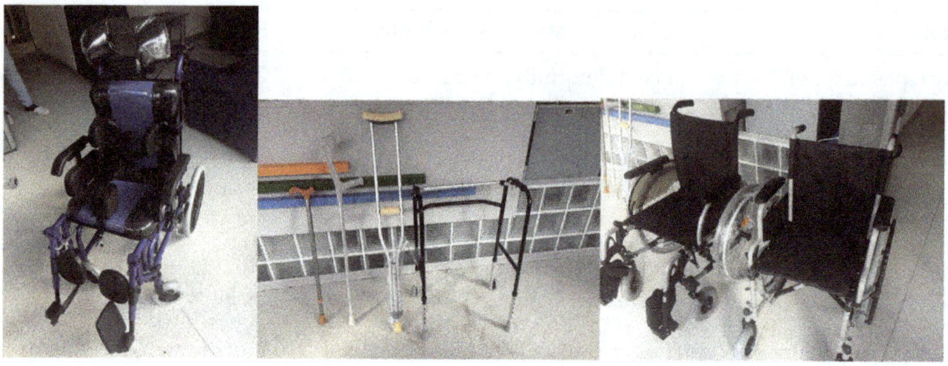

Picture 2. Mobility device for participation of people with disabilities.

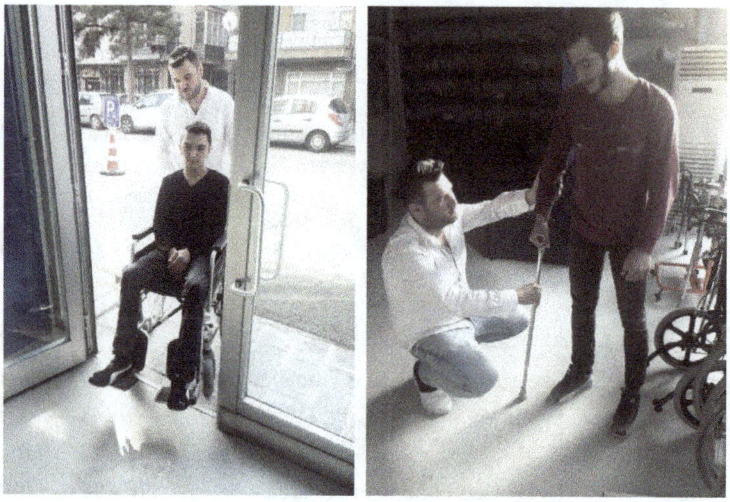

Picture 3. Client's needs for mobility.

4.3. Sensory aids

When a person has a sensory impairment such as seeing and hearing, assistive technology can provide assistance with information entry. In the case of the sensory aid, the human technology interface is a user screen, which depicts the sensory information for the human user. The processed information is presented to the user so that the alternative pathway can also be processed. For the visual pathway, this is a visible display such as a video monitor; for the auditory pathway, it is an audio display such as a speaker; and for the tactile pathway, it is a vibrating pin or electrode array through which pressure or touch data are provided to the user [21].

Hearing impairment is unique among disabilities and does not prevent an individual from performing an activity of daily living nor limit his or her ability to function effectively at a vocation. It is important to evaluate and use appropriate assistive technology for deafness or hearing impairment, because communicating with others affects social development or makes his or her life more difficult [22].

Assistive device for people with hearing impairment and deafness can generally be classified as either alerting devices or communicating devices. An alerting device often communicates some information to the individual, and a communicating device may well need to alert the individual that information is being communicated [23].

Alerting device may use sound, light, vibration, or any combination of these three to provide the alert. The modality selected for a given situation depends on the disability and preferences of the individual who will use the device, as well as on the environmental conditions. If the person's hearing impairment is not great, an amplified sound is impractical or ineffective; a light or vibration alerting device may be necessary. Because a vibration device needs to be contact with the body, a light-based device is preferable for a stationary device in an environment where the hearing impaired individual needs to move around.

Many assistive communication devices consist of a receiver and a transmitter. The person with the hearing impairment wears the receiver. The transmitter either is worn by the speaker or is stationary within a given environment. Three primary methods of transmission are used for these devices: infrared, radio frequency modulation, and inductive coupling.

Devices for daily living activities: these devices are helpful in using the telephone, listening television, and performing other daily living activities. A variety of sound within a home indicate things that require attention; among these sounds are doorbells, smoke alarms, alarm clocks, baby crying, and telephone ringing. Alerting systems similar to those that inform individuals who are hearing impaired or deaf of the ringing of a telephone are available for other sounds. Vibrating and flashing alarm clocks can be used to awaken an individual who cannot hear a standard alarm clock in their whole life.

The technologies produced for blind or low vision are mainly designed to provide access to information or provide safe travel. Determining the time on a watch, identifying money, reading today's mail, reviewing text on a computer screen, differentiating between black and white chess pieces, or preparing dinner without being burned access to information may mean accessing information. The information may be transmitted in tactile form, as synthetic or digitized speech, or through the use of some sort of visual enhancement such as optical or electronic magnification. People who are visually impaired typically have sufficient residual vision to permit them to perform most of their daily activities with the assistance of optical aids.

For people with low vision, increased illumination is frequently essential to their use of residual vision. Small tensor lamps placed near printed text can improve reading. Large bright light illuminates large areas; environmental adaptation or optical filters can help to provide the desired visual contrast. They can read books and magazines using computer technology. It is the most important tool for education, employment, and recreation for people with low vision. Use of Braille notetakers and Braille printers in lessons and exams is important for blind students and their teachers.

4.4. School and work aids

Assistive technologies can prove major benefits for children in education settings through all education life. Postural control or mobility systems allow children for maximal participation in classroom activities. For the use of computer and other electronic devices, special purpose interface can be effective for speaking and writing. There are some manipulatives in education that can be used to independently manipulate real objects. However policy and rules make opportunities or barriers for reaching these technologies; these are the potentials for achieving a positive educational effect.

In order to discuss assistive technology for classroom, we need to understand educational activities first. And secondly necessary appropriate access between occupational therapist and school staffs for all these sources can be used affectively. Reading, writing, math, music, and art, all, require motor, sensory, and cognitive skills.

Reading primarily associated with as motor skills is positioning the material, turning pages, picking up a book, and opening it. If reading material is electronic, tasks include using mouse and keyboard, searching a word, and printing a part of or all text. For sensory tasks we use visual system such as visual field, visual acuity, and oculomotor function. For cognitive tasks, we use word identification, spelling, and comprehension.

Writing can be divided into three groups such as note taking, massaging, and formal writing. There are many alternative methods for writing by hand. Computer-aided writing can do word processing, recognize the screen, and edit and translate the task. Despite all these aids, writing needs more motor control such as pencil grip or producing the letters; sensory skills such as visual, auditory, and tactile monitoring; and cognitive skills such as thinking and reasoning. Thus occupational therapist must need to understand which process, hand use, or electronic alternatives are more affective for client in the education setting.

Music instruction involves basic rhythm and group participation. They need to learn instrument and listen to voice. *Art* activities need to fine motor skills and understand, imagine, and create shapes and colors.

Work is one of the three basic performance areas that many individuals participate daily. However in the community setting, there is barrier to participate in the work activities, it is an important life role to survive in life. There are two types of individuals that need to use assistive technology for access to employment. One is with typical disability such as spinal cord injury, arthritis, cerebral palsy, and visual impairment. Second population is at high risk for injury or has been injured while working. Disabilities most commonly seen in the second population are musculoskeletal disorders such as back pain, carpal tunnel syndrome, and tendonitis and shoulder injuries.

In order to discuss assistive technology applications in the work setting, we must define the activities that are performed in the workplace. There are three major activities that we use in the job: communication, manipulation, and mobility.

Communication includes all various information handling activities which include writing, reading, interacting with others, and using telephone. *Manipulation* also includes a number of different tasks such as filing, sorting, assembling, lifting, and moving objects such as books, documents, and equipment and using office machines such as copiers. Paperless office becomes much easier of this activity output. *Mobility* characteristics involve personal movement to and from the work site and within the workplace. For many individuals, getting to work is the single largest barrier. For wheelchair users, accessible public transportation means booking pickup times with range of an hour or more and paying additional fees. Due to the special tax reduction policy, the modified private transportation means may be more advantageous for individuals with disabilities. Work environment can be a challenge for person with disabilities. Activities include entering and exiting the building safely, opening and closing doors, climbing the stairs, sitting and standing, postural control, pressure management, operating device, and manipulating objects at the same time. All these activities need motor, sensory, and cognitive skills [23].

4.5. Recreation or leisure and play

Recreation, leisure, or play is the last of the three basic performance areas that many individuals participate. It is essential to consider individual interests, goals, skills, and functional abilities in identifying appropriate and satisfying leisure pursuits. The identification of *recreational* interests should focus initially on the features of different types of activity, rather than the naming of specific hobbies or sports. Characteristics of activities may be competitive such as amputee football, creative such as art craft, individual or group, organized or unstructured, physically active or sedentary. One's activity needs to match with individual's ability and desire. A person's motor, sensory, and cognitive functions must be assessed adequately. Then assistive device must be selected for those people. Adaptation can be made to ensure satisfactory participation. Assistive devices for recreation can be categorized as personal, activity-specific, or environmental technologies. Personal technology is an equipment that they wear to participate in a desired activity such as racing wheelchair, dynamic prosthesis; activity-specific technologies enable them to perform specific types of activities such as hand bike, monoski, and tennis grips. Environmental technologies most often function to provide the daily living needs of people such as shelter, food, and water. Additionally environmental technologies also include maps, signs, and other means used to communicate accessible information for each environment [24].

Nowadays, it is common to consider *play* a child's work. For children with physical conditions that limited their opportunities to explore play materials and their play possibilities, the purpose of intervention and assistive technology must bring the opportunities to them not to direct their play but to make intrinsically motivated activities and play pleasurably as possible.

There are two important areas for play: environment (indoor and outdoor) and toys. Every child's bedroom and play areas have the same four things: walls, floors, ceiling, and openings such as windows and doors. There are many ways to match an individual child's developmental needs with the home's physical environment. Most of the following ideas are simple, inexpensive, or free and are just a starting point to stimulate thinking. It is important to keep in mind the child's developmental changes, the family's life style, and the child's siblings and friends. There are many ways to use assistive technology to make an outdoor play area fun for children with a disability. For them there are some important challenges such as safety, gates, water play, ground, trees, and commercial play structures [25].

5. Interaction of setting and context and assistive technology

In the models used before the 1950s, only the disability was focused. Later, with the developing models, it was observed that the person with a disability has environmental factors as obstacles that hinder the person from doing the activity, and the awareness in this subject has increased. It has been seen that the lives of people with disabilities are greatly facilitated by person-environment harmony. In relation to this, there are many approaches that define and regulate the environment. These models include:

- Human Activity Assistive Technology (HAAT) model [5]
- Matching Person and Technology (MPT) model
- Comprehensive Assistive Technology (CAT) Model [26, 27]
- Needs Analysis and Requirements Acquisition (NARA) framework
- USERfit methodology (USERfit) [26]

Accomplishing the procedure of NARA has several loops of four steps: gathering information from users like dealing with groups and interviews, using the information to obtain requirements, producing a paper-based mock-up or low fidelity prototype that carries out the requirements, and evaluating the guidelines for accurate implementation, usability, and relevance. The new groups of assessment activities, which are advanced from procedure that is the former one, are applied to a new sample of end users.

The MPT and USERfit are also having a well-developed questionnaire structure for getting end-user data.

The HAAT and CAT models have a hierarchical structure with four components of person, activity, technology, and context at the top level (**Boxes 1** and **2**). They could be used for knowledge obtained in the format of questionnaires or interviews [27].

The CAT model consists of main categories that are similar to the HAAT model; hence, the CAT model is almost identical to the HAAT model. Both models are appropriate for applications

Context	
Cultural and social context	Wider social and cultural context
	User's social and cultural context
National context	Infrastructure
	Legislation
	Assistive technology context
Local settings	Location and environment
	Physical variables

Box 1. Context in the CAT model.

Context	
Setting	Individual home
	Group home
	Employment
	School
	Community
Social context	Familiar peers
	Familiar nonpeers
	Strangers
	Alone
Cultural context	
Physical context	Light
	Sound
	Heat

Box 2. Context in the HAAT model.

of device design and development, guidance of the service delivery process, and outcome evaluation. However, the supporting description separates both models. The interaction that is more dynamic is hypothesized by HAAT model. The CAT model, on the other hand, presupposes more description of the individual categories.

In this part, we will observe the context closely according to the model of HAAT.

Setting: Setting not only is the location but also a combination of an environment, a set of governing the tasks, tasks to be done, and a level of good feeling.

The settings are listed in **Box 1** and **2**.

Many people with disabilities live in their own homes. In order for these individuals to be able to survive independently, some modifications are required within or outside the home. Group houses are houses where a large number of individuals with the same needs are present unlike individual houses. On the one hand, group houses are not enough for some requirements such as lack of privacy, degree of interaction with other consumers who can help in developing strategies of use, and the availability of organized recreational and educational activities. On the other hand, they have some principles and security system [28]. Thus, all of them should be taken into account.

The three settings that we differentiate significant to the application of assistive technologies outside the living situation are employment, school, and community. Work requires to be completed in a timely and accurate manner, and assistive technologies can influence the conclusion for a handicapped person in a vocational or educational setting. All those places that recreation, leisure, shopping, and entertainment occur are surrounded by the community setting. Why it is hard to characterize it specifically is that this setting is so different. In this setting, the variety also causes requirements being placed on the assistive technology. For instance, the use of an assistive device affects mobility of blind people in order to observe the type of terrain and existence of obstacles. In a home or employment setting that travel paths are used regularly and objects are fixed in, obtaining this orientation is relatively straightforward. However, ignorance of environment and travel is more difficult in a shopping mall, restaurant, or theater, which is an unusual place to visit for blind person. The type of setting dictates the characteristic of the assistive technology system, and a system is successful in one environment, whereas the system is not successful in another [29]. Additionally, the requirements of devices change according to terrain such as a manual wheelchair is okay around the house with hard rubber tires, but it is not for rough outdoor terrain.

5.1. Social and cultural contexts

We should deal with the social context that this performance takes place in because we deal with helping human performance in communication, manipulation, and mobility, so social context is important. Handicapped people may be stigmatized by reason of their disability; thus, using the assistive devices may cause further isolation and contribute to the labeling. For instance, a person who has hearing handicap may not want to wear a hearing aid, but the person is unlikely to have same claim not to wear glasses for reading. In the environments that the activity will be well performed, why it is crucial to conduct assessments and technology trials is that main subject in assistive technology use is likely social context.

Social and cultural contexts may be almost identical; especially, it is for people who form part of dominant cultural and social contexts except members of minority groups, including people with disabilities. Variables of interest in both the user's and wider social and cultural context include language, other cultural factors, and attitudes to people with disabilities, and attitudes to assistive technology. Why language and other cultural factors are very important is that many features of assistive technology devices that can be used are only provided in English and sometimes a small number of European languages, whereas both speech output, if any, and documentation and manuals need to be in the local language. Furthermore, the device requires designing and presenting in a way that is culturally relevant. This consists of the choice of symbols or other labels for controls that are simple in the cultural context.

5.2. Physical context

Physical context is simply environmental situation that means the system is used. Heat, sound, and light are the usual measured parameters that most directly influence the success of the assistive technologies. The temperature influences some materials. For instance, the features of gels and foams used in seat pillows can alter under hot or cold conditions. The temperature influences monitoring of liquid crystal like existing light.

In the environment of classrooms or work, the use of assistive technologies depends on existing light. In situation of bright light, some display reverse light and are better. On the other hand, others give out light and are better in low light.

Penetrability of voice recognition systems or speakers can be affected by existing sound. For instance, in a classroom, some devices that generate sound such as powered wheelchairs, computers, and printers may upset classroom attention.

The occupational therapy approaches are not considered without context. Because the occupations is affected by context is no static. The assistive technology is used in education or work that are most important occupational areas. The assistive technology is important for people with disabilities to facilitate the changing life.

6. The use of assistive technology for the people with disabilities: sensory, perceptual, cognitive, and motor control and other functions

Assistive technology is an umbrella term for assistive, adaptive, and rehabilitative devices for people with disabilities. It also includes the process of selecting, positioning, and using these devices. It is used to provide transportation to the house, to the interiors, or to the buildings. They provide access to community spaces, home, education, recreation areas, transportation, and jobs. By changing or improving the tasks that people have failed before, they are able to greatly increase their independence and contribute to health and well-being. Greatly increase their independence, and contribute to health and well-being. It can be used to protect, maintain, or increase the independence of people. Assistive technology allows people to learn, play, act, work, communicate, and participate as their peers [30, 31]. In short, it opens the gates of the world to the people.

Assistive technology can be any tool or product that enhances the individual's involvement and functions. These devices may be particularly developed for the use of a specific person or may be accessible to the whole community, developed for all, that can also be used by persons with disabilities. These tools may be products that are simple to design and use (such as clothing aids) and may also be very high-tech (bioelectrical orthoses) products. It facilitates interaction with the environment for everyone. The proper use of assistive technology reduces the help from other people to minimal level and can support people's independent living in the community. Assistive technology transport greatly enhances the quality of life for both people with and without disabilities. In addition to the people with physical, sensorial, and cognitive impairment, disadvantaged populations such as seniors and pregnant women are the most beneficiaries [31–35].

It is a common mistake to consider the assistive technology as equipment, which compensates the impaired body parts and/or functions. In the leadership of one of the mainstream occupational therapy models, Person-Environment-Occupation (PEO) model [36], an occupational therapist must remember that it is not only the personal factors that have a contribution on occupational performance but the contexts of the environment and the occupation itself. This leads us to two points: (1) expanding the assistive technology assessment and interventions, including environmental, and occupation, and (2) personal factors are not the only reason of decreased activity performance and/or participation. The first aspect is being argued in the future part of this chapter. The latter aspect, however, is the point that has to be stressed in this case. An individual who so called "healthy" may be suffering from decreased occupational performance due to either environmental or occupational factors. Although it is ideal to have a universal design in the physical environment, which is something that makes the surrounding available for the individuals in the community, the universal designed tools are not the most suitable media for everyone since they are not created for individual. And of course it has an impact on the performance of the people. Last but not least, the occupation itself can lead to the need of assistive technology. Tasks such as requiring inactivity, putting too much pressure to the human body, and forcing human body's function boundaries make the assistive technology support indispensable. Imagine an office worker, who is a 25-year-old female, consults an occupational therapy practitioner complaining about excessive fatigue and tiredness in her back during her working hours. A neurologist referred her and there was no specific problem with the medical examination. The role of occupational therapist as an assistive technology practitioner is to evaluate the both physical environment and the tasks in occupations besides the personal factors [35, 37–39].

There is something very important that needs to be underlined when talking about this subject. Assistive technology is not all about the recovery but a protection and maintenance, too. That is, assistive technology should not only be regarded as a method in the rehabilitation phase but should also take place in the previous phases of healthcare systems [31, 35, 40].

6.1. Assistive technology types

As mentioned above, wide range of devices could be applied to improve and maintain performance and functionality. In literature, there are different ways of classification for all of these products [31, 35, 41, 42]. These could be:
Low tech: communication cards made from cards
High technology: special purpose computers
Hardware: prostheses, mounting systems, or positioning tools
Computer hardware: special keys, keyboards, and pointing devices
Computer software: screen readers and communication programs

If assistive technology is available and appropriate for the people, they can benefit from living independently, enjoy self-management and decision-making skills, and be able to benefit from educational facilities, carrying on a meaningful career, being fully involved in general economic, political, social, cultural, and educational contexts.

Benefits of assistive technology in individuals can be summarized as follows [42]:

- Reduce or eliminate participation restrictions.
- Promote inclusion.
- Equal opportunity to participate.
- Contribution to quality of life.

- Increase independence and self-care.
- Provide an environment free of hindrances at home, at school, at work, and in communal areas.
- Build confidence and self-confidence.

Assistive technology seems quite useful for both children and adults. However, every assistive technology tool received is unfortunately not always used for a long time. One of the main reasons of this consequence is ignoring to get the opinion of the client. And also, some machines are easy to get. This can lead to quick purchases, without having to worry much enough when making a purchase [43]. No matter how easily a device can be reached, the occupational therapist must make a detailed assessment in order to be able to combine and meet the advantages of the assistive technology to the needs of the person. Another reason is that a person thinks they can get this device easily without consulting the therapist for evaluation and application. In addition, evaluation and training are also important to make use of and benefit from the purchase of the product. And of course, a change in the priorities of the client may cause the disuse. At that point, it is important to remember an assistive technology is a tool that fills the gap among the person, environment, and occupation. Any change in them may cause a change in the need for assistive technology. For example, a child using a wheelchair, who is a student, would be in need of a ramp builder for the stairs in front of the school building until the elevator is built. When the building becomes available for that child, there will be no need for that specific tool, but rather a need auditory support for the use of the elevator.

7. Service and maintenance in assistive technologies

The steps of the service process in assistive technology (AT) are referral, need analyses, recommendations, implementation, and follow-up. In referral step, the person specifies a need about assistive technology intervention and consults a therapist or AT provider. The need analyses step is an evaluation phase of human's need, skills, and functions. In recommendation step, it is important to justify funding and make the recommendations based on the results of assessments. In implementation step, fitting and training of the AT device or system should be done. Finally, in follow-up, maintenance and repair needs of AT device or system should be considered, and the effect of AT use should be evaluated [44, 45]. If these steps of the service process in AT are not considered by the therapist or provider of AT, the barriers to use the AT device may occur [44–49]. Below, you can find barriers, which may affect the use of AT device (**Table 3**).

7.1. Assistive technology assessment and intervention principles

The first step of the AT intervention is assessment of the person. Because through results of the assessment, the person is understood and analyzed by the therapist, and then the intervention plan is conducted. For the assistive technology process, many models are developed and used [49–51]. You can find these models in the AT field below (**Table 4**).

Barriers to use AT
• Staff training issues • Training of consumer issues • Availability problem of AT • Funding problem of AT • AT assessment issues (all components should be assessed) • Planning issues such as nonstructural programs • Selection of inappropriate AT device

Table 3. Barriers which may affect the use of assistive technology.

Matching Person and Technology (MPT) model	It was developed for use in persons with disability aged 15 years and older. The purpose of the model is to facilitate the selection of the suitable AT in regard to the human's perspectives and abilities, the details of the AT, and the environmental conditions [49–52]
Framework for modeling the selection of ATD	There are no instruments directly based on this framework. The aim of the model is looking for a good outcome in terms of the best match between AT, the person, and the environment [49–53]
Human Activity Assistive Technology (HAAT) model	In this model, AT is defined as extrinsic enablers. It has four components: the human, the activity, the context, and AT. It does not provide any assessment [49, 50]
Model of AT user's career	This model focuses on the different phases during time-dependent AT use and the factors that may influence the use or nonuse of AT. It does not provide any assessment, and it is not an appropriate model for the selection of AT [49, 54]
Social cognition model	This model is not an AT-specific model. Therefore, it is not an appropriate model for the selection of AT directly [49, 54]
The social cognitive model of assistive device (AD) used in older persons	It is a social cognitive model adapted to the AT field. It is not an appropriate model for the selection of AT [49, 54, 55]
Perceived attributes theory	It is a social cognitive theory and it is not an AT-specific model. This theory defines AT as a new product for a person to adapt daily life [49, 54]

Table 4. Models are used in assistive technology field.

According to a research study, we are focusing on environmental components especially physical environment much more in the AT studies [56]. Therefore, these models are important for focusing all parameters related to AT. Consequently, principles which are important for systematizing assessment and intervention in AT are represented below. These principles may provide significant support for the aim, selection of the models, standards, and types of assistive technology [50].

- Assistive technology assessment and intervention should include all components such as person, activity, and environment.
- The aim of AT should be maintaining the function which is impaired, not remediating the function. So AT should be an enabler for the function.
- Assistive technology assessment and intervention should be collaborative.
- Assistive technology assessment should be perpetual.
- Interpreting the assessment and the outcomes of intervention is important for the selection of AT [44, 50].

7.2. The Human Activity Assistive Technology (HAAT) model

The Human Activity Assistive Technology (HAAT) model, which is designed by Cook and Hussey in 1995, is a framework about assistive technology for people with disability. The model is created to guide assessment and clinical intervention and evaluate the outcomes. The HAAT model is a well-known model in assistive technology (AT) field [50, 57].

Some of the research studies mentioning the HAAT model suggest its extensive use in research and clinical applications [45]. According to a survey which is done to rehabilitation clinicians and by Friederich et al. [51], even though clinicians expressed that they are not using any framework for their practice, it was found that HAAT model was the only specific assistive technology model which is used [53]. Also the model is used as a reference in several research studies [56, 58–61].

7.3. Components of the HAAT model

There are four components in the model: the human, the activity, the assistive technology, and the context (**Figure 2**). There is a dynamic relation between three components, and the context has effect on these three components.

The human component contains cognitive, physical, and emotional elements. Cognitive abilities include problem solving, attention, alertness, and concentration, and they have effect on emotional abilities. Physical abilities include balance, range of motion, strength, and coordination. It is very important to know these abilities about human because they probably affect the use of assistive technology. Therefore for the effective use of assistive technology, a match between human abilities and the requirements of assistive technology is needed. Also AT may provide assistance in the area, which the person has problems such as hearing or visual. For example, in hearing problems AT can provide a device for hearing and provide the person to maintain this ability again.

The activity component contains self-care, productivity, and leisure activities. Self-care activities include dressing, eating, hygiene, mobility, and communication. Productive activities are educational and vocational activities and home management. Leisure activities include relaxation or enjoyment such as watching TV, resting, reading books, or dancing. These activities may require many abilities such as cognitive and physical. If the person has no capacity to

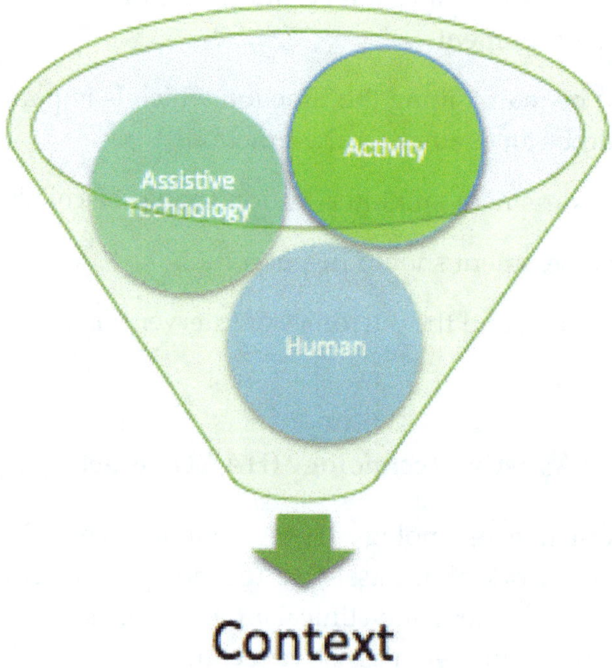

Figure 2. HAAT model [5].

do an activity, with the use of an assistive technology system, the person may gain his/her performance on this activity again.

The context contains cultural (pattern of behaviors, values, attitudes) physical (natural and built surroundings such as home, school, workplace, or parks), institutional (religious, educational institutions), and social (family, friends, strangers). Facilitators and barriers in the environment are very important for the selection, evaluation, and use of the assistive technology system.

The assistive technology is described as extrinsic enablers because they provide the performance, which is blocked by disability. Choosing or designing an AT system should be done through considering needs, skills, and goals of the person. Therefore a detailed assessment about functions, activities, and environment is needed before determining the AT system for the person [50, 57].

8. Funding assistive technology services and systems

Most consumers have problem about evaluation, implementation, and maintenance and repair of assistive technologies because of not having the adequate financial resources available to purchase the necessary services and equipment. Funding by third-party sources is appropriate for individuals to procure assistive technology services and equipment. Funding for many assistive technology services and devices is widely available, and accessing that funding is generally a matter of following a straightforward process. As a service provider, the occupational therapist's role is assisting with the acquisition of this funding.

In most countries assistive technology services and devices are financed by numerous sources instead of by a system only dedicated to the funding of assistive technology services and equipment. For any given individual, equipment and services may be financed only by one source or a combination of sources. Funding for assistive technology is usually rendered through agencies that have been primarily developed for the provision of other types of health, education, or social services programs.

In this part funding for assistive technologies in several countries (the United States, Australia, Canada, and Turkey) is described. Funding programs in these countries are representative of those in many other countries with local modifications of elements of the programs. The various funding sources can be categorized as public and private.

8.1. Public sources of funding

8.1.1. US public sources of assistive technology funding

Public funding sources for assistive technology in the United States include federal, state, and local government agencies; several public sources of funding are listed in **Box 3** [62].

Public programs

Medicare

Medicaid

Required and optional services

Intermediate care facilities for persons who are mentally retarded

Early and periodic screening, diagnosis, and treatment

Home- and community-based waivers

Community-supported living arrangements

Maternal and child health

Maternal and child health block grant to states

Children with special healthcare needs

Special projects of regional and national significance

Education

Individuals with Disabilities Education Act state grants (Part B)

IDEA programs for infants and toddlers with disabilities and their families (Part H)

State-operated programs

Vocational education

Head start

Vocational Rehabilitation

Low-interest loans

Private foundations

Service clubs

Special state appropriations

State bond issues

Employee accommodations program

Equipment loan program

Corporate-sponsored loans

Charitable organizations

US TAX CODE

Medical care expense deduction

Business deductions

Employee business deductions

Americans with Disabilities Act credit for small business

Credit for architectural and transportation barrier removal

Targeted jobs tax credit

Charitable contribution deduction

Private health insurance

Health insurance

State grants	Workers' compensation
Supported employment	Casualty insurance
Independent living Parts A, B, and C	Disability insurance
Social security benefits	Civil rights
Title II: Social Security Disability Insurance	Americans with Disabilities Act
Title XVI: Supplemental Security Income	Rehabilitation Act, Section 504
Work incentive programs	Universal access
Developmental disability programs	Rehabilitation Act, Section 508
Department of Veterans Affairs programs	Decoder Circuitry Act
Older Americans Act programs	Telecommunications
Alternative financing	Telecommunications for the People with disabilities Act of 1982
Revolving loan fund	Telecommunications Accessibility Enhancement Act of 1988
Lending library	
Discount program	

*Received from Cook and Polgar [5].

Box 3. The public funding sources in the United States*.

8.1.2. Canadian provincial and territorial sources of assistive technology funding

In Canada the delivery of health services is the responsibility of the provinces and territories. Although there are federal programs, most of assistive technology funding is allocated and managed at the provincial/territorial level. Most of the federal programs have clauses about funding only what the provinces and territories do not fund. The Canadian federal programs that fund assistive technologies were listed in **Table 5**. Canadian public funding sources by province or territory are changed by funded assistive device, special conditions, or program features and eligibility [62].

8.1.3. Australian state government funding schemes

The funding programs that are provided through the state governments of Australia have been designed specifically to provide for people with disabilities and include assistive technology in the lists of approved items. The state programs have evolved quite independently in each Australian state or territory and therefore are not uniform. The schemes are administered through various state government departments and are funded from state/territory sources. Although all these programs have similar objectives, there is variation in the level and range of assistance that they provide to people with disabilities. These programs also vary in their level of means testing. The Australian state funding schemes are summarized in **Table 6** [62].

Program	Assistive devices funded	Special conditions or program features	Eligibility
Aging and seniors	Depends on province or territory	Benefits related to provincial/ territorial programs	
Workers' compensation board	Devices necessary for return to work	One for each province and territory	Workplace injuries including work-related accidents or diseases that require medical treatment or time away from work
Health Canada-First Nations and Inuit Health: noninsured health benefits	A variety of mobility devices, aids to daily living items not listed on the benefit list may be considered on a case-by-case basis with written medical justification	Device is listed by program; intended for use in a home or other ambulatory care settings; not available through any other federal, provincial territorial, or private health or social program; prescribed by health professional licensed to prescribe; provided by a recognized provider	Canadian resident and one of the following: (1) registered Native Canadian according to the Indian Act, (2) Inuk recognized by one of the Inuit Land Claim Organizations, or (3) infant less than 1 year of age whose parent is an eligible recipient
Veterans' affairs	Aids to daily living, canes, walkers; foot boards, over bed tables, raised toilet seats, bath benches	Available devices may vary by province	Group "A" clients: pension from Veterans Affairs CanadaGroup "B" clients: established eligibility for treatment of non-pensioned conditions, established health need, benefits not covered by the province

*Received from Cook and Polgar [5].

Table 5. Canadian Federal Programs That Fund Assistive Technologies*.

State	Assistive technology funding program name	Managing authority
New South Wales	Program of Appliances for People with disabilities	New South Wales Department of Area Health and Community Services
Victoria	Victorian Aids and Equipment Program	Department of Human Services
Western Australia	Community Aids and Equipment Program	Disability Services Commission
Queensland	Medical Aids Subsidy Scheme	Queensland Health
South Australia	Independent Living Equipment Program	Disability Services South Australia
Tasmania	Community Equipment Scheme	Department of Health and Human Services
Northern Territory	Territory Independence and Mobility Scheme	Department of Health and Community Services
Australian Capital Territory	Australian Capital Territory Equipment Subsidy Scheme	Aged Care and Rehabilitation Service

*Received from Cook and Polgar [5].

Table 6. Australian funding programs by state*.

8.2. Turkey state government funding

In Turkey, the assistive technology is termed as medical device which means any instrument, apparatus, appliance, software, material, or other articles, whether used alone or in combination, including the software intended by its manufacturer to be used specifically for diagnostic and/or therapeutic purposes and necessary for its proper application and intended by the manufacturer to be used for human beings for the purpose of (1) diagnosis, prevention, monitoring, treatment, or alleviation of disease; (2) diagnosis, monitoring, treatment, alleviation, or compensation for an injury or handicap; (3) investigation, replacement, or modification of the anatomy or of a physiological process; and (4) control of conception, which does not achieve its principal intended action in or on the human body by pharmacological, immunological, or metabolic means, but which may be assisted in its function by such means [63].

Health Application Notification (HAN) (Sağlık Uygulama Tebliği—SUT) is a document in which price ratio is listed. The HAN was issued within the framework of the Social Security Institution Law No. 5502, the Social Insurance and General Health Insurance Law No. 5510, and the General Health Insurance Transactions Regulation published in the Official Gazette dated August 28, 2008 and numbered 26981. The purpose of HAN is services related to health insurance, social security institution, general health insurance and establishment obligations, health services financed by the institution, methods for utilizing the road, and daily and attendant expenses, and the procedures related to the procedures are stated in the Health Services Pricing Commission [64].

8.2.1. Private sources of funding

In addition to public sources, there are private sources of funding such as self-funding, private health insurance, and others. These vary by economic condition or person. For instance, the Solidarity Association for the people with physical disabilities in Turkey provides their citizens who have physical disabilities or financial difficulties in order to facilitate their lives and to participate in life and to be liberated by making wheelchair aids with the priority needs. World Eye Foundation in Turkey provided 300 "smartphones" designed for the high school students with visually impaired to help them function independently and utilize information in their daily lives easily, support their educations and facilitate their access to information.

8.2.2. Private health insurance in Turkey

Financing of the public health insurance system in Turkey is covered by employee and employer premium. Participation in the general health insurance system, which has been implemented since January 10, 2008, is mandatory and essential. The private health insurance that "completes and supports" the general health insurance is a voluntary insurance type and secondary. In Turkey, there is no possibility of making a substitute private health insurance. For this reason, private health insurance in our country can be referred to as "voluntary health insurance" or "complementary and supportive health insurance." Health insurance is defined in article 1513 of the Turkish Commercial Code No. 6102. According to this, health insurance and insurer give a guarantee for (1) the end of the disease if necessary, including any medicinal treatment, pregnancy, and birth; (2) for costs determined for the early diagnosis of diseases, including consecutive studies, (3) in cases where it is necessary to perform medically inpatient treatment, (4) for the daily allowance for the insured's unavailability of earnings due to ill-treatment, (5) if the insured is in need of care, costs incurred due to care, or agreed daily care allowance [65].

Author details

Gokcen Akyurek*, Sinem Kars, Zeynep Celik, Ceren Koc and Özge Buket Cesim

*Address all correspondence to: gkcnakyrk@gmail.com

Department of Occupational Therapy, Faculty of Health Science, Hacettepe University, Ankara, Turkey

References

[1] Technology Related Assistance for Individuals with Disabilities Act of 1988, Pub. L. No. 105-394, Sec (3) (a) 3-4

[2] American Occupational Therapy Association. Specialized knowledge and skills in technology and environmental interventions for occupational therapy practice. American Journal of Occupational Therapy. 2010;**64**:44-56

[3] Murphy EF, Cook AM, Harvey RF. Neuromuscular prosthetics and orthotics. Englewood Cliffs, NJ: Prentice Hall; 1982

[4] McKechnie JL. Webster's New Twentieth Century Dictionary of the English Language. New York: Simon and Schuster; 1983

[5] Introduction and overview. In: Cook AM, Polgar JM, editors. Cook and Hussey's Assistive Technologies: Principles and Practice. 3rd ed. St. Louis, MO: Mosby Elsevier; 2008. pp. 3-33

[6] Bevan N. International standards for HCI and usability. International Journal of Human-Computer Studies. 2001;**55**(4):533-552

[7] Bevan N. Quality in use: Meeting user needs for quality. Journal of Systems and Software. 2001;**49**(1):89-96

[8] Earthy J. The improvement of human-centred processes—Facing the challenge and reaping the benefit of ISO 13407. International Journal of Human-Computer Studies. 2001;**55**:553-585

[9] RESNA. Code of Ethics. [Internet]. 2016. Available from: http://www.resna.org/sites/default/files/legacy/certification/RESNA_Code_of_Ethics.pdf [Accessed: 21 February 2017]

[10] RESNA. Standards of Practice. [Internet]. 2016. Available from: http://www.resna.org/sites/default/files/legacy/certification/Standards_of_Practice_final_10_10_08.pdf [Accessed: 21 February 2017]

[11] Tarvydas VS, Cottone RR. Ethical responses to legislative, organizational, and economic dynamics: A four level model of ethical practice. Journal of Applied Rehabilitation Counseling. 1991;**22**:11-18

[12] Peterson DB, Murray GC. Ethics and assistive technology service provision. Disability and Rehabilitation: Assistive Technology. 2006;**1**(1-2):59-67

[13] Anson D. Assistive technology. In: Pendleton HM, Schultz Krohn W, editors. Pedretti's Occupational Therapy Practice Skills for Physical Dysfunction, 6th ed. St. Louis, MO: Mosby Elsevier; 2006. pp. 349-371

[14] American Occupational Therapy Association (AOTA). Commission on Practice: Occupational therapy practice framework: Domain and process. American Journal of Occupational Therapy. 2002;**56**:609-639

[15] Alves de Oliveira AI, Lourenço JMQ, Garoti MF. Tecnologia Assistiva: pesquisa e pratica. Belém: EDUEPA; 2008. p. 184

[16] Neistadt ME, Crepeau EB. In: Willard & Spackman's Occupational Therapy. 9th ed. Rio de Janeiro: Guanabara Koogan; 2002. p. 888

[17] Enders A, Leech P. Low technology aids for daily living and do it yourself device. In: Galvin JC, Scherer MJ, editors. Evaluating, Selecting and Using Appropriate Assistive Technology. Gaithersburg, Md.: Aspen publishers. 1996. pp. 27-50

[18] A framework for assistive technologies. In: Cook AM, Polgar JM, editors. Cook and Hussey's Assistive Technologies: Principles and Practice. 3rd ed. St. Louis, MI: Mosby; 2008. pp. 34-53

[19] Technologies that enable mobility. In: Cook AM, Polgar JM, editors. Cook and Hussey's Assistive Technologies: Principles and Practice. 3rd ed. St. Louis, MI: Mosby; 2008. pp. 408-442

[20] Akyürek G, Bumin G. Investigation of factors that affect community participation of people with disabilities. The 13th International Conference on Mobility and Transport for Elderly and People with disabilities Persons (TRANSED 2012); September 17-20, 2012; New Delhi, India

[21] Sensory aids for persons with visual or auditory impairments. In: Cook AM, Polgar JM, editors. Cook and Hussey's Assistive Technologies: Principles and Practice. 3rd ed. St. Louis, MI: Mosby; 2008. pp. 310-334

[22] Enders A, Leech P. Aids for hearing impairment and deafness. In: Galvin JC, Scherer MJ, editors. Evaluating, Selecting and Using Appropriate Assistive Technology. Gaithersburg, Md.: Aspen publishers. 1996. Pp. 144-161

[23] Assistive technologies in the context of work. In: Cook AM, Polgar JM, editors. Cook and Hussey's Assistive Technologies: Principles and Practice. 3rd ed. St. Louis, MI: Mosby; 2008. pp. 525-544

[24] Longmuir P E and Axelson P. Assistive technology for recreation. In: Galvin JC, Scherer MJ, editors. Evaluating, Selecting and Using Appropriate Assistive Technology. Gaithersburg, Md.: Aspen publishers. 1996. pp. 162-190

[25] Greenstein DB. It' child's play. In: Galvin JC, Scherer MJ, editors. Evaluating, Selecting and Using Appropriate Assistive Technology. Gaithersburg, Md.: Aspen publishers. 1996. pp. 198-213

[26] Hersh MA, Johnson MA. On modelling assistive technology systems part 1: Modelling framework, Technology and Disability. 2008;**20**(3):193-215

[27] Hersh MA, Johnson MA. On modelling assistive technology systems part 2: Applications of the comprehensive assistive technology model. Technology and Disability. 2008;**20**(4):251-270

[28] Activity, human, and context: The human doing an activity in context. In: Cook AM, Polgar JM, editors. Cook and Hussey's Assistive Technologies: Principles and Practice. 4th ed. St. Louis, MO: Mosby Elsevier; 2015. pp. 40-67

[29] Disability and assistive technology systems. In: Hersh MA, Johnson MA, editors. Assistive Technology for Visually Impaired and Blind People. London, Guildford, UK, Springer Verlag; 2008. pp. 1-47

[30] Bryant DP, Bryant BR. Assistive Technology for People with Disabilities. Boston: Allyn &Bacon/Pearson; 2011

[31] Technologies that assist people who have disabilities. In: Cook AM, Polgar JM, editors. Cook and Hussey's Assistive Technologies: Principles and Practice. 4th ed. St. Louis, MO: Mosby Elsevier; 2014. pp. 16-39

[32] Miskelly FG. Assistive technology in elderly care. Age and Ageing. 2001;**30**(6):455-458

[33] Wright VC, Chang J, Jeng G, Macaluso M, Control CfD, Prevention. Assisted reproductive technology surveillance—United States, 2005. MMWR Surveillance Summaries. 2008;**57**(5):1-23

[34] Borg J, Larsson S, Östergren PO. The right to assistive technology: For whom, for what, and by whom? Disability & Society. 2011;**26**(2):151-167

[35] Gitlin LN, editor. International Handbook of Occupational Therapy Interventions. Springer International Publishing; 2015, p. 165-175 11p.

[36] Law M, Cooper B, Strong S, Stewart D, Rigby P, Letts L. The person-environment-occupation model: A transactive approach to occupational performance. Canadian Journal of Occupational Therapy. 1996;**63**(1):9-23

[37] Scherer MJ. Assistive Technology: Matching Device and Consumer for Successful Rehabilitation. Washington, DC, American Psychological Association; 2002

[38] Ivanoff SD, Iwarsson S, Sonn U. Occupational therapy research on assistive technology and physical environmental issues: A literature review. Canadian Journal of Occupational Therapy. 2006;**73**(2):109-119

[39] Rose DH, Hasselbring TS, Stahl S, Zabala J. Assistive technology and universal design for learning: Two sides of the same coin. Handbook of Special Education Technology Research and Practice. 2005. pp. 507-518. Whitefish Bay, WI: Knowledge by Design.

[40] Schoonover J, Norton-Darr S. Adapting books: Ready, set, read!: EAT: Equipment, adaptations, and technology. Journal of Occupational Therapy, Schools & Early Intervention. 2016;**9**(1):19-26

[41] Lancioni G, Sigafoos J, O'Reilly MF, Singh NN. Assistive Technology: Interventions for Individuals with Severe/Profound and Multiple Disabilities. Newyork: Springer; 2012

[42] Association ATIA. AT Resources. ATİA; 2017. https://www.atia.org/at-resources/what-is-at/

[43] Phillips B, Zhao H. Predictors of assistive technology abandonment. Assistive Technology. 1993;**5**(1):36-45

[44] Occupational therapy practice framework: Domain and process. The American Journal of Occupational Therapy. 2014;**68**:1-48

[45] Phillips B, Zhao H. Predictors of assistive technology abandonment. Assistive Technology. 1993;**5**(1):36-45

[46] Lesar S. Use of assistive technology with young children with disabilities. Journal of Early Intervention. 1998;**21**(2):146-159

[47] Riemer-Reiss ML, Wacker RR. Factors associated with assistive technology discontinuance among individuals with disabilities. Journal of Rehabilitation. 2000;**66**(3):44-50

[48] Copley J, Ziviani J. Barriers to the use of assistive technology for children with multiple disabilities. Occupational Therapy International. 2004;**11**(4):229-243

[49] Bernd T, Van Der Pijl D, De Witte LP. Existing models and instruments for the selection of assistive technology in rehabilitation practice. Scandinavian Journal of Occupational Therapy. 2009;**16**(3):146-158

[50] Principles of assistive technology: Introducing the human activity assistive technology model. In: Cook AM, Polgar JM, editors. Assistive Technologies: Principles and Practice. 4th ed. St. Louis, MO: Mosby Elsevier; 2015. pp. 1-15

[51] Friederich A, Bernd T, De Witte L. Methods for the selection of assistive technology in neurological rehabilitation practice. Scandinavian Journal of Occupational Therapy. 2010;**17**(4):308-318

[52] Scherer MJ, Frisina DR. Characteristics associated with marginal hearing loss and subjective well-being among a sample of older adults. Journal of Rehabilitation Research and Development. 1998;**35**(4):420-426

[53] Scherer M, Jutai J, Fuhrer M, Demers L, Deruyter F. A framework for modelling the selection of assistive technology devices (ATDs). Disability and Rehabilitation Assistive Technology. 2007;**2**(1):1-8

[54] Lenker JA, Paquet VL. A review of conceptual models for assistive technology outcomes research and practice. Assistive Technology. 2003;**15**(1):1-15

[55] Roelands M, Van Oost P, Depoorter A, Buysse A. A social-cognitive model to predict the use of assistive devices for mobility and self-care in elderly people. The Gerontologist. 2002;**42**(1):39-50

[56] Ivanoff SD, Iwarsson S, Sonn U. Occupational therapy research on assistive technology and physical environmental issues: A literature review. Canadian Journal of Occupational Therapy [Revue canadienne d'ergotherapie]. 2006;**73**(2):109-119

[57] Giesbrecht E. Application of the Human Activity Assistive Technology model for occupational therapy research. Australian Occupational Therapy Journal. 2013;**60**(4):230-240

[58] Wiart L, Darrah J. Changing philosophical perspectives on the management of children with physical disabilities—Their effect on the use of powered mobility. Disability and Rehabilitation. 2002;**24**(9):492-498

[59] van der Woude LHV, de Groot S, Janssen TWJ. Manual wheelchairs: Research and innovation in rehabilitation, sports, daily life and health. Medical Engineering & Physics. 2006;**28**(9):905-915

[60] Giesbrecht EM, Ripat JD, Quanbury AO, Cooper JE. Participation in community-based activities of daily living: Comparison of a pushrim-activated, power-assisted wheelchair and a power wheelchair. Disability and Rehabilitation Assistive Technology. 2009;**4**(3):198-207

[61] Arthanat S, Nochajski SM, Lenker JA, Bauer SM, Wu YW. Measuring usability of assistive technology from a multicontextual perspective: The case of power wheelchairs. The American Journal of Occupational Therapy. 2009;**63**(6):751-764

[62] Funding assistive technology services to the consumer. In: Cook AM, Polgar JM, editors. Cook and Hussey's Assistive Technologies: Principles and Practice. 3rd ed. St. Louis, MO: Mosby Elsevier; 2008. pp. 143-176

[63] Turkish Medicines and Medical Devices Agency (TMMDA). Available from: http://www.titck.gov.tr/TıbbiCihaz/TıbbiCihazHakkında [Accessed: 25 February 2017]

[64] Health Application Notification (Sağlık Uygulama Tebliği-SUT). 2008. Available from: http://www.resmigazete.gov.tr/eskiler/2008/09/20080929M1-1.htm [Accessed: 25 February 2017]

[65] Complementary and Supportive Health Insurance Model Recommendations for Turkey. 2013. Available from: www.tsb.org.tr/Document/Yonetmelikler/TSS_Rapor_16.05.14.docx [Accessed: 25 February 2017]

9

Efficacy of a Stress Management Module in Managing Stress and Clean Time in Dual Diagnosis (Mental Illness and Substance Misuse) Clients

Patricia Precin

Abstract

A 1-year pilot quasi-experimental efficacy study of the Stress Management for Recovery Module (SM) was performed with 37 dual diagnosis (DD) clients from a DD outpatient clinic in the United States. It was hypothesized that clients who received the SM would show more improvement in their ability to manage stress and clean time than controls and when compared to themselves before and after the SM intervention. Outcome data showed that clients who received the SM learned new material and used it to make changes in their lives. Results from paired sample t tests demonstrated that clients who received the SM showed a significant improvement in their number of clean days during intervention as compared to before ($p = 0.008$). Clients showed a significant improvement in their knowledge of stress after the intervention as compared to before (pre- versus post-test) ($p = 0.033$), but there was no significant difference when compared to the control group. These results indicate that this SM is an effective method for improving stress management skills and clean time in DD clients at this clinic and a need for future randomized and controlled experimentation.

Keywords: living skills, occupational therapy, addiction

1. Introduction and literature review

Over the last 30 years, clinical researchers have been establishing best practices for dual diagnosis (DD) clients (clients diagnosed with a chronic major mental illness and substance abuse or dependence). Treatment techniques often involved motivational enhancement, peer support, harm minimization, and relapse prevention. Group treatment usually focused on psychoeducation on drug use and mental health, reasons for drug use, reasons to change, harm reduction strategies, planning for the future, assertiveness training to cope with high risk situations [1–3], leisure activity development [4], and skills training (stress management, time management, and social skills including assertiveness training) with an emphasis on problem solving [5, 6], refusal of drugs, and coping with cravings throughout topics. Treatment facilities included both inpatient and outpatient programs. Most of these researchers used an intervention group that ran anywhere from 2 to 18 months [7] with a closed cohort group, or an open group of ongoing duration where clients were discharged after meeting the group's objectives. Timko, Dixon, and Moss [8] reported 70% of the 298 nationwide *psychiatric* residential Veterans Affairs treatment facilities in their study offered some form of stress management treatment for their DD clients and 90% out of 114 nationwide *substance abuse* residential Veterans Affairs treatment facilities they studied offered some form of stress management treatment for their DD clients.

Even though the efficacy studies above all included some form of stress management to help clients develop alternative ways to manage their problems, there have been few studies published to date that examine the effects of a treatment group focused exclusively on stress management training for DD clients. Yet, many clinician/authors have stated that the inclusion of stress management training in a DD rehabilitation program is imperative. Hodgson et al. [4] stated that DD clients need to develop alternative coping behaviors to substance misuse. Lindsay [9] believed that one of the major roles of a therapist working in alcohol treatment facilities is to help clients identify daily problems and learn to cope with them in new ways that do not include substance misuse. Patrick [10] stated that persons with schizophrenia and substance misuse are particularly susceptible to stress, both perceived and anticipated, and that stress management helps prevent relapse in these clients. Goldman and Barr [11] offered an explanation for increased anxiety and depression upon drug cessation, the rapid decrease in abnormally high (from substance misuse) levels of dopamine. Gutman [12] recommended stress management to deal with these intense initial emotions but also ongoing emotions, since addiction effects neurological pathways throughout the lifespan even after drug cessation. Buijsse et al. [13] suggest stress management training to teach techniques that can be used to decrease the effects of environmental stress on people who misuse substances.

The Living Skills Recovery Curriculum (LSRC) [14] is a treatment intervention that helps DD clients acquire basic living skills. It contains four different modules: Activities of Daily living for Abstinence, Social Skills for Sobriety, Time Management for 12-Step Treatment, and Stress Management for Recovery. Each skill is taught in relation to how it aids in relapse prevention and recovery for each client's personal lifestyle and pattern of addiction.

The purpose of this study was to examine the efficacy of the Stress Management Recovery training module on reducing substance misuse and increasing the ability to manage stress in DD clients with the hope that it can be utilized in other settings by occupational therapists. A reduction in substance misuse is defined as an increase in the number of days sober, or a decrease in the length of drug relapses, or a decrease in the number of drug relapses. The ability to manage stress is defined as the use of healthy coping skills to manage daily stressors. The hypothesis is that clients who received the LSRC's SM would show more improvement in their ability to manage stress and clean time than controls and when compared to themselves before and after SM intervention.

2. Method

2.1. Sample

The subjects in this 1-year quasi-experimental efficacy study (both experimental and control) were adults (over 18 years of age) from a DD outpatient clinic in a metropolitan hospital in the United States where the average length of stay was 5 years. The clinic was in operation Monday through Friday from 9:00 am to 2:00 pm. Both experimental and control group clients received treatment through the DD clinic as clinically necessitated. Treatment for both groups included the possibility of substance misuse groups, vocational groups, task groups, music therapy, nursing intervention, and psychiatric services. All received once-a-week case management services and random drug screens. All gave written consent to be in the study.

The total number of subjects in the experimental group (those that received the LSRC's SM) was 21. For their demographics, see **Tables 1** and **2**. Some of the clients' clean time data were not available before the SM began because these clients started the SM when they started the program. For some other clients, clean time measures could not be obtained 4 months after the SM because they graduated from the program. Therefore, when statistical analyses on clean time were performed, the number of clients (N) in the groups varied. Occasionally, some of the clients preferred not to take the pre- or post-test; so the N was adjusted accordingly and reported separately for each outcome. The total number of subjects in the control group was 16. Their demographics are also reported in **Tables 1** and **2**.

	Experimental		Control	
Demographic	#	%	#	%
Median age	18	37	16	36
Male	12	67	11	66
Female	6	33	5	34
African-American	12	67	11	68.75
Caucasian	3	12	2	12.5
Hispanic	2	11	2	12.5
Other	1	9	1	6.25
Mean # psychiatric hospitalizations	18	6	16	6
Mean # detoxifications	18	1	16	1
Mean # of rehabilitations	18	0.5	16	1

Table 1. Demographics of experimental and control groups.

	Experimental		Control	
Diagnoses	#	%	#	%
Schizophrenia with				
Polysubstance	5	28	8	50
Crack	3	17	4	25
Alcohol & crack	3	17		
Alcohol & cocaine	1	5.5		
Alcohol & marijuana	1	5.5	1	6.25
Cocaine	1	5.5		
Alcohol	1	5.5	2	12.5
Marijuana	1	5.5		
Marijuana & crack	1	5.5		
Other	1	5.5	1	6.25
Total	18	100	16	100

Table 2. Diagnostic Statistical Manual diagnoses.

2.2. Treatment

The SM of the LSRC included 16 topic areas dealing with stress management for recovery. The topics provided a structured skeleton useful to elicit personal information from clients on their strengths and problem areas in coping with stressful recovery situations and identifying stressful situations and their personal signs of stress. Topics also provided stress management techniques that had to do with recovery, such as developing alternative coping strategies that did not involve drugs, managing raw emotions (anger management), identifying triggers and warning signs, relaxation skills, stretching exercises, biofeedback, nutrition, music, poetry, crafts, and how to work through relapses. The SM utilized a cognitive behavioral approach to recovery and living skills acquisition. Paradigms of treatment included peer support (universality from group intervention), harm minimization, and relapse prevention. Goal setting and problem solving skills were emphasized throughout all topics.

2.3. Measures

2.3.1. Pre-test

A pre-test was administered to both the experimental group and control group the day before the SM began in order to determine the clients' knowledge of stress management prior to intervention. The pre-test used was a paper and pencil open-ended questionnaire with six questions on stress management that was replicated from Precin's *Living Skills Recovery Workbook* [14] for this population. No reliability or validity studies have yet been published using this questionnaire. Clients completed the questionnaire in 5–10 min.

2.3.2. *Post-test*

A post-test was administered to both the experimental group and control group the day after the SM ended in order to determine how much of the SM material was learned and/or relearned, stored, and recalled after 4 months of SM intervention. The post-test was the same as the pre-test, and clients were able to complete it in 5–10 min.

2.3.3. *Outcome measures*

2.3.3.1. *Attendance*

Attendance was a measure of the number of sessions attended per client in the experimental group.

2.3.3.2. *Objectives*

Each session of the SM had approximately 4–6 objectives to be learned by each client as listed in the LSRC Group Leader Plans [14]. Scores were percentages of total possible objectives that a client met on the days he or she attended the SM. This was a measure of the amount of material learned each session and only gathered for the experimental group.

2.3.3.3. *Goals*

Goals were the number of SM related goals that the clients in the experimental group achieved during the 4-month treatment period. This is a measure of how well material generalized to the outside.

2.3.3.4. *Members report that they learned new material (MRLNM)*

At the end of the intervention, each client in the experimental group completed a satisfaction questionnaire [14] in which he or she stated whether or not they learned new material.

2.3.3.5. *Members report that they made changes in their lives (MRMCL)*

At the end of the intervention, each client in the experimental group completed a satisfaction questionnaire [14] in which he or she stated whether or not they made changes in their lives due to the SM intervention.

2.3.3.6. *Staff observations (SO)*

At the end of the 4-month intervention period, staff members not involved in the LSRC reported whether they thought their clients in the experimental group's skills in stress management improved, stayed the same, or got worse during the 4-month intervention period.

2.3.3.7. *Clean time*

Clean time was collected three different ways to increase the accuracy of measuring substance use. The number of clean days (#CD), the number of relapses (#R), and the average length of relapse (ALR) were counted 4 months before, during, and 4 months after intervention. To control for the influence of other aspects of treatment taking place in the dual diagnosis clinic, the same clean time measures (#CD, #R, ALR) were gathered at enrollment. Clean time measures were obtained from the clients' charts through the substance abuse counselor's documentation of drug screen results.

2.4. Procedures

Treatment began after the facility's Internal Review Board approved this study under an exempt status because no risks were involved and no invasive procedures were used. The LSRC's SM was run in the DD clinic by an occupational therapist for 4 months three times consecutively in 1 year. Clients attended twice-a-week. Each time, the module was run with seven clients in the group, so that at the end of a year, a total of 21 clients received the SM and constituted the experimental group.

The control group consisted of clients in the DD clinic not currently assigned to the module who gave consent to be in the study through their case managers. There were three control groups of six, five, and five clients each with a total of 16 clients. Each time, outcome measurements were taken from the SM experimental group, and the same outcome measures were gathered from each control group. Data were gathered, recorded, and analyzed by the author.

2.5. Statistical and data analysis

Statistical data were analyzed using the Statistical Package for the Social Sciences (SPSS) program. Percentages were calculated by the author. In order to examine the effectiveness of the LSRC SM, a within subjects, paired t-test was used to compare the difference in post-test scores from the pre-test scores. In addition, an independent t-test was used to compare the participants of the SM to controls to see whether the change in score was due to the intervention or to participation in the program. The data distribution was evaluated using Leven's test for Equality of Variance. For non-normal data, the Mann-Whitney U test (a nonparametric statistic) was employed. Findings with a p value < or = to 0.05 were considered statistically significant. To further examine the effectiveness of the LSRC, percentages of the number of objectives met, attendance, MRLNM, MRMCL, and SO, along with the number of goals met were calculated for clients in the experimental group. Within subjects analyses, using paired t tests were performed to investigate whether the DD members significantly increased their clean time during and after receiving the SM as compared to their previous amount of clean time before intervention began. Correlations using a Pearson-product moment correlation coefficient were used to answer the following investigative questions. Was newly learned material lost over time? Was attendance a factor in clients' progress? Did staff's observations correlate with members' self-reports of progress and/or objective findings? Did members' self-report of progress correlate with other objective findings? Did the number of goals met on the outside correlate with the amount of material each patient learned throughout the session? Do patients who report having learned new material also tend to report that they made changes in their lives due to the SM? Pearson-product moment correlation coefficients were also used to see whether there were any correlations between demographics and the ability to utilize the SM.

3. Results

3.1. Change in pre- and post-test values

The change in pre- and post-test values between experimental and control groups over time is presented in **Table 3**. For 18 members in the SM experimental group, the mean pre-test in SM was 0.30 ($SD = 0.16$). This increased to a 0.46 ($SD = 0.26$) post-SM score. This increase in value was statistically significant ($p = 0.033$) within the experimental group as per a paired samples t test. For the 16 individuals in the control group, the mean pre-test in SM was 0.15 ($SD = 0.19$). This increased to a 0.22 ($SD = 0.21$) post-SM score. This increase in value was not statistically significant ($p = 0.331$) within the control group as per a paired samples t test. The rate of change between pre- and post-test scores was compared in the experimental group with the control group. The average change from pre- to post-test for the experimental group was 0.16, whereas the average change for the control group was 0.07. The resulting p value of 0.92 ($t[19] = -0.10$) generated from an independent t test reflecting the magnitude of change per groups (experimental verses control) was not statistically significant. The 95% confidence interval for the mean difference between the two was −1.91 to 1.73.

Treatment				**Control**				***p*-Value**
Pre-test		Post-test		Pre-test		Post-test		
N	*M (SD)*	*N*	*M (SD)*	*N*	*M (SD)*	*N*	*M (SD)*	
18	0.30 (16)	18	0.46 (0.26)	16	0.15 (0.19)	16	0.22 (0.21)	0.92

Note: *p*-Value is derived from unpaired t test on the mean change from pre-test to post-test and reflects a paired analysis reflecting the magnitude of change per groups.

Table 3. Average change from pre- to post-test values between treatment and control groups over time.

3.2. Effectiveness of SM on the experimental group

The 21 clients in the SM experimental group achieved an average of 77% of the total number of objectives possible in SM on the days they attended. The average number of goals related to stress management achieved by each client during the SM was four. The average attendance throughout the 4 months was 63%. Ninety-one percent of the clients reported that they learned new material, and 86% reported that they made changes in their lives as a result of the SM training. The staff observed that 73% of the clients showed improvement in their ability to manage stress during the intervention.

3.3. Substance use

3.3.1. *Clean days*

For the results of the #CD, see **Table 4**. For 18 individuals in the SM, the mean #CD 4 months before treatment was 84.4 ($SD = 44.1$). This increased to 108.9 ($SD = 23.6$) during intervention. This increase in value was statistically significant ($t[17] = -3.01$, $p = 0.008$) within the experimental group as per paired samples t test. The 95% confidence interval for the mean difference between the two was −41.58 to −7.30. There was a slight drop in the #CD 4 months after intervention ($M = 102.2$, $SD = 38.1$). This drop was not significant when compared to the #CD 4 months before treatment ($t[17] = 1.69$, $p = 0.11$, 95% CI −4.46 to 40.02) or the #CD during intervention ($t[17] = -0.76$, $p = 0.46$, 95% CI −25.07 to 11.74).

Measure	Clean time					
	4MB	4MD	4MA	P1	P2	P3
	M (SD)	*M (SD)*	*M (SD)*			
Clean days	84.40 (44.10)	108.90 (23.60)		0.008**		
		108.90 (23.60)	102.20 (38.10)			0.460
	84.40 (44.10)		102.20 (38.10)		0.110	
# Relapses	0.94 (1.40)	0.389 (0.698)		0.067		
		0.389 (0.698)	0.50 (0.86)			0.682
	0.94 (1.40)		0.50 (0.86)		0.104	
ALR	30 (43.9)	8.2 (19.3)		0.017*		
		8.2 (19.3)	16.1 (37.4)			0.343
	30 (43.9)		16.1 (37.4)		0.217	

Notes: P1 = the magnitude of difference (p) between 4MB and 4MD, P2 = the magnitude of difference (p) between the magnitude of difference between 4MD and 4MA, P3 = the magnitude of difference (p) between 4MB an 4MA, 4MB = 4 months before treatment began, 4MD = 4 months during treatment, 4MA = 4 months after treatment, * = significant at the $p < 0.05$ level, ** = significant at the $p < 0.01$ level.

Table 4. Clean time comparisons before, during, and after treatment through paired t tests, $N = 18$.

3.3.2. Relapses

For the results of the #R, see **Table 4**. For 18 individuals in the SM experimental group, the mean #R 4 months before intervention was 0.944 ($SD = 1.4$). This decreased to 0.389 ($SD = 0.698$) during intervention. This decrease in value was marginally significant ($t[17] = 1.97$, $p = 0.066$) within the experimental group as per paired samples t test. The 95% confidence interval for the mean difference between the two was −0.04 to 1.15. The mean #R 4 months after intervention was 0.500 ($SD = 0.857$). The difference between the average #R 4 months before intervention and 4 months after intervention was not significant ($t[17] = -1.72$, $p = 0.104$, 95% CI −0.99 to 0.10), nor was the difference between the average #R during intervention as compared to 4 months after intervention ($t[17] = 0.42$, $p = 0.682$, 95% CI −0.452 to 0.674).

3.3.3. Average length of relapses

For the results of the ALR, see **Table 4**. For 18 individuals in the SM experimental group, the ALR 4 months before intervention was 30 days ($SD = 43.9$). This decreased to 8.2 ($SD = 19.3$) days during intervention. This decrease in value was statistically significant ($t[17] = 2.65$, $p = 0.017$) within the experimental group as per paired samples t test. The 95% confidence interval for the mean difference between the two was 4.45 to 39.1. The ALR 4 months after intervention was 16.1 days ($SD = 37.4$). The difference between the ALR 4 months before intervention as compared to after intervention was not significant ($t[17] = -1.28$, $p = 0.217$, 95% CI −36.87 to 8.98), nor was the difference between the ALR during intervention and 4 months after intervention ($t[17] = 0.97$, $p = 0.343$, 95% CI −9.12 to 24.78).

3.4. Correlations

For the results of correlations between SM outcomes in the experimental group see **Table 5**. In the SM experimental group, the following positive correlations were significant at the $p < 0.05$ level: attendance and number of objectives met, attendance and number of goals met, attendance and MRLNM, attendance and MRMCL, number of objectives met and MRLNM, number of objectives met and SO, MRLNM and MRMCL, MRLNM and SO, MRMCL and SO. All other correlations in the stress management experimental group were not significant at the $p < 0.05$ level. There were no significant correlations between the demographics of the experimental group and any of the outcome measures.

	Attendance	Objectives	Goals	MRLNM	MRMCL
Attendance					
Objectives	$r = 0.553$**				
	$N = 21$				
	$p = 0.009$				
Goals	$r = 0.723$**	$r = 0.292$			
	$N = 22$	$N = 18$			
	$p = 0.000$	$p = 0.240$			

	Attendance	Objectives	Goals	MRLNM	MRMCL
MRLNM	$r = 0.710$**	$r = 0.618$**	$r = 0.330$		
	$N = 21$	$N = 18$	$N = 21$		
	$p = 0.000$	$p = 0.006$	$p = 0.144$		
MRMCL	$r = 0.645$**	$r = 0.414$	$r = 0.393$	$r = 0.795$**	
	$N = 21$	$N = 18$	$N = 21$	$N = 22$	
	$p = 0.002$	$p = 0.09$	$p = 0.078$	$p = 0.000$	
SO	$r = 0.274$	$r = 0.535$**	$r = 0.226$	$r = 0.513$*	$r = 0.647$**
	$N = 22$	$N = 18$	$N = 22$	$N = 21$	$N = 21$
	$p = 0.218$	$p = 0.022$	$p = 0.311$	$p = 0.017$	$p = 0.002$

Notes: **Correlation is significant at the 0.01 level (2-tailed). *Correlation is significant at the 0.05 level (two-tailed). MRLNM = members report that they learned new material as a result of SM, MRNCL = members report that they made changes in their lives as a result of SM, and SO = staff observations.

Table 5. Correlation matrix of LSRC outcomes using Pearson-product moment coefficient.

4. Discussion

The experimental group significantly increased their knowledge of stress management information after completing the SM, demonstrating the ability to learn, store, and recall new information, whereas the control group did not show a significant increase. However, the increase noted in the experimental group when compared to the control group was no longer significant. Since there were improvements in so many other aspects of stress management in the experimental group, it could be that stress management is best learned and utilized through hands on experience and talking about feelings instead of obtaining knowledge about the subject. It is one thing to "know about" stress reduction, but a different experience to "feel it in one's bones." The fact that the SM does both could account for the difference in outcomes. For instance, the objectives for each session of the SM incorporate knowledge about stress management with hands on experience. The objective for day 26, "clients will use biofeedback as a stress management technique," presents the knowledge of how to count breaths and gives the client the physical experience that respiration rate can be controlled and decreasing respiration rate can be calming. Clients did very well in achieving the objectives for each session (an average of 77% of the objectives was met in the SM). The fact that clients achieved on the average of four stress management goals that they set during the SM demonstrates that the material learned and experienced generalized to their lives outside the clinic.

The other outcome measures also support the efficacy of the LSRC's SM. Clients in the experimental group (91%) reported that they learned new material and 86% reported that they made changes in their lives as a result of the SM. This is consistent with staff members reporting that 73% of their clients in SM were better able to manage stress. Clients who participated in the SM significantly improved their #CD and their ALR. Four months after SM ended, they experienced a slight decrease in #CD and ALR. Although this decrease was statistically insignificant when compared to their clean time during SM, it was also statistically insignificant when compared to before SM, indicating that clients were almost back to where they started before intervention. In order for stress management for recovery intervention to be effective, it should be longer than 4 months. Clients showed no significant change in the #R before, during, or after SM. This could be because the average #R was and remained one, so there was not a lot of improvement to be made. Correlations indicated that newly learned material was not lost over time (percentage of objectives met x post-test scores). This may be due to repetition, review, and multiple modes of training (visual, auditory, bodily sensations, and eliciting prior experiences), which have been built into the curriculum. Attendance was an important factor in clients' progress. The more clients came to SM, the more objectives and goals they met, the more they reported that they learned new material, and the more staff observed improvements in their ability to manage stress. Even though the attendance rate of 63% achieved by the experimental group is standard for what is reported in psychiatric clinics, it may be beneficial, given the significance of attendance, to generate ways to improve it.

Staff's observations correlated positively with members' self-report of progress and the number of objectives met. Staff's sensitivity to improvement is necessary to encourage and provide positive feedback to clients and provide continuity across intervention modalities throughout the clinic, just as their sensitivity to ongoing needs of the clients can be helpful in referring future clients to the LSRC. Members' self-report of progress correlated with one of two objective findings. There was a positive correlation between member's reporting that they learned new material and achieving objectives, but not with the number of goals met outside the clinic. Perhaps the clients in answering this question did not consider goal achievement an indicator of change. If so, this would be an important connection to help the clients make in order for their self-esteem to fully benefit from their progress. The number of goals met on the outside did positively correlate with the amount of material each patient learned throughout the session. Patients who report having learned new material also tend to report that they made changes in their lives due to the SM.

4.1. Limitations

This study was a quasi-experiment. The author used a sample of convenience that followed the selection/referral procedure found in most clinics. Although the demographic profile of these clients closely approximated those in the literature for dual diagnosis outpatient clinics, caution should be used if generalizing the results to other settings because of a possible sample bias. Validity and reliability of the pre-/post-test had not been established.

4.2. Conclusion

The LSRC's SM is an effective method for improving stress management skills and clean time in DD clients in this DD clinic. Clients significantly increased their number of clean days, decreased their average length of relapse, and were able to learn, store, and recall information on stress management. They achieved over three-fourths of the daily objectives, reported learning new material, and were able to make changes in their lives by generalizing what they learned/experienced to their environment outside the clinic. These results lend support for future randomized controlled experiments to investigate the efficacy of this SM with DD clients and also for the use of this module by occupational therapists working with the DD population.

Acknowledgements

This research was supported by a grant from the Metropolitan New York District of the New York State Occupational Therapy Association.

Author details

Patricia Precin

Address all correspondence to: patricia.precin@touro.edu

Occupational Therapy at Touro College, Licensed Psychoanalyst in Private Practice, Faculty of the National Psychological Association for Psychoanalysis and Stony Brook University, New York, NY, USA

References

[1] Chaney E, O'Leary M, Marlatt G. Skill training with alcoholics. Journal of Consulting Clinical Psychology. 1976;**46**:1092-1104. DOI: 10.1037/0022-006X.46.5.1092

[2] Jones S, Kanfer R, Lanyon R. Skills training with alcoholics: A clinical extension. Addictive Behavior. 1982;**7**:285-290. DOI: 10.1016/0306-4603(82)90057-0

[3] Marlatt G, Gordon J, editors. Relapse Prevention: Maintenance Strategies in the Treatment of Addictive Behavior. New York: Guilford; 1985

[4] Hodgson S, Lloyd C, Schmid T. The leisure participation of clients with a dual diagnosis. British Journal of Occupational Therapy. 2001;**64**(10):487-492. DOI: 10.1177/030802260106401003

[5] Abrams D. Psychosocial assessment of alcohol and stress interactions: Bridging the gap between laboratory and treatment outcome research. In Pohorecky L, Brick J, editors. Stress and Alcohol Use. New York: Elsevier Biomedical; 1983. pp. 61-86.

[6] Monti P, Abrams D, Kadden R, Cooney N.. Treating Alcohol Dependence: A Coping Skills Guide. New York: Guilford; 1990

[7] Jerrell JM, Ridgely MS. Comparative effectiveness of three approaches to serving people with severe mental illness and substance abuse disorders. The Journal of Nervous and Mental Disease. 1995;**183**(9):566-576. DOI: 10.1097/00005053-199509000-00002

[8] Timko C, Dixon K, Moos RH. Treatment for dual diagnosis patients in the psychiatric and substance abuse systems. Mental Health Services Research. 2005;**7**(4):229-242. DOI: 10.1007/s11020-005-7455-9

[9] Lindsay W. The role of the occupational therapist: Treatment of alcoholism. American Journal of Occupational Therapy. 1983;**37**:36-43. DOI: 10.5014/ajot.37.1.36

[10] Patrick DD. Dual diagnosis: Substance-related and psychiatric disorders. Nursing Clinics of North America. 2003;**38**(1):67-73. DOI: 10.1016/S0029-6465(02)00066-X

[11] Goldman D, Barr CS. Clinical implications of basic research. Restoring the addicted brain. New England Journal of Medicine. 2002;**347**:843-845.

[12] Gutman, S. Why addiction has a chronic, relapsing course. The neurobiology of addiction: implications for occupational therapy practice. Occupational Therapy in Mental Health. 2006;**22**:1-29. DOI: 10.1300/J004v22n02_01

[13] Buijsse N, Woody C, Davis SF. Occupational therapy in the treatment of addictive behaviors. British Journal of Therapy and Rehabilitation. 1999;**6**:300-307. DOI: 10.12968/bjtr.1999.6.6.13973

[14] Precin P. Living Skills Recovery Workbook. Brattleboro, VM: Echo Point Books and Media, LLC; 2015

10

Arthritis/Rheumatoid Arthritis

Zeynep Bahadır Ağce, Esma Özkan and Barkın Köse

Abstract

Rheumatoid arthritis is a progressive, chronic, and degenerative disease that adversely affects the quality of life of individuals. Depending on the individual's symptoms of rheumatoid arthritis, basic and instrumental daily life activities are restricted, and participation of life is adversely affected. Occupational therapy interventions for rheumatoid arthritis rehabilitation include self-management programs (e.g., arthritis self-management program, bone up on arthritis, self-management arthritis treatment physical activity), splinting techniques for rheumatoid arthritis, and vocational rehabilitation. In this chapter, updated information about these approaches is brought together and presented to the reader.

Keywords: coping with rheumatoid arthritis, health education, joint protection, energy conservation, occupational therapy, rheumatoid arthritis

1. Introduction

Arthritis is a very common health problem which is cause activity of daily living (ADL)–related and instrumental activity of daily living (IADL)–related functional disability, restriction of work and social participation, and fulfilling their life roles [1–6]. Arthritis is characterized by inflammation, autoimmune cell activation, and tissue destruction in the joints [7–9]. The patients typically complain about joint pain, stiffness, generalized fatigue, and reduced quality of life [2, 9–12]. Symptoms are seen in exacerbations and remissions [9]. Arthritis has many different types, such as rheumatoid arthritis (RA), psoriatic arthritis, systemic lupus erythematosus, ankylosing spondylitis, reactive arthritis, and juvenile idiopathic arthritis [8].

This chapter focuses on the rheumatoid arthritis and influences person's life. Rheumatoid arthritis (RA) prevalence ranges from 0.3 to 1% of the adult population, and female-to-male prevalence ratio was 4:1 [10, 13, 14]. It is related to low- and middle-income countries [10, 15, 16].

Rheumatoid arthritis affects people's life balance and their ability to perform work, leisure, self-care, and rest and sleep decreased [17–19]. In addition, they lose values of activity for their life so feel anxious and depressed and influence their health related quality of life [20–22].

Occupational therapist works with not only pain or symptoms management in rheumatoid arthritis but also the prevention of functional limitations and adaptation to lifestyle changes improve emotional state and social participation to maintain independence in daily living activities [11, 19, 23]. Occupational therapy (OT) interventions especially focus on improving occupational performance which is negatively affected by rheumatoid arthritis. For this reason, occupational therapists use some approaches for improving occupational performance such as using behavioral change approach, energy conservation approach, relax renovation and pain control, fatigue management, maintain ındependence, adaptive device, and home adaptations in rheumatoid arthritis [9, 24].

2. Prevalence and incidence

Arthritis includes approximately over 150 diseases and syndromes, and arthritis is the common problem and reason of substantial pain, limitation of activity, work, and social participation [2, 25, 26]. Rheumatoid arthritis is the most common variety among arthritis types [27]. Rheumatoid arthritis is typically diagnosed in adults between the ages 30 and 50, though it can develop at any age [28]. It is related to low- and middle-income countries, and one study showed high education level is influenced by positive feel pain and functional capacity [15, 25, 29]. At least 50% of the patients who live in developed countries have lost their ability to work in 10 years [25]. Family history is an important risk to occurrence of RA, the risk rate of twins increased approximately three to five [27]. The incidence of rheumatoid arthritis is thought to be influenced by geographical conditions, the prevalence of rheumatoid arthritis according to studies conducted in various nations is: in Turkey 0.57%, in Italy 0.48%, in France 0.29%,in Lithuania 0.50%, in Serbia 0.35%, in Argentina 0.329%, in Sweden 0.41%, in the USA 0.5–1.0% of general population [14, 30–33]. According to the 2010 classification criteria, countries' incidence rates are different from each other, for instance, the rate in Catalonia 0.20/1000 person/years, in Argentina 18.5/100,000 person/years, in Sweden 41/100,000 person/years, in Italy 68/100,000 person/years, in the UK 79/10,000 person/years, and in the USA 41/100,000 person/years [14, 30–32, 34].

3. Pathology

Rheumatoid arthritis is a chronic progressive disease that affects joints and systems [35]. Due to the presence of autoantibodies [seropositivity] in rheumatoid arthritis, which is an autoimmune disease, many symptoms have occurred, such as joints and bone destruction and mortality [27, 36, 37]. Although the pathophysiology of rheumatoid arthritis is not clearly explained, it is known that genetic and environmental factors affect the development of the illness [27, 35, 37]. Environmental effects such as recurrent exposure to exogenous, endogenous, commensal viral, bacterial, silica, alcohol, or smoking are factors that support the development of rheumatoid arthritis [27, 35, 38]. T cells, B cells, and pro-inflammatory cytokines have a key role in the development of the disease [35, 39]. The presence of HLA-DRB1, particularly HLA-DRB1, is associated with disease progression by affecting peptides [27]. Genetic factors affecting the development of rheumatoid arthritis have been associated with anti-citrullinated protein antibody (ACPA) positive [40]. When ACPA is positive, the risk of developing rheumatoid arthritis is increased [37]. The presence of ACPA was detected 10 years before the diagnosis of rheumatoid arthritis, and it indicated that there is an increase in ACPA, such as serum cytokine concentrations, especially before the onset of joint involvement [27]. In a study conducted on twins, it was reported that the stochastic factors, lifestyle and environmental effects, may be more effective than genetic factors in ACPA positivity. It is stated that there is a significant relationship between ACPA positivity and smoking in the study of smokers who have the DRB1 allele gene [41]. When rheumatoid arthritis is treated effectively, there is a decrease in RF and ACPA [27].

4. Diagnosis and special tests

Diagnostic tests play an important role in the diagnosis of RA, but diagnosis is based on clinical findings [28]. For the diagnosis of rheumatoid arthritis, especially autoantibodies, such as RF and anti-citrullinated protein antibody (ACPA) (tested as anti-cyclic citrullinated peptide (anti-CCP)), have been used for many years [42]. RF is frequently used in the diagnosis and follow-up of rheumatoid arthritis but is not a distinctive diagnostic parameter because it is also detected in other rheumatic diseases [28, 43]. Rheumatoid arthritis causes destruction in joints and causes disability, so early diagnosis is very important [43, 44]. Anti-cyclic citrullinated peptide/protein (anti-CCP) is especially used for early diagnosis [44]. The most widely used and most reliable test, anti-ccp2, was accepted as the gold standard in ACPAs in 2010 [42]. But ACPA is not positive for every rheumatoid arthritis patient [43]. Individuals with ACPA positive are 90% estimated to be diagnosed with rheumatoid arthritis within 3 years, while 30% of those with ACPA positive [45]. As a result of a joint study by American College of Rheumatology (ACR) and European League Against Rheumatism (EULAR) for rheumatoid arthritis diagnostic criteria, ACPA has been included in the current 2010 rheumatoid arthritis diagnostic criteria (**Table 1**) [42].

5. Living with rheumatoid arthritis

In rheumatoid arthritis, loss of function is seen in daily life due to symptoms such as degeneration, pain, swelling in joints, morning impairment, and fatigue based on joint inflammation [46]. In addition, especially effects on hand joints of rheumatoid arthritis also influence independence by causing problems in the individual's daily life activities [47, 48]. Gradually,

	Score
Target population (who should be tested?): patients who	
1. Have at least 1 joint with definite clinical synovitis (swelling)	
2. With the synovitis not better explained by another diseas	
Classification criteria for RA (score-based algorithm: add score of categories a–d;	
A score of ≥6/10 is needed for classification of a patient as having definite RA)	
A. Joint involvement	
1 large joint	0
2–10 large joints	1
1–3 small joints (with or without involvement of large joints)	2
4–10 small joints (with or without involvement of large joints)	3
>10 joints (at least one small joint)	5
B. Serology (at least one test result is needed for classification)	
Negative RF and negative ACPA	0
Low-positive RF or low-positive ACPA	2
High-positive RF or high-positive ACPA	3
C. Acute-phase reactants (at least one test result is needed for classification)	
Normal CRP and normal ESR	0
Abnormal CRP or abnormal ESR	1
D. Duration of symptoms	
<6 weeks	0
≥6 weeks	1

Table 1. The 2010 American College of Rheumatology/European League against rheumatism classification criteria for rheumatoid arthritis [42].

changes in the health of individuals lead to limitations in their ability to participate in everyday life, such as individual roles, work, school, self-care, leisure time activities, home work, and family functioning, so the quality of life of an individual is reduced [6, 32, 48–51]. The daily life of women on rheumatoid arthritis is more affected than men because of the complex roles such as motherhood, spouse, and nursing [52, 53]. It is a very difficult process to live with a chronic disease like rheumatoid arthritis [54]. After the diagnosis, the individual learns to live with rheumatoid arthritis in three stages, namely "becoming aware," "learning to live with," and finally "mastery." The first stage involves the initiation of medical treatment for the twinges problem. In the second stage, as physical life and emotional manifestations emerge, there is living with the experience of coping with multiple physical and emotional symptoms in daily life. Finally, it increases the quality of life of individuals by learning how to set goals and expectations, how to use energy, how to maintain the relationship between family and society, and how to manage the medical routine with doctors [53]. İndividuals' disease experience is different from others, and individual responses are influenced by the individual's spiritual characteristics, his/her view of the disease, biological, social, and environmental factors [49, 53, 55]. The person not only that burden from clinical symptoms, but also the physical weakness effected her/his life, so it is important that the individual maintains his/her independence in social and recreational areas [46, 53]. For this reason, although the individual has effective treatment, the level of pain, fatigue, and functionality may be low [55]. Individuals may lose physical well-being, independence, privacy, autonomy, control of cynicism, restriction of social roles, loss of opportunity to plan for the future, and decrease in family and friends relations [54]. Maintaining independence in the lives of individuals with rheumatoid arthritis is important for quality of life and well-being [48].

6. Occupational therapy evaluation

In progress of time, rheumatoid arthritis leads to a decline in well-being and quality of life, depending on the individual's functional capacity and decreased mobility, decreased productivity, and difficulties in daily life performance [6, 51, 56, 57]. For this reason, it is very important to implement the evaluation with an interdisciplinary approach [58]. As stated in the "International Classification of Functioning, Disability And Health" (ICF), the body structure and functions of the individual, as well as the level of activity and life participation and the personal and environmental factors affecting it, must be approached with a holistic perspective [59]. Rheumatoid arthritis focuses on evaluating the individual's disease management, compliance, self-efficacy, comprehension, and range of motion; due to pain and fatigue effect, the individual's functional ability to be restricted and participation in social life is affected [11, 59, 60]. Symptoms of individuals with rheumatoid arthritis may be fluctuating, so how the individual occupational performance affected by symptoms such as morning stiffness, pain and fatigue, and how to deal with it and the use of assistive devices should be evaluated [26]. In addition, how rheumatoid arthritis affects the individual's life and treatment goals and expectations should also be assessed [60].

6.1. Client history

In the past medical history of the individual, age, gender, date of diagnosis, medication and adherence, current clinical symptoms, second complications, deformities due to rheumatoid arthritis, and previous treatments should be questioned. In the assessment, personal factors such as the individual's point of view of the illness, his/her values, his/her knowledge of the illness, self-efficacy, problem-solving skills, spiritual activities, his/her feelings should be taken into consideration. In addition, the individual's personal, environmental, and social experiences, current activity level, activities restricted by rheumatoid arthritis, difficulties in work, leisure activities, family, and friends relations should be questioned [6, 9, 17, 46, 49, 55].

6.2. Occupational profile

Occupation is defined as everything that a person does in his life, such as physical, mental, social, and rest occupations, and occupations for productivity, leisure, and self-care [61]. Everybody's priority and meaningful occupations are different from others. For this reason, it is important to determine the occupation and occupational profile of the individuals who are affected by the clinical symptoms of rheumatoid arthritis [9, 53]. The individual's ability to cope with stress, where he lived or worked, family and socio cultural expectations, community resources, and transport opportunities affect his occupational performance [9, 62]. In-depth interviews with open-ended questions provide information on individual roles, meaningful activities, occupational activity level, priorities, occupational profile, activity-rest balance, individual's stress perception, social stress, relationship with health professionals, comorbidity, and physical fitness [6, 55]. Another effective method for determining the occupational profile of an individual is the typical day assessment. Typical day assessments can provide important information about how a person lives a day, such as habits and routines, sleeping, diet, exercise habits, and activity rest periods [6, 55].

6.3. Occupational performance

Occupational therapists work to improve the occupational performance of individuals who are affected by the person, environment and occupations from themselves [59]. Occupational performance can be evaluated by interviewing and observing the Canadian Occupational Performance Measure (COPM) [6, 63]. COPM is revealed by the occupational performance and satisfaction of the individual in self-care, leisure, and productivity activities [26, 64–66]. Individual self-efficacy, stress, sleep posture, use of assistive technology, and exercise habits should be considered because they may affect symptoms of rheumatoid arthritis [26]. In addition, the person-centered approach should be used to understand the individual experiences in daily life due to rheumatoid arthritis [17, 63]. Activity requirements such as work-house ergonomic conditions, tools and equipment should be assessed while assessing the factors that limit the individual's activities [6, 26]. It should not be forgotten that during the evaluation of the activity, the symptoms that the individual struggles with may change day by day or day to day [23]. For instance, which activity increased the fatigue or pain, or when it is more intense, the way the individual follows in the fight with it should be evaluated [67–70].

6.4. Evaluation of body structure

Rheumatoid arthritis is characterized by swelling in the joints, tenderness on palpation, morning stiffness, decreased range of motion, and weakening in the muscles due to them [71–73]. Therefore, the presence of posture, atrophy, swelling, scar tissue, skin changes, and deformity should be observed with the inspection [74, 75]. The increased inflammation symptom can be detected such as tenderness and swelling of the joint with palpation in rheumatoid arthritis [9, 76]. Goniometer is used to determine whether there are any limitations by evaluating passive and active ranges of motion [75]. Hand joints are particularly affected by rheumatoid arthritis, so manual muscle testing can be used to assess muscle strength; in addition, power grip, pinch grip, and tripod grip strength can be evaluated for both hands using Jamar Dynamometer [77].

The use of manual muscle testing is indicated in the general muscle strength instead of the isokinetic devices because they may provoke inflammation [9]. Surrounding measurement or water immersion methods can be used to assess swelling around the joint [77].

7. Patient education

Development of early and progressive treatment for rheumatoid arthritis (RA) made interventions to occupational therapy, physiotherapy, and patient education be done earlier [78].

The multidisciplinary teamwork consisting of rheumatologists, occupational therapists, physiotherapists, surgeons, and other contributing professionals is rather important for obtaining positive results in RA. Occupational therapy is defined as a treatment method that aims to treat and compensate the limited functions of the patients. Occupational therapy helps patients manage their daily life activities and improves their self-care skills [79].

In rheumatoid arthritis, personalized treatment programs consisting of arthritis education (individual or group), ADL education, joint protection, fatigue management and exercise (especially for the hands and arms), splinting (for the wrist/hand, foot, and neck), assisting devices, work and free time counsel, sexual advice, pain relaxation, and stress management and self-management education as required are developed by occupational therapists [3].

OT involves both therapeutic and educational interventions and aims to increase the performance of daily life duties, to facilitate successful organization of the lifestyle, and to prevent function loss. Therapists also aim to improve psychological organization of living with arthritis by helping individuals have the sense of controlling the symptoms more by means of using self-management methods and developing self-efficiencies of the individuals [79–81].

For individuals with RA, a preventive approach is adopted in order to maintain optimum participation to normal activities, to minimize dysfunction, to protect and help improve health by means of providing knowledge about the disease and facilitating positive behavior regarding effective learning strategies in improving self-management skills [81].

Patient education can be defined as planned, organized learning experiences that are developed in order to enable and support individuals to organize their health and well-being and to manage living with their condition. Education of the patient is proposed as an inseparable part of the management in RA because the individual gets prepared for self-management activities with patient education [82, 83].

A comprehensive review of studies on patient education in patients with arthritis showed a positive change in more than one factor in 77–87% of studies [84]. Another comprehensive review examined the effectiveness of patient education interventions on health status (disease activity, patient global assessment, joint counts, pain, functional disability, and psychological well-being) in patients with RA. At the end of the study was found a small beneficial effect of patient education at first follow-up for psychological status, joint counts functional disability, depression, and patient global assessment [85]. A meta-analysis of psychoeducational interventions in arthritis showed that the intervention groups experienced 22% greater advancement in depression score, 16% advancement in pain over control groups, and an 8% greater advancement in disability [86].

Patient education programs are developed based on psycho-behavioristic theories and holistic approaches in order for the patients to assume their self-care and to acquire problem-solving skills. The attitudes that reduced the risks regarding health were examined, and the fact that educational approaches aimed at individuals required behavioral change was emphasized by the World Health Organization [9]. In patient education programs, health belief model, social cognitive theory, and transtheoretical model are widely used [80, 87].

7.1. Models of health behavior

7.1.1. Health belief model

Health belief model is structured in order to clarify which beliefs are to be targeted in the communicational interventions that result in positive health behaviors. According to the health belief model, probability of a person changing his/her behavior in order to prevent the disease depends on the person's realization of the facts that he/she can also catch the disease (perceived sensitivity), the consequences of the disease may be serious (perceived seriousness), cautious behavior will prevent the disease effectively (perceived benefit) and that the benefit of reducing the dangers/risks is greater than the damage of getting into the act. The basic structures and application proposals for the health belief model are briefly given in **Table 2** [88, 89].

Basic structures	**Application proposals**
Perceived sensitivity expresses the person's belief regarding the possibility of catching the disease.	Define the population at risk and the level of risk. Personalize the risks based on an individual's characteristics or behavior. Synchronize the perceived sensitivity of the individual with the real risk.
Perceived seriousness is defined as the belief about how serious a situation and its sequels are.	Indicate the consequences of the risks and conditions.
Perceived benefit expresses the belief regarding the effectiveness of a recommended action to reduce the risk or seriousness of a disease.	Clarify when, where, and how a person should behave, and what the expected positive effects of these behaviors will be.
Perceived barrier is defined as the belief about the moral and material cost of the proposed action.	Reduce the perceived barrier by giving assurance, correcting misinformation, giving courage, and helping.
Action hints indicate the strategies based upon increasing the state of readiness.	Provide information regarding how behavioral change could be made, increase awareness and use appropriate reminding systems.
Self-efficacy reflects the confidence of the individual in his/her skill of getting into action.	Provide education and guidance during the recommended action. Set goals gradually. Give verbal support. Show sample for desired actions. Reduce the anxiety.

Table 2. Basic structures of the health belief model and application proposals [89].

Other variable factors in the application of the health belief model (age, gender, ethnic background, personal characteristics, socioeconomic condition, and educational status) influence the individual's perception of sensitivity, seriousness, benefit, and prevention and thus his/her behaviors [90].

7.1.2. *Social cognitive theory*

Social cognitive theory adopted concepts from sociology and political sciences in order to understand the functions and capacity of a group. The theory also integrated concepts of humanistic psychology by means of analyzing the processes that formed the basis of self-will, self-sacrifice, and moral behavior. Moreover, it highlights the fact that perceived targets, perceived environmental barriers and promoters, outcome expectations, and self-efficacy influence the organization of human behavior, motivation, and well-being. Perceived self-efficacy is the most important key consideration in this causative structure with the effect of other determiners. According to the social cognitive theory, social structure is also effective on health as much as personal determiners [91, 92].

Social cognitive theory added new concepts to the list of behaviors regarding health that are excluded from health belief model. First, it highlighted the motivational role of support and role of observational learning through modeling (imitating) others' behavior [93].

Second significant contribution is the definition of the concept of self-efficacy (efficacy expectations), which is distinct from the concept of outcome expectations. Outcome expectations are known as predictions of the individual regarding specific actions that would bring ultimate results, and it is quite similar to the concept of perceived benefit in the health belief model. Efficacy expectations are defined as the belief that the actions required to bring results can be managed successfully. Both efficacy and outcome expectations are required for the behavior (**Figure 1**) [94].

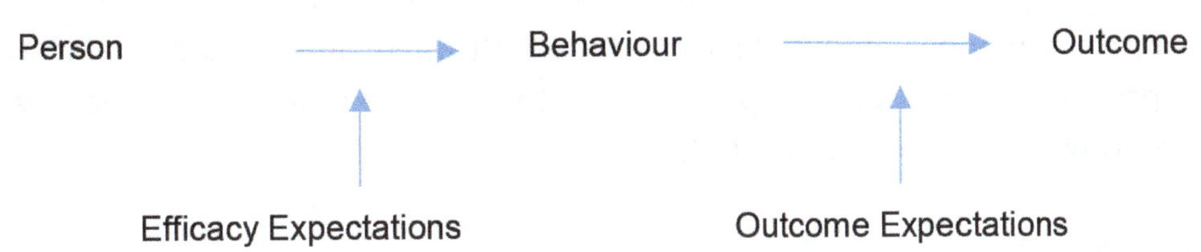

Figure 1. The effect of self-efficacy on behavior [95].

In the figure mentioned above, Bandura demonstrates this relation [95]. For instance, a woman with RA (person) wants to lose weight (behavior) to be healthier (outcome). For the woman to achieve this, she has to believe in the fact that both losing weight is beneficial for her health (outcome expectation) and that she has the ability to lose weight (efficacy expectation).

7.1.3. *Transtheoretical model*

The model consists of stages of pre-contemplation, contemplation, preparation, action, maintenance, and termination. At the pre-contemplation stage, individuals are either very little aware or not aware at all of the problems; thus, they are unwilling to make a change in these problems. Behavioral change within the next 6 months is out of question for the individuals at this stage. Contemplation stage is when both the problem and change are evaluated and addressed. Individuals at this stage are more open to feedback and information regarding their behaviors, and they think of changing their behaviors within the next 6 months. In the preparation stage, individuals are usually determined to change their behaviors within the next 30 days. These people have tried changing in the past and have put some effort in getting prepared for the change. Stage of action is when behavioral change or the change occurs and at this stage some explicit changes have occurred in the last 6 months in the lifestyles of the individuals. Maintenance stage is when the unlimited period begins as the first 6 months of the change begin as well. Changes have already turned into habits and recurrence risk of the behavior is decreased. In the termination stage, individuals do not have the desire to return to unhealthy behaviors, and the efficacy level is 100% [96, 97].

Stages of change clarify the time of changes in individuals' intention, attitude, and behavior. The process of change, on the other hand, helps to understand which experiences individuals use in order to change their problematic behaviors. Ten variables consisting of five cognitive and five behavioral variables were found to facilitate change. The cognitive ones are emotions, values, and factors regarding awareness of the individuals, while behavioral processes indicate which behaviors individuals do choose on the path to change. Processes guide the studies on change, significantly [97, 98].

During the practice of TTM applications, it should be taken into account that not all the individuals in the study group are ready for the change, and even if they are thought to be ready, not everyone is at the same stage; thus, personalized interventions are required. At the first two stages, providing more information regarding change and how it is to be made and giving motivational support are very important. At the third and fourth stages, suggestions aiming at providing support about their self-efficacy may be made and discussed about, and motivational prizes may be benefitted from. At the fifth stage, determination of the conditions in order to prevent recurrence and planning of the required steps in order to sustain the change in the long term are necessary [98].

7.2. Self-management

In the last 20 years, self-management interventions in chronic diseases have gained significance. Self-management education programs highlight the role of patient education in protective and therapeutical health-care activities and consist of organized learning experiences usually designed to facilitate the adoption of health-promoting behaviors. Self-management interventions often involve various skills regarding the disease, including problem solving, decision-making, and relations with health professionals [99, 100]. Self-management interventions are person-centered, and they focus on encouraging active participation of the individuals in order for them to develop their well-being and to manage the symptoms [101].

Self-management training programs include three main topics: information sharing, behavioral change (skills development), and psychosocial counseling. Information about the diagnosis and symptoms of the disease is provided, and training is provided to develop self-management skills to manage these symptoms. The individuals are expected to participate actively in these trainings. Self-management skills are taught through observation and role-play within educational groups. Considering the individual needs, individuals are trained about joint protection, fatigue management, exercise, pain-related factors, and sleep adjustment [102, 103]. Psychosocial counseling can be provided to help individuals feel stronger about their self-efficacy and help them cope with arthritis to enable them to acquire a functional and socially active lifestyle [101].

The first step needs evaluation of self-management programs in RA. The first assessment is conducted via face-to-face interview. The interview is very important for recognizing the strong aspects of the individual and the aspects to be supported. A needs evaluation provides information about individual's notice, abilities, obstacles, strong sides, and motivation for self-management. It should also be addressed in demographic and environmental factors that may be effective in the behavioral change of the individual during evaluation interview. Arthritis patient education programs aim to teach the individual how to organize daily activities that are affected by the symptoms of the disease after the initial assessment interview with the patient. In other words, the patient is taught how to approach situations related to arthritis and how to arrange each individual needs [104, 105].

7.2.1. Self-management intervention programs for arthritis

7.2.1.1. Arthritis self-management program

Although there are many different models, perhaps the most well-known program is the arthritis self-management program (ASMP) developed by Lorig and his colleagues. Arthritis self-management program (ASMP), also known as the arthritis self-help course (ASHC), is the arthritis education program. First developed by Kate Lorig, DrPH, at Stanford University, arthritis foundation adopted the program in 1981. The ASMP is a 6-week series of classes for 2–2.5 h per session (total 12 h). Standardized course materials have been developed to assess pain, fear, depression, and disability in arthritic individuals. It focuses on what people need to know about arthritis concerns and aims to learn problem-solving skills so that individuals can adapt to fluctuations in disease activity and disorder levels [106].

Problem-solving, decision-making, communication with providers, exercise, relaxation, and energy-saving techniques are utilized in training how to deal with illnesses during the program. Self-efficacy strategies (goal setting/contract, role modeling, peer support and persuasion, reinterpretation of symptoms), experiential training methods (problem-solving discussions, brainstorming, demonstration, and feedback), behavioral change techniques (behavior shaping, repetitive implementation and feedback, self-monitoring/diaries, environmental sign), and social support strategies (important other people's involvement, time sharing, and feedback for group sharing) are used during the program [107, 108].

7.2.1.2. *Bone up on arthritis*

The bone up on arthritis (BUOA) program is a home-based self-management education program. It consists of six 2-h lessons on audiocassettes, supplemented by illustrated print materials. The program, the contents of which are similar to the arthritis self-management program, was adopted by the arthritis foundation in 1989. The BUOA concept is based on basic disease information, communication, disease management skills, and problem-solving strategies. Coping with depression, sleep regulation and pain management techniques, relaxation techniques, and exercise are taught. Self-efficacy strategies and behavioral strategies (promoting the repeated application of self-care behaviors, problem-solving), similar to ASMP training, are used in the training process [109].

7.2.1.3. *Self-management arthritis treatment*

Self-management arthritis treatment (SMART)] program was developed by Healthtrac, Inc. and is also known as the arthritis home health program. Course materials including self-management plan, self-care books, relaxation audiotapes, and an exercise videotape are uploaded to attendees' personal computers. The letter created in the computer environment is transmitted via e-mail and communication is provided in this way. The program is intended to teach individuals improve in order to use self-care activities and problem-solving skills, and enhance their self-efficacy, and to use health-care services to reduce side effects of medication [109].

7.2.1.4. *Physical activity*

Physical activity is a core self-management activity for people with arthritis. The recommendation for early treatment of arthritis recommends a professional-directed therapeutic exercise for arthritic individuals. In 2002, the American Rheumatism Academy (ARA) recommended physical activity involving individuals exercising aerobic activity and lower extremities for 2–3 days per week for 30–60 min [34, 110]. People with arthritis can exercise (PACE) program developed by the arthritis foundation in 1987 and revised in 1999, is a group exercise program, preferably 1–3 times a week. It is applied in two levels according to the skills of the individuals. The advanced level includes more aerobic activities. The trainer selects 72 exercises that are appropriate to the needs of the group. The program includes endurance exercises and relaxation techniques [109].

8. Joint protection and energy conservation

When the changes that patients with rheumatoid arthritis experienced during the course of the disease are examined, permanent and progressive changes have a direct impact on maintaining joint independence in daily life, such as joint limitations, edema, general or regional pain complaints, and fatigue. From this point of view, ergotherapists use joint and energy conservation techniques in the treatment process in order to ensure the independence of the individual in daily life, to protect the joints in order for the activities to be performed by the individual, and to perform the activity in the most effective manner [39, 79, 111].

Why should we protect the joints?

8.1. In inflammatory arthritis, the aims of joint protection are to:

- Reduce pain during activity and at rest resulting from pressure on nociceptive endings in joint capsules from inflammation and mechanical forces on joints.
- Reduce forces on joints: internal (i.e., from muscular compressive forces, e.g., during strong grip) or external (i.e., forces applied to joints while carrying or pulling/pushing objects).
- Help preserve joint integrity and reduce risk of development and/or progression of deformities.
- Reduce fatigue by reducing effort required for activity performance and improve or maintain function [19].

8.2. What can be done in this situation?

- Informing the patient about his/her progress and living conditions.
- Patient joint and energy conservation techniques can be taught.
- Patient splinting techniques can be applied to reduce pain and maintain ideal mechanical position; assistive device and physical environment modification can be applied to make the daily life activities of the patient easier, to provide pain control, and to achieve fatigue.
- Depending on the current capacity of the individual, activities at home and at work can be re-organized [19].

9. Joint protection and energy conservation principles

Different authors have identified a variety of principles. A consensus was published by the College of Occupational Therapy specialist section in rheumatology [19].

9.1. Joint protection

- Respect pain: use this as a signal to change activities, distribute load over several joints.
- Reduce the force and effort required to perform activities by altering working methods.
- Using assistive devices and reducing the weight of objects.
- Use each joint in its most stable anatomic or functional plane.
- Avoid positions of deformity and forces in their direction.
- Use the strongest, largest joint available for the job.
- Avoid staying in one position for too long.

- Avoid gripping too tightly.
- Avoid adopting poor body positioning, posture, and using poor moving and handling techniques.
- Maintain muscle strength and range of movement [19].

9.2. Energy conservation

- Pace activities by balancing rest and activity, alternating heavy and light tasks, and performing activities more slowly.
- Use work simplification methods, for example, planning ahead, prioritizing, using labor-saving gadgets, and delegating to others when necessary.
- Avoid activities that cannot be stopped immediately if it proves to be beyond the person's ability.
- Modify the environment to suit ergonomic/joint protection practices [19].

10. Assistive technology and reorganization of living areas

When the disease prognosis of the individual is taken carefully, it is necessary to support the individual's maximum independence in life and to be able to cope with pain and fatigue in a place where the occupational therapists should primarily emphasize (**Table 3**) [20]. At this point, it is important that the living space of the individual is arranged and a suitable auxiliary device is proposed. The term "assistive technology" has replaced the expression disability equipment to describe products and services used by people of all ages to gain increased autonomy and maximize their occupational performance [19]. Evaluation is made within the scope of the concept when a suitable auxiliary device is suggested. This assessment is effectively an interaction with each other similar to successive gear wheels. Moreover, it is impossible for this interaction process to be isolated from the living environment of the individual (**Figure 2**).

The arrangements to be made in the living environment of the individual are made by changes in the physical environment and adaptations of assistive devices. This intervention is called inclusive design. In other words, "inclusive design" is the term used to describe a design process whereby designers "address the needs of the widest possible audience by including the needs of groups who are currently excluded from or marginalised by mainstream design practices" [112]. The purpose here is to provide a maximum benefit by intervening in a holistic way to individuals who are not in normal life events. Given the external forces that individuals are exposed to in the home and work environment, interventions made with a holistic view are important at the point of raising quality of life and ensuring pain control. The following are a combination of living room regulations and ancillary technology recommendations applied to various problems (**Tables 4–6**) [19].

Person	Technology	Social environment
Age/gender	Quality of performance	Physical environment in which it will be used
		E.g., home, workplace
Functional abilities		Cultural issues
Functional needs	Comfort	Attitudinal factors
Lifestyle		
Occupational adaptation	Appearance	Political environment
Personal preferences	Cost	
Feelings about self	Availability	Economic environment
Feelings about devices	Support requirements	

Table 3. An example of relationship between person, social environment, and technology.

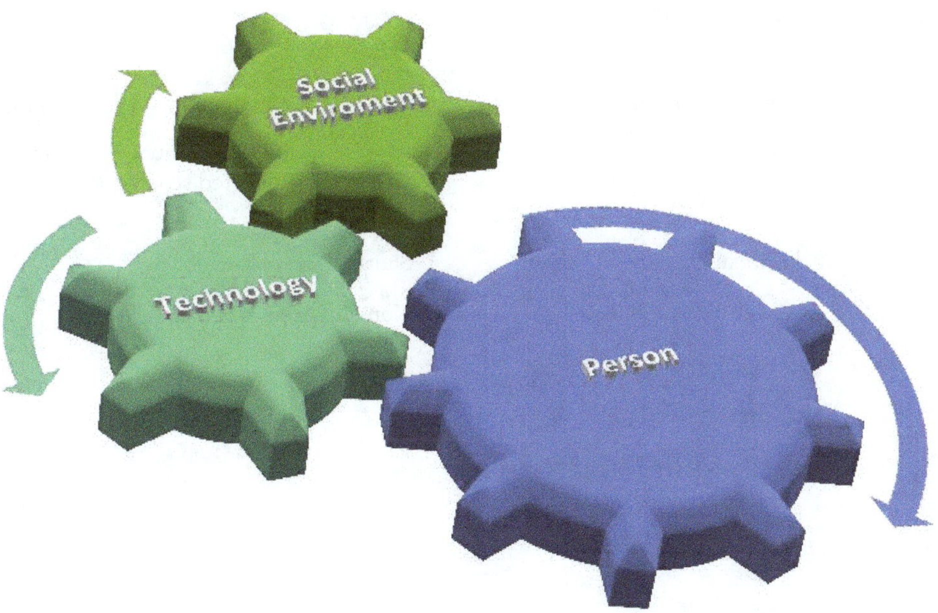

Figure 2. The dynamic relationship between person, social environment, and technology.

Activity limitation	Mainstream design	Assistive technology	Home adaptation
Bathing	Modern wet room area	Portable bath lift	Level access shower with shower seat
Toileting	Wall-mounted toilet installed at the appropriate height	Raised toilet seat	Toilet plinth fitted between floor and toilet to raise height
Personal hygiene	Bidet	Bottom wiper	Electric bidet with wash/dry facility
Personal care	Powered toothbrush/shaver	Tubing to enlarge grip, easy grip handles	

Table 4. Personal care and hygiene.

Activity limitation	Mainstream design	Assistive technology	Home adaptation
Standing tolerance	Energy-saving kitchen layout	Perching stool	It would be unusual for a major kitchen adaptation to be undertaken for a person with a rheumatic condition
Carrying	Continuous worktops and limited distances between key work areas	Wide range of small devices, for example, trolley, cooking baskets	
Lifting	Consideration of weight of household appliances, for example, irons, and products, for example, saucepans		
Reduced reach	Organization of cupboards, pull out/Down shelving in units	Wide range of small devices, for example, helping hand, cleaning products with extended handles	
Bending	Plug sockets at relevant height		
Grip	Attention to controls on appliances	Large handled plugs	

Table 5. Food preparation and household tasks.

Activity limitation	Mainstream design	Assistive technology	Home adaptation
Mobility	Intercom	Small mobility aids manual wheelchair, powered scooter or wheelchair	Intercom
Steps and stairs	Additional rails	Stairlift, ramped access	
Communication	• Large button phones • Use of Skype with headset • Ergonomic computer keyboard • Voice-activated computer software	Non-slip grips for pens	

Table 6. Mobility and other activities.

11. Splinting techniques for rheumatoid arthritis

There are various important wrist and hand structures that may be affected by the inflammatory and degenerative process experienced by people with rheumatic conditions. Therefore, hand splints are a recommended conservative option for occupational therapists to prescribe to support vulnerable structures, reduce pain, and optimize function, and they have been used for many years [113]. Evidence continues to emerge regarding the clinical effectiveness of splints with the most robust evidence reporting their ability to reduce levels of the wrist and hand pain when worn [62].

The splints given to individuals must be made appropriately to the client. Because splinting is aimed at improving activity performance by reducing the pain and fatigue of individuals. Splints that are made of standard uniform type may damage the client [114].

There are two types of splint therapy according to the prognosis of the disease. The aim of correcting the deformities that occur when the primary disease is chronic is the deformity orthoses given to provide pain control and to increase the fatigue tolerance of the patient. These are ulnar deviation orthoses, swan necks, and ring orthoses for thumb hypertension. The second group of splints is the resting orthoses that are given to prevent pain and inflammation in the acute phase of the disease and to help the individual to rest while protecting the function. These are volar wrist orthosis, static wrist orthosis, metacarpophalangeal joint stabilization orthosis, static volar and dorsal wrist orthoses, and air pressure splint. The splints given to treat deformity should be used intensively throughout the day. Resting orthoses should be worn during the rest of the day and after exercises during the day, provided that they are removed at night [114–116].

12. Vocational rehabilitation

Rate of erythrocyte sedimentation, which is also known as patient activity, and sensitive joints causes structural harms such as joint destruction and deformation. Structural harms emerged in RA result in limitation of physical functions such as force, endurance, mobility, and manual skills. Work disability may develop at early stages for this reason [117, 118].

Work disability in individuals with RA depend on factors related to both work and RA; physical effort demands at work being too high and keeping work pace under control are factors related to work. On the other hand, factors related to the disease may differ among individuals. Unlike factors related to the disease, factors such as functional capacity, high age, educational status, and stress management skill are also related with work disability [117].

One of the goals of rehabilitation in rheumatoid arthritis is ensuring return to work. It may require job modification, vocational training, and vocational rehabilitation in order to achieve this goal. Vocational rehabilitation helps an individual with a health problem for continuing to work, returning to work, or getting a new job. Occupational therapists play an important role in individuals' continuation to work and getting a new job by means of increasing the capacity of the individual with RA. Moreover, occupational therapists aim to maximize the level of individual-environment occupation harmony and to develop work performance [26].

In vocational rehabilitation, the occupational therapy process is based on interview, observation, and individual evaluations made through standardized procedures. A comprehensive starter interview that gathers detailed information regarding the individual's medical record, performance level of daily life activities and work activities, and work background is held. Furthermore, participation of the individual to the daily life activities, leisure activities, and productive activities is evaluated. Positive factors supporting individual's participation and negativities preventing him/her from participating are determined. This process is important in order to rely on the strengths of the individual during the intervention. Moreover, during the evaluation, person's roles, abilities, interests, and needs regarding work performance and work task demands are determined. In occupational therapy evaluations, functional capacity analysis to determine the suitability of the individual and the work that he/she desires to do;

work analysis to detect the task demands expected from the individual in the corresponding work; and work place analysis including ergonomic assessment and assessment of the equipment, work routine, and accessibility in order to determine the factors related to the work place, are considerably important [26, 119, 120].

After the interviews and evaluations, short- and long-term intervention plans are formed. These formed plans should be suitable to the roles, habits, functional capacity, life choices, and the living environment of the individual. The interventions should be aimed at bringing educational performance skill and developing daily life skills, preparation to work skills and work performance. In vocational rehabilitation, education about occupational therapy, RA, and medication involves education on employee rights, employer rights, ergonomic recommendations, prevention of injury in order to reduce disability regarding injuries, stress management, sleep posture and hygiene, choice of shoe, and splinting. Moreover, occupational activity training in order to develop producer behaviors, employee roles, and skills; work modifications and adaptations in order to develop the work performance, and personalized programs on transition to work are also quiet significant in occupational therapy interventions [26, 120].

Author details

Zeynep Bahadır Ağce[1]*, Esma Özkan[2] and Barkın Köse[2]

*Address all correspondence to: fztzeynepbahadir@gmail.com

1 Faculty of Health Sciences, Occupational Therapy Department, Üsküdar University, Turkey

2 Faculty of Health Sciences, Occupational Therapy Department, Hacettepe University, Turkey

References

[1] Loyola-Sanchez A, Richardson J, Pelaez-Ballestas I, Alvarez-Nemegyei J, Lavis JN, Wilson MG, et al. The impact of arthritis on the physical function of a rural Maya-Yucateco community and factors associated with its prevalence: A cross sectional, community-based study. Clinical Rheumatology. 2015:1-10

[2] Hootman JM, Helmick CG, Barbour KE, Theis KA, Boring MA. Updated projected prevalence of self-reported doctor-diagnosed arthritis and arthritis-attributable activity limitation among US adults, 2015-2040. Arthritis & Rheumatology. 2016

[3] Mann WC, Hurren D, Tomita M. Assistive devices used by home-based elderly persons with arthritis. American Journal of Occupational Therapy. 1995;**49**(8):810-820

[4] Griffith LE, Raina P, Levasseur M, Sohel N, Payette H, Tuokko H, et al. Functional disability and social participation restriction associated with chronic conditions in middle-aged and older adults. Journal of Epidemiology and Community Health. 2016;**71**. DOI: 10.1136/jech-2016-207982

[5] Theis KA, Furner SE. Shut-in? Impact of chronic conditions on community participation restriction among older adults. Journal of Aging Research. 2011;**2011**

[6] Deshaines L. Arthritis. In: Khron HMPWS, editors. Pedretti's Occupational Therapy Practice Skills for Physical Dysfunction. 6th ed. California: Mosby/Elsevier; 2005. pp. 950-982

[7] Cavalli G, Koenders M, Kalabokis V, Kim J, Tan AC, Garlanda C, et al. Treating experimental arthritis with the innate immune inhibitor interleukin-37 reduces joint and systemic inflammation. Rheumatology. 2016;**55**(12):2220-2229.

[8] Sandles L. Occupational Therapy in Rheumatology: An Holistic Approach. Campling J, editor. London: Springer; 2013. 1-10 p

[9] Dziedzic K, Hammond A. Rheumatology: Evidence-Based Practice for Physiotherapists and Occupational Therapists. Elsevier Health Sciences; 2011

[10] Organization WH. Chronic Diseases and Health Promotion 2016 [Available from: http://www.who.int/chp/topics/rheumatic/en/

[11] Steultjens EE, Dekker JJ, Bouter LM, Schaardenburg DD, Kuyk MAM, Van den Ende EC. Occupational therapy for rheumatoid arthritis. The Cochrane Library. 2004

[12] Okely JA, Cooper C, Gale CR. Wellbeing and Arthritis Incidence: The Survey of Health, Ageing and Retirement in Europe. Annals of Behavioral Medicine. 2016;**50**(3):419-426

[13] Roy N, Tanner K, Merrill RM, Wright C, Miller KL, Kendall KA. Descriptive epidemiology of voice disorders in rheumatoid arthritis: Prevalence, risk factors, and quality of life burden. Journal of Voice. 2016;**30**(1):74-87

[14] Di WT, Vergara F, Bertiller E, de los Angeles Gallardo M, Gandino I, Scolnik M, et al. Incidence and prevalence of rheumatoid arthritis in a health management organization in Argentina: A 15-year study. The Journal of Rheumatology. 2016;**44**. DOI: 10.3899/jrheum.151262

[15] Rudan I, Sidhu S, Papana A, Meng SJ, Xin–Wei Y, Wang W, et al. Prevalence of rheumatoid arthritis in low–and middle–income countries: A systematic review and analysis. Journal of Global Health. 2015;**5**

[16] Kraus VB. Editorial [Hot topic: Waiting for action on the osteoarthritis front (Guest Editors: Virginia Byers Kraus and Thomas Aigner)]. Current Drug Targets. 2010;**11**(5):518-20

[17] Dubouloz C-J, Laporte D, Hall M, Ashe B, Smith CD. Transformation of meaning perspectives in clients with rheumatoid arthritis. American Journal of Occupational Therapy. 2004;**58**(4):398-407

[18] Poole JL, Chiappisi H, Cordova JS, Sibbitt W. Quality of life in American Indian and White women with and without rheumatoid arthritis. American Journal of Occupational Therapy. 2007;**61**(3):280-289

[19] Goodacre L, McArthur M. Rheumatology Practice in Occupational Therapy: Promoting Lifestyle Management. John Wiley & Sons; 2013

[20] Poole JL, Cordova JS, Sibbitt WL, Skipper B. Quality of life in American Indian women with arthritis or diabetes. American Journal of Occupational Therapy. 2010;**64**(3):496-505

[21] Matcham F, Rayner L, Steer S, Hotopf M. The prevalence of depression in rheumatoid arthritis: a systematic review and meta-analysis. Rheumatology. 2013;**52**(12):2136-2148

[22] Klaassen K, Nyklíček I, Traa S, de Nijs R. Distressed personality is associated with lower psychological well-being and life satisfaction, but not disability or disease activity in rheumatoid arthritis patients. Clinical Rheumatology. 2012;**31**(4):661-667

[23] de Almeida PHTQ, Pontes TB, Matheus JPC, Muniz LF, da Mota LMH. Occupational therapy in rheumatoid arthritis: What rheumatologists need to know?. Revista Brasileira de Reumatologia (English Edition). 2015;**55**(3):272-280

[24] Law M, Cooper B, Strong S, Stewart D, Rigby P, Letts L. The person-environment-occupation model: A transactive approach to occupational performance. Canadian Journal of Occupational Therapy. 1996;**63**(1):9-23

[25] WHO. Chronic Diseases and Health Promotion World Health Organization: WHO: World Health Organization: WHO; 2016 [Available from: http://www.who.int/chp/topics/rheumatic/en/

[26] Macedo AM, Oakley SP, Panayi GS, Kirkham BW. Functional and work outcomes improve in patients with rheumatoid arthritis who receive targeted, comprehensive occupational therapy. Arthritis Care & Research. 2009;**61**(11):1522-1530

[27] Smolen JS, Aletaha D, McInnes IB. Rheumatoid arthritis. The Lancet. 2016;**388**

[28] Ağıllı M, Ekinci Ş, Aydın FN, Şener İ, Parlak A, Yaman H. Anti-siklik Sitrüllinlenmiş Peptid/Protein (Anti-CCP) ve Romatoid Artrit Tanısındaki Değeri. TAF Preventive Medicine Bulletin. 2014;**13**(1)

[29] Jiang X, Sandberg ME, Saevarsdottir S, Klareskog L, Alfredsson L, Bengtsson C. Higher education is associated with a better rheumatoid arthritis outcome concerning for pain and function but not disease activity: Results from the EIRA cohort and Swedish rheumatology register. Arthritis Research & Therapy. 2015;**17**(1):1

[30] Rossini M, Rossi E, Bernardi D, Viapiana O, Gatti D, Idolazzi L, et al. Prevalence and incidence of rheumatoid arthritis in Italy. Rheumatology International. 2014;**34**(5):659-664

[31] Eriksson JK, Neovius M, Ernestam S, Lindblad S, Simard JF, Askling J. Incidence of rheumatoid arthritis in Sweden: A nationwide population-based assessment of incidence, its determinants, and treatment penetration. Arthritis Care & Research. 2013;**65**(6):870-878

[32] Ma VY, Chan L, Carruthers KJ. Incidence, prevalence, costs, and impact on disability of common conditions requiring rehabilitation in the United States: Stroke, spinal cord injury, traumatic brain injury, multiple sclerosis, osteoarthritis, rheumatoid arthritis, limb loss, and back pain. Archives of Physical Medicine and Rehabilitation. 2014;**95**(5):986-995. e1

[33] Zlatkovic-Svenda M, Saraux A, Tuncer T, Dadoniene J, Miltiniene D, Gilgil E, et al. FRI0558 rheumatoid arthritis prevalence in Europe, a eular-endorsed survey. Annals of the Rheumatic Diseases. 2016;**75**(Suppl 2):643

[34] Fina-Aviles F, Medina-Peralta M, Mendez-Boo L, Hermosilla E, Elorza J, Garcia-Gil M, et al. The descriptive epidemiology of rheumatoid arthritis in Catalonia: a retrospective study using routinely collected data. Clinical Rheumatology. 2016;**35**(3):751-757

[35] Choy E. Understanding the dynamics: Pathways involved in the pathogenesis of rheumatoid arthritis. Rheumatology. 2012;**51**(suppl 5):v3-v11

[36] Smolen JS, Emery P, Fleischmann R, van Vollenhoven RF, Pavelka K, Durez P, et al. Adjustment of therapy in rheumatoid arthritis on the basis of achievement of stable low disease activity with adalimumab plus methotrexate or methotrexate alone: The randomised controlled OPTIMA trial. The Lancet. 2014;**383**(9914):321-332

[37] Kurowska W, Kuca-Warnawin E. New evidence for a role of bone marrow in the pathogenesis of rheumatoid arthritis. Reumatologia. 2016;**54**(5):215-216

[38] Seegobin SD, Ma MH, Dahanayake C, Cope AP, Scott DL, Lewis CM, et al. ACPA-positive and ACPA-negative rheumatoid arthritis differ in their requirements for combination DMARDs and corticosteroids: Secondary analysis of a randomized controlled trial. Arthritis Research & Therapy. 2014;**16**(1):1

[39] Furst DE, Emery P. Rheumatoid arthritis pathophysiology: Update on emerging cytokine and cytokine-associated cell targets. Rheumatology. 2014;**53**. DOI: 10.1093/rheumatology/ket414

[40] Padyukov L, Seielstad M, Ong RT, Ding B, Rönnelid J, Seddighzadeh M, et al. A genome-wide association study suggests contrasting associations in ACPA-positive versus ACPA-negative rheumatoid arthritis. Annals of the Rheumatic Diseases. 2010:annrheumdis126821

[41] Lundström E, Källberg H, Alfredsson L, Klareskog L, Padyukov L. Gene–environment interaction between the DRB1 shared epitope and smoking in the risk of anti–citrullinated protein antibody–positive rheumatoid arthritis: All alleles are important. Arthritis & Rheumatism. 2009;**60**(6):1597-1603

[42] Aletaha D, Neogi T, Silman AJ, Funovits J, Felson DT, Bingham CO, et al. 2010 rheumatoid arthritis classification criteria: An American College of Rheumatology/European League Against Rheumatism collaborative initiative. Arthritis & Rheumatism. 2010;**62**(9):2569-2581

[43] Kim S, Hwang J, Xuan J, Jung YH, Cha H-S, Kim KH. Global metabolite profiling of synovial fluid for the specific diagnosis of rheumatoid arthritis from other inflammatory arthritis. PLoS One. 2014;**9**(6):e97501

[44] Aggarwal R, Liao K, Nair R, Ringold S, Costenbander KH. Anti–citrullinated peptide antibody assays and their role in the diagnosis of rheumatoid arthritis. Arthritis Care & Research. 2009;**61**(11):1472-1483

[45] van der Helm-vanMil AH, le Cessie S, van Dongen H, Breedveld FC, Toes RE, Huizinga TW. A prediction rule for disease outcome in patients with Recent-onset undifferentiated arthritis: How to guide individual treatment decisions. Arthritis & Rheumatism. 2007;**56**(2):433-440

[46] Dür M, Coenen M, Stoffer MA, Fialka-Moser V, Kautzky-Willer A, Kjeken I, et al. Do patient-reported outcome measures cover personal factors important to people with rheumatoid arthritis? A mixed methods design using the International Classification of Functioning, Disability and Health as frame of reference. Health and Quality of Life Outcomes. 2015;**13**(1):1

[47] Manning VL, Hurley MV, Scott DL, Coker B, Choy E, Bearne LM. Education, self-management, and upper extremity exercise training in people with rheumatoid arthritis: A randomized controlled trial. Arthritis Care & Research. 2014;**66**(2):217-227

[48] Dellhag B, Bjelle A. A five-year followup of hand function and activities of daily living in rheumatoid arthritis patients. Arthritis Care and Research. 1999;**12**:33-41

[49] Keefe FJ, Affleck G, Lefebvre J, Underwood L, Caldwell DS, Drew J, et al. Living with rheumatoid arthritis: The role of daily spirituality and daily religious and spiritual coping. The Journal of Pain. 2001;**2**(2):101-110

[50] Hammond A, Tyson S, Prior Y, Hawkins R, Tennant A, Nordenskiold U, et al. Linguistic validation and cultural adaptation of an English version of the Evaluation of Daily Activity Questionnaire in rheumatoid arthritis. Health and Quality of Life Outcomes. 2014;**12**(1):1

[51] Suurmeijer TP, Waltz M, Moum T, Guillemin F, Van Sonderen F, Briançon S, et al. Quality of life profiles in the first years of rheumatoid arthritis: results from the EURIDISS longitudinal study. Arthritis Care & Research. 2001;**45**(2):111-121

[52] Lapsley H, March L, Tribe K, Cross M, Courtenay B, Brooks P. Living with rheumatoid arthritis: Expenditures, health status, and social impact on patients. Annals of the Rheumatic Diseases. 2002;**61**(9):818-821

[53] Shaul MP. From early twinges to mastery: The process of adjustment in living with rheumatoid arthritis. Arthritis & Rheumatism. 1995;**8**(4):290-297

[54] Ziarko M, Mojs E, Kaczmarek Ł, Warchol-Biedermann K, Malak R, Lisinski P, et al. Do urban and rural residents living in Poland differ in their ways of coping with chronic diseases? European Review for Medical and Pharmacological Sciences. 2015;**19**(22):4227-4234

[55] Walter MJ, van't Spijker A, Pasma A, Hazes JM, Luime JJ. Focus group interviews reveal reasons for differences in the perception of disease activity in rheumatoid arthritis. Quality of Life Research. 2016:**1-8**

[56] Janssens X, Decuman S, De Keyser F, group BRADAs. Assessment of activity limitations with the health assessment questionnaire predicts the need for support measures in patients with rheumatoid arthritis: A multicenter observational study. PloS One. 2014;**9**(9):e106749

[57] Nordgren B, Fridén C, Jansson E, Österlund T, Grooten WJ, Opava CH, et al. Criterion validation of two submaximal aerobic fitness tests, the self-monitoring Fox-walk test and the Åstrand cycle test in people with rheumatoid arthritis. BMC Musculoskeletal Disorders. 2014;**15**(1):1

[58] Luqmani R, Hennell S, Estrach C, Birrell F, Bosworth A, Davenport G, et al. British Society for Rheumatology and British Health Professionals in Rheumatology guideline for the management of rheumatoid arthritis (the first two years). Rheumatology. 2006;**45**(9):1167-1169

[59] Kirchberger I, Stamm T, Cieza A, Stucki G. Does the comprehensive ICF core set for rheumatoid arthritis capture occupational therapy practice? A content-validity study. Canadian Journal of Occupational Therapy. 2007;**74**(5 suppl):267-280

[60] Strand V, Wright GC, Bergman MJ, Tambiah J, Taylor PC. Patient expectations and perceptions of goal-setting strategies for disease management in rheumatoid arthritis. The Journal of rheumatology. 2015;**42**(11):2046-2054

[61] Stamm TA, Cieza A, Machold KP, Smolen JS, Stucki G. Content comparison of occupation-based instruments in adult rheumatology and musculoskeletal rehabilitation based on the International Classification of Functioning, Disability and Health. Arthritis Care & Research. 2004;**51**(6):917-924

[62] Steultjens EM, Dekker J, Bouter LM, Van Schaardenburg D, van Kuyk MAH, Van Den Ende CH. Occupational therapy for rheumatoid arthritis: a systematic review. Arthritis Care & Research. 2002;**47**(6):672-685

[63] Dubouloz CJ, Vallerand J, Laporte D, Ashe B, Hall M. Occupational performance modification and personal change among clients receiving rehabilitation services for rheumatoid arthritis. Australian Occupational Therapy Journal. 2008;**55**(1):30-38

[64] Phipps S, Richardson P. Occupational therapy outcomes for clients with traumatic brain injury and stroke using the Canadian Occupational Performance Measure. American Journal of Occupational Therapy. 2007;**61**(3):328-334

[65] Carswell A, McColl MA, Baptiste S, Law M, Polatajko H, Pollock N. The Canadian occupational performance measure: A research and clinical literature review. Canadian Journal of Occupational Therapy. 2004;**71**(4):210-222

[66] Ripat J, Etcheverry E, Cooper J, Tate R. A comparison of the Canadian occupational performance measure and the health assessment questionnaire. Canadian Journal of Occupational Therapy. 2001;**68**(4):247-253

[67] Tack BB. Fatigue in rheumatoid arthritis: Conditions, strategies, and consequences. Arthritis & Rheumatism. 1990;**3**(2):65-70

[68] Nikolaus S, Bode C, Taal E, de Laar MA. Fatigue and factors related to fatigue in rheumatoid arthritis: A systematic review. Arthritis Care & Research. 2013;**65**(7):1128-1146

[69] Cramp F, Hewlett S, Almeida C, Kirwan JR, Choy EH, Chalder T, et al. Non-pharmacological interventions for fatigue in rheumatoid arthritis. The Cochrane Library. 2013

[70] Matcham F, Ali S, Hotopf M, Chalder T. 087. Psychological correlates and predictors of fatigue in rheumatoid arthritis: A systematic review. Rheumatology. 2015;**54**(suppl 1):i84–i.

[71] Grassi W, De Angelis R, Lamanna G, Cervini C. The clinical features of rheumatoid arthritis. European Journal of Radiology. 1998;**27**:S18-S24

[72] Shankar V, Sharma P, Mittal R, Mittal S, Kumar U, Gamanagatti S. Effectiveness of arthroscopic elbow synovectomy in rheumatoid arthritis patients: Long-term follow-up of clinical and functional outcomes. Journal of Clinical Orthopaedics and Trauma. 2016;**7**

[73] Häkkinen A, Sokka T, Kotaniemi A, Hannonen P. A randomized two-year study of the effects of dynamic strength training on muscle strength, disease activity, functional capacity, and bone mineral density in early rheumatoid arthritis. Arthritis & Rheumatism. 2001;**44**(3):515-522

[74] Steinbrocker O, Traeger CH, Batterman RC. Therapeutic criteria in rheumatoid arthritis. Journal of the American Medical Association. 1949;**140**(8):659-662

[75] Clarkson HM. Musculoskeletal Assessment: Joint Range of Motion and Manual Muscle Strength. Lippincott Williams & Wilkins; 2000

[76] Hwang YS, Moon KP, Kim KT, Kim JW, Park WS. Total knee arthroplasty for severe flexion contracture in rheumatoid arthritis knees. Knee Surgery & Related Research. 2016;**28**(4):325

[77] Fraser A, Vallow J, Preston A, Cooper R. Predicting'normal'grip strength for rheumatoid arthritis patients. Rheumatology. 1999;**38**(6):521-528

[78] Ekelman BA, Hooker L, Davis A, Klan J, Newburn D, Detwiler K, et al. Occupational therapy interventions for adults with rheumatoid arthritis: An appraisal of the evidence. Occupational therapy in health care. 2014;**28**(4):347-361

[79] Rapolienė J, Kriščiūnas A. The effectiveness of occupational therapy in restoring the functional state of hands in rheumatoid arthritis patients. Medicina. 2006;**42**(10):823-828

[80] Hammond A, Young A, Kidao R. A randomised controlled trial of occupational therapy for people with early rheumatoid arthritis. Annals of the Rheumatic Diseases. 2004;**63**(1):23-30

[81] Hammond A. The Elizabeth Casson Memorial Lecture 2014: Changing ways; changing times. British Journal of Occupational Therapy. 2014;**77**(8):392-399

[82] Ndosi M, Johnson D, Young T, Hardware B, Hill J, Hale C, et al. Effects of needs-based patient education on self-efficacy and health outcomes in people with rheumatoid arthritis: A multicentre, single blind, randomised controlled trial. Annals of the Rheumatic Diseases. 2015;**75**:10.1136/annrheumdis-2014-207171

[83] Hill J, Bird H, Johnson S. Effect of patient education on adherence to drug treatment for rheumatoid arthritis: A randomised controlled trial. Annals of the Rheumatic Diseases. 2001;**60**(9):869-875

[84] Hirano PC, Laurent DD, Lorig K. Arthritis patient education studies, 1987-1991: A review of the literature. Patient Education and Counseling. 1994;**24**(1):9-54

[85] Riemsma RP, Taal E, Kirwan JR, Rasker JJ. Systematic review of rheumatoid arthritis patient education. Arthritis Care & Research. 2004;**51**(6):1045-1059

[86] Mullen PD, Laville EA, Biddle AK, Lorig K. Efficacy of psychoeducational interventions on pain, depression, and disability in people with arthritis: A meta-analysis. The Journal of Rheumatology Supplement. 1987;**14**:33-39

[87] Iversen M. Arthritis Patient Education and Team Approaches to Management. Rheumatology Philadelphia: Elsevier. 2011:427-432

[88] Harrison JA, Mullen PD, Green LW. A meta-analysis of studies of the health belief model with adults. Health Education Research. 1992;**7**(1):107-116

[89] Glanz K, Rimer BK, Viswanath K. Health behavior and health education: Theory, research, and practice. John Wiley & Sons; 2008

[90] Carpenter CJ. A meta-analysis of the effectiveness of health belief model variables in predicting behavior. Health Communication. 2010;**25**(8):661-669

[91] McAlister AL, Perry CL, Parcel GS. How individuals, environments, and health behaviors interact. Health Behavior. 2008;**169**

[92] Bandura A. Health promotion from the perspective of social cognitive theory. Psychology and Health. 1998;**13**(4):623-649

[93] Bandura A. Health promotion by social cognitive means. Health Education & Behavior. 2004;**31**(2):143-164

[94] Rosenstock IM, Strecher VJ, Becker MH. Social learning theory and the health belief model. Health Education & Behavior. 1988;**15**(2):175-183

[95] Bandura A, Walters RH. Social Learning Theory. 1977

[96] Prochaska J, Marcus B, Dishman R. Advances in Exercise Adherence. 1994

[97] Prochaska JO, Velicer WF. The transtheoretical model of health behavior change. American Journal of Health Promotion. 1997;**12**(1):38-48

[98] Prochaska JO. Decision making in the transtheoretical model of behavior change. Medical Decision Making. 2008;**28**(6):845-849

[99] Ackerman IN, Ngian G-S, Van Doornum S, Briggs AM. A systematic review of interventions to improve knowledge and self-management skills concerning contraception, pregnancy and breastfeeding in people with rheumatoid arthritis. Clinical Rheumatology. 2016;**35**(1):33-41

[100] Warsi A, Wang PS, LaValley MP, Avorn J, Solomon DH. Self-management education programs in chronic disease: A systematic review and methodological critique of the literature. Archives of Internal Medicine. 2004;**164**(15):1641-1649

[101] Iversen MD, Hammond A, Betteridge N. Self-management of rheumatic diseases: State of the art and future perspectives. Annals of the Rheumatic Diseases. 2010;**69**:annrheumdis129270

[102] Hammond A, Badcock L. Improving education about arthritis. Rheumatology. 2002;**41**:87

[103] Hammond A, Bryan J, Hardy A. Effects of a modular behavioural arthritis education programme: A pragmatic parallel-group randomized controlled trial. Rheumatology. 2008;**47**(11):1712-1718

[104] Schwarze M, Kirchhof R, Schuler M, Musekamp G, Nolte S, Jordan J, et al. Ein blick down under. Zeitschrift für Rheumatologie. 2008;**67**(3):189-198

[105] Riemsma RP, Kirwan JR, Taal E, Rasker J. Patient education for adults with rheumatoid arthritis. The Cochrane Database of Systematic Reviews. 2003;**2**

[106] Lorig K, Holman H. Arthritis self-management studies: A twelve-year review. Health Education Quarterly. 1993;**20**(1):17-28

[107] Lorig K, González VM, Laurent DD, Morgan L, Laris B. Arthritis self-management program variations: Three studies. Arthritis & Rheumatology. 1998;**11**(6):448-454

[108] Lorig K, Ritter PL, Plant K. A disease-specific self-help program compared with a generalized chronic disease self-help program for arthritis patients. Arthritis Care & Research. 2005;**53**(6):950-957

[109] Brady TJ, Kruger J, Helmick CG, Callahan LF, Boutaugh ML. Intervention programs for arthritis and other rheumatic diseases. Health Education & Behavior. 2003;**30**(1):44-63

[110] Bartlett SJ. Clinical care in the rheumatic diseases: Association of Rheumatology Health Professionals; 2006

[111] Tonga E, Uysal SA, Karayazgan S, Hayran M, Düger T. Development and reliability of a Turkish version of the short form-joint protection behavior assessment (JPBA-S). Journal of Hand Therapy. 2016;**29**(3):275-280

[112] Yang C-W, Yen Z-S, McGowan JE, Chen HC, Chiang W-C, Mancini ME, et al. A systematic review of retention of adult advanced life support knowledge and skills in healthcare providers. Resuscitation. 2012;**83**(9):1055-1060

[113] Williams A, Lee P, Kerr A. Scottish intercollegiate guidelines network (SIGN) guidelines on tonsillectomy: A three cycle audit of clinical record keeping and adherence to national guidelines. The Journal of Laryngology & Otology. 2002;**116**(06):453-454

[114] Kaya T. İnflamatuvar Romatizmal Hastalıkların Ortezle Tedavisi. Turkish Journal of Rheumatology. 2009;**24**(1)

[115] Günendi Z, Göğüş F, Keleş Z, Durukan T. Romatoid Artritli Hastaların El-El Bileği İstirahat Splinti Kullanımına Uyumu. Turkiye Klinikleri Journal of Medical Sciences. 2010;**30**(1):213-217

[116] Taşkıran ÖÖ. Romatoid El. Journal of Physical Medicine & Rehabilitation Sciences/ Fiziksel Tup ve Rehabilitasyon Bilimleri Dergisi. 2011;**14**

[117] de Buck PD, Schoones JW, Allaire SH, Vlieland TPV, editors. Vocational Rehabilitation in Patients with Chronic Rheumatic Diseases: A Systematic Literature Review. Seminars in Arthritis and Rheumatism. Elsevier; 2002

[118] De Croon E, Sluiter J, Nijssen T, Dijkmans B, Lankhorst G, Frings-Dresen M. Predictive factors of work disability in rheumatoid arthritis: A systematic literature review. Annals of the Rheumatic Diseases. 2004;**63**(11):1362-1367

[119] Désiron HA, de Rijk A, Van Hoof E, Donceel P. Occupational therapy and return to work: A systematic literature review. BMC Public Health. 2011;**11**(1):615

[120] Wenborn J, Challis D, Pool J, Burgess J, Elliott N, Orrell M. Assessing the validity and reliability of the Pool Activity Level (PAL) checklist for use with older people with dementia. Aging and Mental Health. 2008;**12**(2):202-211

11

Virtual Reality and Occupational Therapy

Orkun Tahir Aran, Sedef Şahin, Berkan Torpil,
Tarık Demirok and Hülya Kayıhan

Abstract

Virtual reality is three dimensional, interactive and fun way in rehabilitation. Its first known use in rehabilitation published by Max North named as "Virtual Environments and Psychological Disorders" (1994). Virtual reality uses special programmed computers, visual devices and artificial environments for the clients' rehabilitation. Throughout technological improvements, virtual reality devices changed from therapeutic gloves to augmented reality environments. Virtual reality was being used in different rehabilitation professions such as occupational therapy, physical therapy, psychology and so on. In spite of common virtual reality approach of different professions, each profession aims different outcomes in rehabilitation. Virtual reality in occupational therapy generally focuses on hand and upper extremity functioning, cognitive rehabilitation, mental disorders, etc. Positive effects of virtual reality were mentioned in different studies, which are higher motivation than non-simulated environments, active participation of the participants, supporting motor learning, fun environment and risk-free environment. Additionally, virtual reality was told to be used as assessment. This chapter will focus on usage of virtual reality in occupational therapy, history and recent developments, types of virtual reality technologic equipment, pros and cons, usage for pediatric, adult and geriatric people and recent research and articles.

Keywords: virtual reality, rehabilitation, occupational therapy, ICF

1. Introduction

Enhancement of functional ability and the realization of greater participation in community life are the two major goals of rehabilitation science. Improving sensory, motor, cognitive functions and practice in everyday activities and occupations to increase participation with intensive rehabilitation may define these predefined goals [1, 2]. Intervention is based primarily on the different types of purposeful activities and occupations with active participation [3–5]. For many injuries and disabilities, the rehabilitation process is long, and clinicians face the challenge of identifying a variety of appealing, meaningful and motivating intervention tasks that may be adapted and graded to facilitate this process [5].

Occupational therapy (OT), which is one of the rehabilitation professions, is a client-centered profession that helps people who are suffering participation and occupational performance limitations. OT offers a wide range of rehabilitation strategies in different medical and social diagnosis [2]. The common point of all these strategies in rehabilitation is that OT assesses and supports enhancing functional ability and participation throughout participating in meaningful activities in a person's lifespan. To enhance participation, OT, like the rest of the health professions, uses World Health Organization's International Classification of Functioning, Disability and Health (ICF) to understand function in a biopsychosocial manner. In ICF framework, function is defined as the interactions between an individual, their health conditions and the social and personal situations in which they thrive. The complex interactions between these variables define function and disability [1].

ICF classifies health and health-related fields in two groups. These groups are "body functions" and "body structures" and "activity and participation." Sub heading of these groups is considered as body function and structures (physical, physiological etc), activities (daily tasks) and participation (life roles) [1]. When these groups taken into account in rehabilitation, occupational therapists focus on all areas to enhance a client's activity participation, social participation, etc. However, in current literature, there are various rehabilitation approaches that are being used for this aim. Advancements in technology in the twenty-first century create great opportunities for people working in different areas. In particular, in health practices like rehabilitation, technology supports therapists' to rehabilitate their clients in too many different ways like robotics, stimulation devices, assessment tools and virtual reality [6–10].

2. Virtual reality

Virtual rehabilitation is the use of VR and virtual environments (VE) within rehabilitation. VR and VE can be described as a simulation of real world environments through a computer and experienced through a "human-machine interface" [11]. VR rehabilitation, since the 1980s, technology has become widespread with rapid developments in computer technology, and nowadays, many commercial uses have come into play with relatively affordable costs. In addition to its use in the field of health sciences, is used for industrial design, production processes and training purposes [12]. VR rehabilitation can be classified in several ways. The first is the classification method according to the specific patient population. Rehabilitation practices in this class can be classified as musculoskeletal disorders, post-stroke and cognitive and psychological disorders. The second classification method concerns the priority of the applied rehabilitation protocol. VR practice in the rehabilitation protocol can only be used as an adjunct or as the basis of a rehabilitation program to retain the place of classical exercise or activity programs. Therapeutic approaches include education approaches through examples, video games and educational approaches or rehabilitation approaches through "exposure" used in psychological disorders. The training method with examples is frequently used in stroke rehabilitation. For example, a system that perceives the arm movements of a patient reflects arm movements on a computer screen as a motion of an object and is required to control movement of the patient. In the approach used by video games, the client tries to control the objects in the ball with a certain joint or body movement. To apply this method, patients are required to have a higher cognitive level. Finally, VR rehabilitation can be classified according to the proximity or distance of the therapist. Therapist and client are in the same room in VR and in tele-rehabiltation method, in tele-rehabilitation method is participating in a remote location in the rehabilitation process of the patient therapist [3, 11, 12].

As virtual reality in its broad definition can be dated as far as the wall-to-wall frescoes of late Roman Republic era [12], the following text will emphasize the recent technological aspect of the phenomenon and its use in rehabilitation research, which aims to expand the reader's intervention choices in occupational therapy practice. The use of computer systems has become an accepted practice in the clinical setting. VR applications are frequently used in different disease groups for this purpose. VR applications are used in a variety of areas, such as neurological, orthopedic, cognitive function, sensory-perceptual and mental health disorders in basic/instrumental daily life activities [13–16]. Following sections will include these areas.

2.1. Virtual reality in pediatric rehabilitation

VR is defined in pediatric rehabilitation as 'An interactive simulation allowing users to feel experiences similar to real-life environments or objects ones with systems which consist in computer hardware and software, [17]. Virtual reality systems (VRS) are mostly used in pediatric rehabilitation program due to these properties. Pediatric rehabilitation is a concept that covers a wide range of applications and includes treatments for various diagnoses or disorders, such as children with neurological, orthopedic or developmental disabilities.

Children with neurologic or neurocognitive impairments may experience decreased functioning in multiple domains including: physical, psychosocial, cognitive or emotional. Such impairments represent significant obstacles to the child's activities of daily life [18]. Holistic approaches to the treatment of all impairments that children may encounter are implemented through a joint study of many disciplines in rehabilitation program. The use of VR by trained therapists enables to cope with these impairments [19].

Play is described as both the earliest and the most important occupation in the childhood [20, 21]. In order to be defined as play, it must contain these five essential domains: intrinsic motivation, pleasure, free choice, non-literal and active engagement [20, 22]. A few theories have proposed the contributions of play to the developing child. Some of them thought play was a tool for intellectual growth, whereas others thought it was necessary for skills development [23–25]. Children with various disabilities have a more restricted play experience than healthy children [26].

VR potentially offers children with disabilities the opportunity to participate in games otherwise inaccessible. It provides a three-dimensional spatial the degree of the movement between the real world and the computer. Children can also practice intensely and simultaneously receive positive visual, proprioceptive, tactile and auditory sense feedbacks in VR [11, 27]. The use of it in children with disabilities provides motor learning, postural and motor control and improves sensorial-perceptual-motor-cognitive-communication skills. So that children become more independent individuals in their daily lives [28].

2.1.1. *The advantages and disadvantages of VR in pediatric rehabilitation*

The virtual reality system is separated according to immersion degree and how the users interact with the system [29]. VR systems can be grouped under two main headings such as immersion VR and desktop VR. Immersion VR is a type of application that involves the use of various materials to make the virtual environment feel like it is a real. Specially, users wear a head mounted display that brings them into a 3D virtual environment. Thus, all movements are controlled by head movement. Second type of system is desktop VR. Images appear on a device such as a computer or a television [30]. The users play with the help of various tools such as keyboard, mouse, speaker, glove etc. Systems also connected to the internet (tele-rehabilitation) have the potential to reach out to children who are in distant areas or in their home [11].

VR has many advantages for pediatric rehabilitation. Firstly, VR is a goal-directed method so that it can be used for training and education to increase of skills like sense, perception, motor, cognitive and social in children [31]. Secondly, it was functional, motivational and fun for children [20]. Because of that, it is one of the most preferred treatment methods for therapists and children. Thirdly, VR can be used both in single and in group activity programs that may be included in more than one person. VR applications involving more than one person can be made up of their family members or peer children who can be practiced in the same ergotherapy session. It is also an advantage to promote therapy sessions. Lastly, VR game systems like Nintendo Wii, Wii sport games, Wii fit or Kinect Xbox are common, low, simple and available in both the occupational therapy departments and children's home [32].

VR also has some disadvantages. Technology is rapidly advancing, and the systems and games developed for children are changing day by day. It is not easy to follow and reach for most citizens of the country. Additionally, current virtual reality systems like Interactive Rehabilitation Exercise System (IREX) are also too expensive for the majority of the population [33].

Knowing the advantages and disadvantages of the systems is important in determining appropriate virtual reality systems for clinical use and academic research. For example, all marketed games are not appropriate for all individual, especially for children. Because of their functions, skills, needs or motivations are difference with each other. The games may increase their functional activity, but rather facilitate the appearance of some unwanted symptoms or movement patterns [20]. For this reason, be careful in the preference and use of the game, preferences should be made to the therapist control.

2.1.2. *Studies on VR in pediatric rehabilitation*

All studies aimed to improve function or quality of movement in upper and lower limbs in order to increase of social participation and achieve better performance in daily life activities. A great majority of the investigations on this field are children with neurological impairments such as cerebral palsy. Most of the researches showed improvement upper limb functions via VR interventions. For example, Chen et al. showed the benefit of VR use for reaching activity in four children with CP between the ages of 4 and 8. Children were treated with the Sony Eye-Toy system for 4 weeks at 2 hours per week. The quality of reaching was shown to improve after individual training [34]. Jannink et al., in 2007, investigated to evaluate upper extremity training with a Sony Eye-Toy. They randomly included in 12 children with CP. Upper extremity functions were evaluated with Melbourne. The results showed the Eye-Toy to be a motivational education tool that developed upper extremity function in children with CP for 6 weeks at 30 minutes twice a week [35]. Similarly, You et al. investigated in VR-based cortical reorganization and functional motor development with hemiparetic CP. The Bruininks-Oseretsky Test of Motor Proficiency (BOTMP), the Modified Pediatric Motor Activity Log (PMAL) tests and functional magnetic resonance imaging (fMRI) were used pre-/post-measurements. Children treated with IREX for 60 minutes 5 times a week for 1 month.

According to the results, functional motor skills, amount of use in affected upper extremities and the quality of the motion, active movement, control and coordination of upper extremity motor performance were increased. Thus, it might be said that VR applications can be used to enhance motor skills [36].

Reid et al. included in 31 children aged between 8 and 12 years. They randomly divided into two: 19 study (VR) and 12 control group. Treatment for 1.5 hours per week for 8 weeks was implemented for the children. Canadian occupational performance measurement (COPM) and Quality of *Upper Extremity* Skills Test (QUEST) were used to evaluate the effect of VR treatment. All results were improved after the treatment, while there was no significant functional difference was found between the groups. According to the results, there were significantly increased social acceptance and motivation in the study group [37]. These results indicated an important point in rehabilitation which treatment is an extensive concept that has not only physical component but also emotional and social components.

Also, home-based treatment approaches are important to integrate effectiveness of VR intervention in daily life. Winkels et al. included 15 children with CP [Manual ability classification system (MACS) Levels I and II] between the age of 6 and 15 in their study. The children were evaluated with the Melbourne Assessment of Upper Limb Function and ABILHAND-Kids and had upper extremity function training using Wii games. They reported to increase in the performance of daily living activities with VR.

Activities of daily living involve in not only upper but also lower extremity. On the other hand, walking ability or strength is generally researched according to lower extremity activity. Recent studies focused on combination with VR system and robot-assisted gait training (RAGT), and they are emphasized the useful interventions which applies together [38, 39].

The other investigation area in disabilities with children about VR is Down syndrome and autism and attention deficit. These studies were showed to increase of sensorimotor functions and motor proficiency by using VR in these disabilities [27, 40].

As a result, these studies proved that VR systems are motivational, evidenced based and useful for children in pediatric rehabilitation interventions. It can be used for improving upper limb function and proficiency, sensorimotor and cognitive functions, activity of daily living, participation of therapy and motivation level in rehabilitation.

2.2. Virtual reality rehabilitation for adult population

VR is being used in adult rehabilitation by therapists for many years. Groups that being focused most are stroke survivors, Parkinson's disease and geriatric population who needs repetitive rehabilitation approaches with active participation. However, current approaches that were being used had some issues about repetition with fun part. VR had a new perspective to the repetitive rehabilitation approaches after its initial use. Studies showed that VR suggests higher dosage of repetition than traditional approaches [41–43]. Initially, VR was being used with flight simulators, surgery training etc.; within the use in health practices, it spreads its use in the area of post-traumatic stress disorder and body image disorders [3]. VR is advantaged with its goal-oriented tasks and repetition. Repetition, task-oriented movements and fun are needed to achieve neuromotor changes which will lead motor enhancements in client's task. The term goal oriented and repetitive tasks are in a collaboration with neuroplasticity terms which of one is the repetition of the task that is needed to be practice must be trained in rich and fun environments. VR offers a great opportunity for therapist who seeks for these terms in their approaches.

VR offers simulation systems, safe activity training etc for OT. OT comes from real-life situations and lives and develops itself in the community. Being this related to the life, OT needed to adapt itself with the technological developments. Nowadays, mobile phones, internet, phone applications and lots of other software and hardware are common worldwide. OT uses this to involve geriatrics, rehabilitate stroke survivors and other disability causes to rehabilitate.

Daily life activities are being studied for stroke survivors using environments such as driving rehabilitation and market simulations [44]. Akinwuntan et al. [45] used STISIM Drive System (Systems Technology Inc., United States) in their research with people with stroke which had real size computer images, visual angle of 45° and adaptations such as left-sided accelerator and steering wheel spinner. In this study, researchers compared virtual driving rehabilitation with conventional rehabilitation which found to be no different from each other

Barcala et al. [46] used Wiifit (Nintendo, Japan) on balance training with people with stroke. The equipment that is commercially available and serves mainly for entertainment and home exercises could reproduce body movements and give auditory feedback through many display choices such as TVs or projectors. Cho et al. [47] used Interactive Rehabilitation and Exercise System (Vivid Group, Canada) for upper extremity rehabilitation of people with stroke. The system which is specifically aimed to neurorehabilitation programs included video cameras, gloves and virtual games. da Silva Cameirão et al. [48] used Rehabilitation Gaming System (Pompeu Fabra University, Spain) with people with acute stroke. The system uses a motion capturing camera in tandem with motion gloves and has activities (e.g., games) which have gradual difficulties. It aims to functional reorganization of neuronal systems through visual input of virtual extremities on screen combined with task oriented action.

Walking, balance and mobility problems of VR application are made in people with Parkinson's disease. Significant improvements are observed in the individuals in these studies [49]. In addition, studies on motor learning, retention-transfer and cognitive functions are being studied with VR applications in Parkinsonian individuals [50]. VR applications are utilized to improve functional balance, mobility, static-dynamic postural control, and dual-task reaction times [51]. VR technologies are utilized in the treatment of loss of cognitive function skills in geriatric people. In individual attention, alertness, reaction time and the short-/long-term memory due to the stimulation of VR applications are preferred [52, 53]. VR technology is also used in mental health treatment in geriatric people. VR technology can be used as a treatment tool for agoraphobia, social phobia, fear of death, depression, anxiety, posttraumatic stress syndrome, attention deficit, dementia and schizophrenia treatment [54]. One of VR performed on geriatric people, and the most important applications are the study of the fall and after the growing fear of falling. These studies provide postural stability, strengthening of activity muscles, ground sensing, proprioceptive and vestibular sensory training [55].

Lee et al. [56] used K-Pop Dance Festival (Nintendo Inc., Japan) software for Nintendo Wii platform for the rehabilitation program of participants with Parkinson's disease. The hand-held motion controller of the platform was strapped to the participants' hands as a compensation strategy. The software includes songs, and the success of the activity depends on dance movements that match the songs' rhythms. The researchers found that independence in activities of daily living and decrease in depressive symptoms were acquired by VR rehabilitation.

Pichierri et al. [57] used TX 6000 Metal DDR Platinum Pro metal dance pads (Mayflash Limited, China) in tandem with Stepmania Software, a free dance and rhythm game (https://www.stepmania.com). Participants were asked to match the direction of arrows on screen that appear in sync with musical rhythm by stepping on the corresponding arrows on the dance pad. By this approach, participants were asked to participate dual task activities. Researchers suggested that cognitive-motor intervention was appropriate to use to increase strength and balance in elderly. Hoffman et al. [58] used Oculus Rift VR goggles (Facebook Inc., United States) during occupational therapy of a young burn patient. Researchers used SnowWorld (University of Washington, United States), a software developed specifically for pain management of burn patients, with Oculus Rift which showed slightly pain decrease of the client. The goggles can be worn head mounted or worn with an arm mounted apparatus. Faber et al. [59] used Cybermind Hi-Res900$_{ST}$ (Jasandre Pty. Ltd, Australia), a head mounted VR goggles during the treatment of burn patients in tandem with SnowWorld software (University of Washington, United States). Researchers measured pain levels of the participants after every session of the treatment. Yoon et al. [60] used Interactive Rehabilitation and Exercise System (Vivid Group, Canada) along with traditional occupational therapy in their research on patients with brain tumor. Researchers used Birds and Balls, Conveyor, Drums, Juggler, Coconuts, and Soccer VR programs of the system. Jahn et al. [61] used Nintendo Wii (Nintendo, Japan) in their research with inpatient adults with cancer. Participants were able to choose either Wii Sports, Family Trainer, Sports Island or Family Ski and Snowboard programs for each single session. Rohani et al. [62] used Kinect (Microsoft, United States) along with a virtual classroom software. The classroom software had two different tasks, and children were asked to accomplish the tasks, while distractions were presented (e.g., a construction worker entering the classroom).

3. Discussion

VR in rehabilitation is a common approach in current rehabilitation era. The repetition enhancement, moving client away from one's diagnosis/disability, enabling and active participation in rehabilitation, enriched environments and making rehabilitation fun are the greatest motives to use VR for rehabilitation. Lots of studies showed the benefits of using VR in different rehabilitation settings. A therapist with VR access may feel confident to use VR.

Both pediatrics and adult population had fun with their VR rehabilitation, which removes the boring role of rehabilitation. In particular, in pediatrics, using VR opens a wide perspective for the therapists. However, technological improvements must consider rehabilitation-based games or applications to achieve fully adaptable and client-special rehabilitation patterns. Commercially, sold games and applications still have low awareness of disability. Additionally, new coded software are needed to be adaptable for each participant and one's current motor/cognitive/social status related to the disability. Also game types that may used for VR may be gender depended as the children or older participants may not be willing to participate VR session.

As the technology improves, more opportunities are likely to occur; as rehabilitation specialists, we must keep our contact with these developments and develop ourselves according to our client's needs.

Author details

Orkun Tahir Aran*, Sedef Şahin, Berkan Torpil, Tarık Demirok and Hülya Kayıhan

*Address all correspondence to: orkunaran@gmail.com

Faculty of Health Sciences, Occupational Therapy, Hacettepe University, Ankara, Turkey

References

[1] Organization WH. International Classification of Functioning, Disability and Health: ICF: World Health Organization; 2001

[2] Roley SS, Barrows CJ, Susan Brownrigg OTR L, Sava DI, Vibeke Talley OTR L, Kristi Voelkerding B. Occupational therapy practice framework: Domain and process 2nd edition. The American Journal of Occupational Therapy. 2008;**62**(6):625

[3] Schultheis MT, Rizzo AA. The application of virtual reality technology in rehabilitation. Rehabilitation Psychology. 2001;**46**(3):296

[4] Trombly CA. Occupation: Purposefulness and meaningfulness as therapeutic mechanisms. American Journal of Occupational Therapy. 1995;**49**(10):960-972

[5] Weiss PL, Rand D, Katz N, Kizony R. Video capture virtual reality as a flexible and effective rehabilitation tool. Journal of Neuroengineering and Rehabilitation. 2004;**1**(1):12

[6] Ang KK, Guan C, Chua KSG, Ang BT, Kuah C, Wang C, editors. A clinical study of motor imagery-based brain-computer interface for upper limb robotic rehabilitation. In: EMBC Annual International Conference of the IEEE 2009; Minneapolis, Minneota, USA ; IEEE, Engineering in Medicine and Biology Society; 2009.

[7] Jezernik S, Colombo G, Keller T, Frueh H, Morari M. Robotic orthosis lokomat: A rehabilitation and research tool. Neuromodulation: Technology at the Neural Interface. 2003;**6**(2):108-115

[8] Bonato P. Advances in wearable technology and applications in physical medicine and rehabilitation. Journal of Neuroengineering and Rehabilitation. 2005;**2**(1):2

[9] Free C, Phillips G, Galli L, Watson L, Felix L, Edwards P. The effectiveness of mobile-health technology-based health behaviour change or disease management interventions for health care consumers: A systematic review. PLOS Medicine. 2013;**10**(1):e1001362

[10] Rust KL, Smith RO. Assistive technology in the measurement of rehabilitation and health outcomes: A review and analysis of instruments. American Journal of Physical Medicine and Rehabilitation. 2005;**84**(10):780-793

[11] Holden MK. Virtual environments for motor rehabilitation: Review. Cyberpsychology and behavior. 2005;**8**(3):187-211

[12] Burdea G, editor. Keynote address: Virtual rehabilitation-benefits and challenges. In: 1st International Workshop on Virtual Reality Rehabilitation (Mental Health, Neurological, Physical, Vocational) VRMHR; 2002. sn

[13] Merians AS, Jack D, Boian R, Tremaine M, Burdea GC, Adamovich SV. Virtual reality—Augmented rehabilitation for patients following stroke. Physical Therapy. 2002; **82**(9):898-915

[14] Piron L, Turolla A, Agostini M, Zucconi C, Cortese F, Zampolini M. Exercises for paretic upper limb after stroke: A combined virtual-reality and telemedicine approach. Journal of Rehabilitation Medicine. 2009;**41**(12):1016-1020

[15] Rose F, Attree E, Johnson D. Virtual reality: An assistive technology in neurological rehabilitation. Current Opinion in Neurology. 1996;**9**(6):461-468

[16] Saposnik G, Teasell R, Mamdani M, Hall J, McIlroy W, Cheung D. Effectiveness of virtual reality using Wii gaming technology in stroke rehabilitation. Stroke. 2010;**41**(7):1477-1484

[17] Sveistrup H, Thornton M, Bryanton C, McComas J, Marshall S, Finestone H, editors. Outcomes of intervention programs using flatscreen virtual reality. In: Engineering in Medicine and Biology Society, 2004 IEMBS'04 26th Annual International Conference of the IEEE; San Francisco, CA, USA; IEEE; 2004

[18] Halton J. Virtual rehabilitation with video games: A new frontier for occupational therapy. Occupational Therapy Now. 2008;**9**(6):12-14

[19] Chen Y-P, Lee S-Y, Howard AM. Effect of virtual reality on upper extremity function in children with cerebral palsy: A meta-analysis. Pediatric Physical Therapy. 2014;**26**(3):289-300

[20] Harris K, Reid D. The influence of virtual reality play on children's motivation. Canadian Journal of Occupational Therapy. 2005;**72**(1):21-29

[21] Kielhofner G. Model of Human Occupation: Theory and Application. Lippincott Williams & Wilkins, Baltimore; 2008

[22] Rubin KH, Fein GG, Vandenberg B. Play. Handbook of Child Psychology. 1983;**4**:693-774

[23] Bjorklund DF, Brown RD. Physical play and cognitive development: Integrating activity, cognition, and education. Child Development. 1998;**69**(3):604-606

[24] Eppright TD, Sanfacon JA, Beck NC, Bradley JS: Sport psychiatry in childhood and adolescence: An overview. Child Psychiatry and Human Development. 1997;**28**(2):71-88

[25] Piaget J. Play, Dreams and Imitation in Childhood. Routledge; Abbington, Oxon; 2013

[26] Howard L. A comparison of leisure-time activities between able-bodied children and children with physical disabilities. The British Journal of Occupational Therapy. 1996;**59**(12):570-574

[27] Wuang Y-P, Chiang C-S, Su C-Y, Wang C-C. Effectiveness of virtual reality using Wii gaming technology in children with Down syndrome. Research in Developmental Disabilities. 2011;**32**(1):312-321

[28] Gunel MK, Kara OK, Ozal C, Turker D. (2014). Virtual Reality in Rehabilitation of Children with Cerebral Palsy, Cerebral Palsy - Challenges for the Future, Associate Prof. Emira Švraka (Ed.), InTech, p 273-301; DOI: 10.5772/57486. Available from: https://www.intechopen.com/books/cerebral-palsy-challenges-for-the-future/virtual-reality-in-rehabilitation-of-children-with-cerebral-palsy

[29] Sandlund M, McDonough S, Häger-Ross C. Interactive computer play in rehabilitation of children with sensorimotor disorders: A systematic review. Developmental Medicine and Child Neurology. 2009;**51**(3):173-179

[30] Wilson PN, Foreman N, Stanton D. Virtual reality, disability and rehabilitation. Disability and Rehabilitation. 1997;**19**(6):213-220

[31] Gabyzon ME, Engel-Yeger B, Tresser S, Springer S. Using a virtual reality game to assess goal-directed hand movements in children: A pilot feasibility study. Technology and Health Care. 2016;**24**(1):11-19

[32] Galvin J, Levac D. Facilitating clinical decision-making about the use of virtual reality within paediatric motor rehabilitation: Describing and classifying virtual reality systems. Developmental Neurorehabilitation. 2011;**14**(2):112-122

[33] Reid DT. Benefits of a virtual play rehabilitation environment for children with cerebral palsy on perceptions of self-efficacy: A pilot study. Pediatric Rehabilitation. 2002;**5**(3):141-148

[34] Chen Y-P, Kang L-J, Chuang T-Y, Doong J-L, Lee S-J, Tsai M-W. Use of virtual reality to improve upper-extremity control in children with cerebral palsy: A single-subject design. Physical Therapy. 2007;**87**(11):1441

[35] Jannink MJ, Van Der Wilden GJ, Navis DW, Visser G, Gussinklo J, Ijzerman M. A low-cost video game applied for training of upper extremity function in children with cerebral palsy: A pilot study. Cyber Psychology and Behavior. 2008;**11**(1):27-32

[36] You SH, Jang SH, Kim Y-H, Hallett M, Ahn SH, Kwon Y-H. Virtual reality-induced cortical reorganization and associated locomotor recovery in chronic stroke. Stroke. 2005;**36**(6):1166-1171

[37] Reid D, Campbell K. The use of virtual reality with children with cerebral palsy: A pilot randomized trial. Therapeutic Recreation Journal. 2006;**40**(4):255

[38] Brütsch K, Schuler T, Koenig A, Zimmerli L, Mérillat S, Lünenburger L. Influence of virtual reality soccer game on walking performance in robotic assisted gait training for children. Journal of Neuroengineering and Rehabilitation. 2010;**7**(1):15

[39] Cho C, Hwang W, Hwang S, Chung Y. Treadmill training with virtual reality improves gait, balance, and muscle strength in children with cerebral palsy. The Tohoku Journal of Experimental Medicine. 2016;**238**(3):213-218

[40] Parsons TD, Rizzo AA, Rogers S, York P. Virtual reality in paediatric rehabilitation: A review. Developmental Neurorehabilitation. 2009;**12**(4):224-238

[41] Laver K, George S, Thomas S, Deutsch JE, Crotty M. Virtual reality for stroke rehabilitation. Stroke. 2012;**43**(2):e20-e21

[42] Demain S, Burridge J, Ellis-Hill C, Hughes A-M, Yardley L, Tedesco-Triccas L. Assistive technologies after stroke: Self-management or fending for yourself. A focus group study. BMC Health Services Research. 2013;**13**(1):334

[43] Fung V, Ho A, Shaffer J, Chung E, Gomez M. Use of Nintendo Wii Fit™ in the rehabilitation of outpatients following total knee replacement: A preliminary randomised controlled trial. Physiotherapy. 2012;**98**(3):183-188

[44] Ahn H, Ku J, Cho B, Kim H, Jo H, Lee J, editors. The development of virtual reality driving simulator for rehabilitation. Engineering in Medicine and Biology Society. In: Proceedings of the 23rd Annual International Conference of the IEEE; İstanbul, Turkey; IEEE; 2001

[45] Akinwuntan AE, Devos H, Verheyden G, Baten G, Kiekens C, Feys H. Retraining moderately impaired stroke survivors in driving-related visual attention skills. Topics in Stroke Rehabilitation. 2010;**17**(5):328-336

[46] Barcala L, Grecco L, Colella F, Lucareli P, Salgado A, Oliveira CS. Visual biofeedback balance training using Wii fit after stroke: A randomized controlled trial. Journal of Physical Therapy Science. 2013;**25**(8):1027-1032

[47] Cho K, Yu J, Jung J. Effects of virtual reality-based rehabilitation on upper extremity function and visual perception in stroke patients: A randomized control trial. Journal of Physical Therapy Science. 2012;**24**(11):1205-1208

[48] da Silva Cameirão M, Bermúdez i Badia S, Duarte E, Verschure PF. Virtual reality based rehabilitation speeds up functional recovery of the upper extremities after stroke: A randomized controlled pilot study in the acute phase of stroke using the rehabilitation gaming system. Restorative Neurology and Neuroscience. 2011;**29**(5):287-298

[49] Mirelman A, Maidan I, Herman T, Deutsch JE, Giladi N, Hausdorff JM. Virtual reality for gait training: Can it induce motor learning to enhance complex walking and reduce fall risk in patients with Parkinson's disease? The Journals of Gerontology Series A. Biological Sciences and Medical Sciences. 2011;66(2);234-240.

[50] dos Santos Mendes FA, Pompeu JE, Lobo AM, da Silva KG, de Paula Oliveira T, Zomignani AP. Motor learning, retention and transfer after virtual-reality-based training in Parkinson's disease-effect of motor and cognitive demands of games: A longitudinal, controlled clinical study. Physiotherapy. 2012;**98**(3):217-223

[51] Bisson E, Contant B, Sveistrup H, Lajoie Y. Functional balance and dual-task reaction times in older adults are improved by virtual reality and biofeedback training. Cyberpsychology and Behavior. 2007;**10**(1):16-23

[52] Cherniack EP. Not just fun and games: Applications of virtual reality in the identification and rehabilitation of cognitive disorders of the elderly. Disability and Rehabilitation: Assistive Technology. 2011;**6**(4):283-289

[53] Optale G, Urgesi C, Busato V, Marin S, Piron L, Priftis K. Controlling memory impairment in elderly adults using virtual reality memory training: a randomized controlled pilot study. Neurorehabilitation and Neural Repair. 2010;**24**(4):348-357

[54] Gregg L, Tarrier N. Virtual reality in mental health. Social Psychiatry and Psychiatric Epidemiology. 2007;**42**(5):343-354

[55] Suárez H, Suárez A, Lavinsky L. Postural adaptation in elderly patients with instability and risk of falling after balance training using a virtual-reality system. International Tinnitus Journal. 2006;**12**(1):41

[56] Lee N-Y, Lee D-K, Song H-S. Effect of virtual reality dance exercise on the balance, activities of daily living, and depressive disorder status of Parkinson's disease patients. Journal of Physical Therapy Science. 2015;**27**(1):145-147

[57] Pichierri G, Coppe A, Lorenzetti S, Murer K, de Bruin ED. The effect of a cognitive-motor intervention on voluntary step execution under single and dual task conditions in older adults: A randomized controlled pilot study. Clinical Interventions in Aging. 2012;**7**:175-184

[58] Hoffman HG, Meyer III WJ, Ramirez M, Roberts L, Seibel EJ, Atzori B. Feasibility of articulated arm mounted Oculus Rift Virtual Reality goggles for adjunctive pain con-

trol during occupational therapy in pediatric burn patients. Cyberpsychology, Behavior, and Social Networking. 2014;**17**(6):397-401

[59] Faber AW, Patterson DR, Bremer M. Repeated use of immersive virtual reality therapy to control pain during wound dressing changes in pediatric and adult burn patients. Journal of Burn Care and Research: Official Publication of the American Burn Association. 2013;**34**(5):563

[60] Yoon J, Chun MH, Lee SJ, Kim BR. Effect of virtual reality-based rehabilitation on upper-extremity function in patients with brain tumor: Controlled trial. American Journal of Physical Medicine and Rehabilitation. 2015;**94**(6):449-459

[61] Jahn P, Lakowa N, Landenberger M, Vordermark D, Stoll O, editors. InterACTIV: An exploratory study of the use of a game console to promote physical activation of hospitalized adult patients with cancer. Oncology Nursing Forum; 2012

[62] Rohani DA, Sorensen HB, Puthusserypady S, editors. Brain-computer interface using P300 and virtual reality: A gaming approach for treating ADHD. Engineering in Medicine and Biology Society (EMBC), 2014 36th Annual International Conference of the IEEE; Chicago, IL, USA; IEEE; 2014

Permissions

All chapters in this book were first published in OTOFHPR, by InTech Open; hereby published with permission under the Creative Commons Attribution License or equivalent. Every chapter published in this book has been scrutinized by our experts. Their significance has been extensively debated. The topics covered herein carry significant findings which will fuel the growth of the discipline. They may even be implemented as practical applications or may be referred to as a beginning point for another development.

The contributors of this book come from diverse backgrounds, making this book a truly international effort. This book will bring forth new frontiers with its revolutionizing research information and detailed analysis of the nascent developments around the world.

We would like to thank all the contributing authors for lending their expertise to make the book truly unique. They have played a crucial role in the development of this book. Without their invaluable contributions this book wouldn't have been possible. They have made vital efforts to compile up to date information on the varied aspects of this subject to make this book a valuable addition to the collection of many professionals and students.

This book was conceptualized with the vision of imparting up-to-date information and advanced data in this field. To ensure the same, a matchless editorial board was set up. Every individual on the board went through rigorous rounds of assessment to prove their worth. After which they invested a large part of their time researching and compiling the most relevant data for our readers.

The editorial board has been involved in producing this book since its inception. They have spent rigorous hours researching and exploring the diverse topics which have resulted in the successful publishing of this book. They have passed on their knowledge of decades through this book. To expedite this challenging task, the publisher supported the team at every step. A small team of assistant editors was also appointed to further simplify the editing procedure and attain best results for the readers.

Apart from the editorial board, the designing team has also invested a significant amount of their time in understanding the subject and creating the most relevant covers. They scrutinized every image to scout for the most suitable representation of the subject and create an appropriate cover for the book.

The publishing team has been an ardent support to the editorial, designing and production team. Their endless efforts to recruit the best for this project, has resulted in the accomplishment of this book. They are a veteran in the field of academics and their pool of knowledge is as vast as their experience in printing. Their expertise and guidance has proved useful at every step. Their uncompromising quality standards have made this book an exceptional effort. Their encouragement from time to time has been an inspiration for everyone.

The publisher and the editorial board hope that this book will prove to be a valuable piece of knowledge for researchers, students, practitioners and scholars across the globe.

List of Contributors

Hatice Abaoğlu, Özge Buket Cesim, Sinem Kars and Zeynep Çelik
Faculty of Health Sciences, Occupational Therapy Department, Hacettepe University, Ankara, Turkey

Edeltraut Emmerich, Marcus Engelmann, Melanie Rohmann and Frank Richter
Institute of Physiology I/Neurophysiology, University Hospital Jena - Friedrich Schiller University, Jena, Germany

Patricia J. Scott, Kelsey McKinney, Jeff Perron, Emily Ruff and Jessica Smiley
Indiana University, Indianapolis, IN, USA

Michel Probst
Department of Rehabilitation Sciences, KU Leuven, Belgium

Sedef Şahin, Semin Akel and Meral Zarif
Faculty of Health Sciences, Occupational Therapy Department, Hacettepe University, Ankara, Turkey

Gokcen Akyurek and Gonca Bumin
Department of Occupational Therapy, Faculty of Health Sciences, Hacettepe University, Ankara, Turkey

Serkan Pekçetin
Department of Occupational Therapy, Faculty of Health Sciences, Trakya University, Edirne, Turkey

Ayla Günal
Department of Physiotherapy and Rehabilitation, Faculty of Health Sciences Gaziosmanpasa University, Tokat, Turkey

Gokcen Akyurek, Sinem Kars, Zeynep Celik, Ceren Koc and Özge Buket Cesim
Department of Occupational Therapy, Faculty of Health Science, Hacettepe University, Ankara, Turkey

Patricia Precin
Occupational Therapy at Touro College, Licensed Psychoanalyst in Private Practice, Faculty of the National Psychological Association for Psychoanalysis and Stony Brook University, New York, NY, USA

Zeynep Bahadır Ağce
Faculty of Health Sciences, Occupational Therapy Department, Üsküdar University, Turkey

Esma Özkan and Barkın Köse
Faculty of Health Sciences, Occupational Therapy Department, Hacettepe University, Turkey

Orkun Tahir Aran, Sedef Şahin, Berkan Torpil, Tarık Demirok and Hülya Kayıhan
Faculty of Health Sciences, Occupational Therapy, Hacettepe University, Ankara, Turkey

Index